T0227126

Concussion

Assessment, Management and Rehabilitation

Concussion

Assessment, Management and Rehabilitation

BLESSEN C. EAPEN, MD
Chief
Physical Medicine and Rehabilitation Service
VA Greater Los Angeles Healthcare System
Los Angeles, California
United States

Associate Professor
Department of Medicine
University of California, Los Angeles (UCLA)
Los Angeles, California
United States

DAVID X. CIFU, MD
Associate Dean of Innovation and System Integration
Herman J. Flax, MD Professor and Chair
Department of Physical Medicine and Rehabilitation
Virginia Commonwealth University School of Medicine

Senior TBI Specialist
U.S. Department of Veterans Affairs

Principal Investigator
Chronic Effects of Neurotrauma Consortium - Long-term Effects of Mild Brain Injury
program (CENC-LIMBIC 2013-2024), U.S. Departments of Defense and Veterans Affairs

ELSEVIER

Concussion
ISBN: 978-0-323-65384-8

Copyright © 2020 Elsevier Inc. All rights reserved.

No part of this publication may be reproduced or transmitted in any form or by any means, electronic or mechanical, including photocopying, recording, or any information storage and retrieval system, without permission in writing from the publisher. Details on how to seek permission, further information about the Publisher's permissions policies and our arrangements with organizations such as the Copyright Clearance Center and the Copyright Licensing Agency, can be found at our website: www.elsevier.com/permissions.

This book and the individual contributions contained in it are protected under copyright by the Publisher (other than as may be noted herein).

Notices

Practitioners and researchers must always rely on their own experience and knowledge in evaluating and using any information, methods, compounds or experiments described herein. Because of rapid advances in the medical sciences, in particular, independent verification of diagnoses and drug dosages should be made. To the fullest extent of the law, no responsibility is assumed by Elsevier, authors, editors or contributors for any injury and/or damage to persons or property as a matter of products liability, negligence or otherwise, or from any use or operation of any methods, products, instructions, or ideas contained in the material herein.

Publisher: Cathleen Sether
Acquisition Editor: Humayra Rahman
Editorial Project Manager: Sandra Harron
Production Project Manager: Sreejith Viswanathan
Cover Designer: Miles Hitchen

Working together
to grow libraries in
developing countries

www.elsevier.com • www.bookaid.org

List of Contributors

Rachel Sayko Adams, PhD, MPH
Rocky Mountain Mental Illness Research Education
  and Clinical Center (MIRECC)
Rocky Mountain Regional Center
Aurora, CO, United States

Institute for Behavior Health
Heller School for Social Policy and Management
Brandeis University
Waltham, MA, United States

Patrick Armistead-Jehle, PhD, ABPP-CN
Chief
Concussion Clinic
Munson Army Health Center
Fort Leavenworth, KS, United States

Laura Bajor, DO
Mental Health and Behavioral Neurosciences Division
James A. Haley VA
Tampa, FL, United States

Department of Psychiatry
Morsani College of Medicine
University of South Florida
Tampa, FL, United States

Harvard South Shore Psychiatry Residency
Harvard Medical School
Boston, MA, United States

Thomas J. Bayuk, DO
Neurologist
United States Air Force
Fellow, Sports Neurology
Barrow Neurological Institute
Phoenix, AZ, United States

Kathleen R. Bell, MD
Professor and Chair
Department of Physical Medicine and Rehabilitation
  Medicine
University of Texas Medical Center
Dallas, TX, United States

Erin D. Bigler, PhD, ABPP
Department of Neurology
University of Utah School of Medicine
Salt Lake City, UT, United States

Departments of Psychology and Neuroscience
Brigham Young University
Provo, UT, United States

Lisa A. Brenner, PhD
Rocky Mountain Mental Illness Research Education
  and Clinical Center (MIRECC)
Rocky Mountain Regional Center
Aurora, CO, United States

Department of Physical Medicine & Rehabilitation
University of Colorado Anschutz Medical Campus
Aurora, CO, United States

Department of Psychiatry
University of Colorado Anschutz Medical Campus
Aurora, CO, United States

Marcus Institute for Brain Health
University of Colorado Anschutz Medical Campus
Aurora, CO, United States

Department of Neurology
University of Colorado Anschutz Medical Campus
Aurora, CO, United States

Samuel Clanton, MD, PhD
Assistant Professor
Physical Medicine and Rehabilitation
Medical College of Virginia/Virginia Commonwealth
    University Health System
Richmond, VA, United States

Attending Physician
Sheltering Arms Rehab
Richmond, VA, United States

Douglas B. Cooper, PhD, ABPP-CN
Senior Scientific Director
Defense and Veterans Brain Injury Center (DVBIC)
South Texas Veterans Healthcare System
Polytrauma Rehabilitation Center (PRC)
San Antonio, TX, United States

Adjunct Associate Professor
Department of Psychiatry
UT Health
San Antonio, TX, United States

Katherine L. Dec, MD, FAAPMR, FAMSSM
Professor
Department of Physical Medicine and Rehabilitation
    and Department of Orthopaedic Surgery
Virginia Commonwealth University School of
    Medicine
Richmond, VA, United States

Past President
American Medical Society for Sports Medicine
Richmond, VA, United States

Paul Dukarm, PhD, ABPP-CN
Assistant Professor
Neuropsychology and Rehabilitation Psychology
    Service
Department of Physical Medicine and Rehabilitation
Virginia Commonwealth University
Richmond, VA, United States

Blessen C. Eapen, MD
Chief
Physical Medicine & Rehabilitation
VA Greater Los Angeles Health Care System
Los Angeles, CA, United States

Associate Professor
David Geffen School of Medicine at UCLA
Los Angeles, CA, United States

Erica L. Epstein, PsyD
Psychology Fellow
Mid-Atlantic Mental Illness Research
Education, and Clinical Center (MA-MIRECC)
Research and Academic Affairs
Salisbury VA Health Care System
Salisbury, NC, United States

Clinical Instructor
Department of Neurology
Wake Forest School of Medicine
Winston−Salem, NC, United States

Inbal Eshel, MA, CCC-SLP
Neuroscience Clinician
Contractor
General Dynamics Health Solutions (GDHS)
Supporting the Defense & Veterans Brain
    Injury Center
Clinical Affairs Division J-9
Defense Health Agency (DHA)
Silver Spring, MD, United States

Sara Etheredge, PT, DPT, CKTP, CCI, CMTPT
Concussion Care Centre of Virginia, Ltd.
Richmond, VA, United States

Tree of Life Services, Inc.
Richmond, VA, United States

Christopher M. Filley, MD
Behavioral Neurology Section
University of Colorado Anschutz Medical Campus
Aurora, CO, United States

Department of Neurology
University of Colorado Anschutz Medical Campus
Aurora, CO, United States

Department of Psychiatry
University of Colorado Anschutz Medical Campus
Aurora, CO, United States

Marcus Institute for Brain Health
University of Colorado Anschutz Medical Campus
Aurora, CO, United States

Jared B. Gilman, MD
Department of Physical Medicine and
    Rehabilitation
Virginia Commonwealth University
Richmond, VA, United States

Gary Goldberg, BASc, MD
Clinical Adjunct Professor
Physical Medicine and Rehabilitation
Medical College of Virginia/Virginia Commonwealth
University Health System
Richmond, VA, United States

Attending Physician
Polytrauma Rehabilitation System of Care
Hunter Holmes McGuire Veterans Administration
Medical Center
Richmond VA, United States

P.K. Gootam, MD
Mental Health and Behavioral Neurosciences Division
James A. Haley VA
Tampa, FL, United States

Department of Psychiatry
Morsani College of Medicine
University of South Florida
Tampa, FL, United States

Riley P. Grassmeyer, MS
Department of Physical Medicine & Rehabilitation
University of Colorado Anschutz Medical Campus
Aurora, CO, United States

Marcus Institute for Brain Health
University of Colorado Anschutz Medical Campus
Aurora, CO, United States

James W. Hall III, PhD
Professor
Department of Communication Sciences and Disorders
John A. Burns School of Medicine
University of Hawai'i at Mānoa
Honolulu, HI, United States

Professor
Osborne College of Audiology
Salus University
Elkins Park, PA, United States

Nancy H. Hsu, PsyD, ABPP-RP
Virginia Commonwealth University
Richmond, VA, United States

Aiwane Iboaya, MD
Clinical Fellow
Department of Physical Medicine and Rehabilitation
University of Texas Southwestern Medical Center
Dallas, TX, United States

Dorothy A. Kaplan, PhD
Neuropsychologist
Defense and Veterans Brain Injury Center (DVBIC)
Defense Health Agency (DHA)
Research and Development Directorate
Silver Spring, MD, United States

Kassandra C. Kelly, MS, ATC
Department of Physical Medicine and
Rehabilitation
Virginia Commonwealth University
Richmond, VA, United States

Tracy Kretchmer, PhD
Mental Health and Behavioral Neurosciences
Division
James A. Haley VA
Tampa, FL, United States

Russell W. Lacey, MD
Professor
Department of Physical Medicine & Rehabilitation
Virginia Commonwealth University
Richmond, VA, United States

Scott R. Laker, MD
Department of Physical Medicine & Rehabilitation
University of Colorado Anschutz Medical Campus
Aurora, CO, United States

Henry L. Lew, MD, PhD
Chair and Professor
Department of Communication Sciences
and Disorders
John A. Burns School of Medicine
University of Hawai'i at Mānoa
Honolulu, HI, United States

Jeffrey D. Lewis, MD, PhD
Neurologist
United States Air Force; Associate Professor
Neurology
Uniformed Services University of the Health Sciences
Bethesda, MD, United States

Xin Li, DO
Staff Physician
Polytrauma Rehabilitation Center
South Texas Veteran Health Care System
San Antonio, TX, United States

Katherine Lin, MD
Polytrauma Rehabilitation Center
South Texas Veterans Health Care System
San Antonio, TX, United States

Christina L. Master, MD, CAQSM, FACSM
Professor of Clinical Pediatrics
University of Pennsylvania Perelman School of
    Medicine
Philadelphia, PA, United States

Co-Director
Minds Matter Concussion Program
Orthopedics
Sports Medicine and Performance Center
Children's Hospital of Philadelphia
Philadelphia, PA, United States

Division of Orthopaedics
Philadelphia, PA, United States

Amy Mathews, MD
Assistant Professor
Department of Physical Medicine and Rehabilitation
University of Texas Southwestern Medical Center
Dallas, TX, United States

Tamara L. McKenzie–Hartman, PsyD
Polytrauma/Physical Medicine and Rehabilitation
    Service
James A. Haley VA
Tampa, FL, United States

Defense and Veterans Brain Injury Center
Tampa, FL, United States

Lindsay Mohney, DO
Polytrauma Rehabilitation Center
South Texas Veterans Health Care System
San Antonio, TX, United States

Risa Nikase-Richardson, PhD
Mental Health and Behavioral Neurosciences Division
James A. Haley VA
Tampa, FL, United States

Polytrauma/Physical Medicine and Rehabilitation
    Service
James A. Haley VA
Tampa, FL, United States

Defense and Veterans Brain Injury Center
Tampa, FL, United States

Pulmonary and Sleep Medicine Division
Department of Internal Medicine
University of South Florida
Tampa, FL, United States

Justin Otis, MD
Department of Psychiatry
University of Colorado Anschutz Medical Campus
Aurora, CO, United States

Department of Neurology
University of Colorado Anschutz Medical Campus
Aurora, CO, United States

Behavioral Neurology Section
University of Colorado Anschutz Medical Campus
Aurora, CO, United States

Linda M. Picon, MCD, CCC-SLP
Senior Consultant
Rehabilitation and Prosthetic Services
Veterans Health Administration
Department of Veterans Affairs
Washington, DC, United States

Terri K. Pogoda, PhD
Research Health Scientist
Center for Healthcare Organization and
    Implementation Research
VA Boston Healthcare System
Boston, MA, United States

Research Assistant Professor
Department of Health Law
Policy & Management
Boston University School of Public Health
Boston, MA, United States

Robert D. Shura, PsyD, ABPP-CN
Neuropsychologist
Mid-Atlantic Mental Illness Research
Education, and Clinical Center (MA-MIRECC)
Mental Health & Behavioral Science
Salisbury VA Health Care System
Salisbury, NC, United States

Clinical Instructor
Department of Neurology
Wake Forest School of Medicine
Winston–Salem, NC, United States

Marc Silva, PhD
Mental Health and Behavioral Neurosciences
Division
James A. Haley VA
Tampa, FL, United States

Department of Psychiatry
Morsani College of Medicine
University of South Florida
Tampa FL, United States

Department of Psychology
University of South Florida
Tampa, FL, United States

Defense and Veterans Brain Injury Center
Tampa, FL, United States

Caroline Sizer, MD
Alpert Brown Medical School/Lifespan Rhode Island
Hospital
Providence, RI, United States

Attending Physician
Physical Medicine and Rehabilitation
Lifespan Concussion Care Center
Providence, RI, United States

Jason A.D. Smith, PhD
Assistant Professor
Department of Physical Medicine and Rehabilitation
University of Texas Medical Center
Dallas, TX, United States

Eileen P. Storey, AB
Center for Injury Research and Prevention
Children's Hospital of Philadelphia
Roberts Center for Pediatric Research
Philadelphia, PA, United States

Chiemi Tanaka, PhD
Adjunct Assistant Professor
Department of Communication Sciences and
Disorders
John A. Burns School of Medicine
University of Hawai'i at Mānoa
Honolulu, HI, United States

Director
Advanced Audiology Center
Audmet K.K. (Oticon Japan, Diatec Company)
Kanagawa-shi, Kanagawa, Japan

Rebecca Tapia, MD
Section Chief
Assistant Professor
Polytrauma Rehabilitation Center
South Texas Veterans Health Care System
San Antonio, TX, United States

Department of Rehabilitation Medicine
University of Texas Health San Antonio
San Antonio, TX, United States

David F. Tate, PhD
Associate Professor
Missouri Institute of Mental Health
University of Missouri-St. Louis
Berkeley, MO, United States

Department of Neurology
University of Utah School of Medicine
Salt Lake City, UT, United States

William C. Walker, MD
Professor
Department of Physical Medicine & Rehabilitation
Virginia Commonwealth University
Richmond, VA, United States

Elisabeth A. Wilde, PhD
Department of Neurology
University of Utah School of Medicine
Salt Lake City, UT, United States

George E. Whalen VA Medical Center
Salt Lake City, UT, United States

Department of Physical Medicine and Rehabilitation
Baylor College of Medicine
Houston, TX, United States

Gerald E. York, MD
Alaska Radiology Associates
TBI Imaging and Research
Anchorage, AK, United States

Nathan D. Zasler, MD, FAAPM&R, FAADEP, DAAPM, CBIST
Founder
CEO & CMO
Concussion Care Centre of Virginia, Ltd
Richmond, VA, United States

Founder
CEO & CMO
Tree of Life Services, Inc.
Richmond, VA, United States

Professor
Affiliate
Department of Physical Medicine and Rehabilitation
Virginia Commonwealth University
Richmond, VA, United States

Associate Professor
Adjunct
Department of Physical Medicine and Rehabilitation
University of Virginia
Charlottesville, VA, United States

Preface

Concussions in athletics, combat, vehicular trauma, and domestic abuse have been a "silent epidemic" for more than 40 years in the American lay press but have risen in public and scientific awareness since the onset of the recent Middle East military conflicts and the specter of dementia related to involvement in sports in the past 2 decades. Despite the fact that there is growing concern about the acute and chronic assessment and management of these mild traumatic brain injuries and the potential association with long-term neurodegeneration, there continues to be significant misinformation about what is known scientifically about concussions, how acute injuries should be evaluated and treated, and what steps can and should be taken to limit ongoing symptoms and potential linkages with dementias. With the establishment of the Chronic Effects of Neurotrauma Consortium (CENC) in 2013 and the continuation of CENC with the Long-term Effects of Mild Brain Injury Consortium (2019–24), the Departments of Veterans Affairs and Defense demonstrated the importance of better understanding the short- and long-term effects and course of recovery of single and repeated concussions and identified a way forward on better understanding both neurodegenerative risks related to concussion and blast and established a clinical intervention network to develop improved management and preventative strategies. In this spirit, this clinically focused text provides a much-needed update across the spectrum of concussive topics, with a clear focus on practical applications. A team of the world's leading neuroscientists and brain injury practitioners have collaborated to provide cutting-edge, evidence-based information and recommendations across the range of concussive injuries, from acute to chronic, and for a wide spectrum of concussed populations. This handbook can be used by students, academics, and clinicians alike to enhance their knowledge, to provide useful assessment and treatment approaches, and to stimulate ideas for ongoing research. Most importantly, this comprehensive text offers a standardized approach to the oftentimes confusing field of concussion that may benefit the individuals who have sustained one or more injuries, so that they may be provided better information on their short- and long-term courses of recovery.

Introduction

This practical text provides the latest scientific, clinical, and practical information regarding the assessment, management, and prognoses for children and adults who have sustained concussions in sports, vehicular trauma, domestic abuse, and combat, with a particular focus on the most commonly seen postconcussive sequelae. The nation's leading researchers and clinicians from academics, Veterans Health affairs, the military, and the private sector have collaborated to bring this comprehensive handbook together. The book begins with the key aspects of overall assessment after mild traumatic brain injury (mTBI), including Dr. Bell's update on acute management and diagnostic criteria, Dr. Hsu and Dukarm's information on neuropsychological assessment, and Dr. Tate's chapter on neuroimaging. Then, the text summarizes key evaluative approaches, management strategies, and anticipated outcomes for postconcussive syndrome (Walker), psychiatric symptoms (Brenner), headache (Zasler), sleep disturbance (Richardson and Bajor), cognitive dysfunction (Picon, Kaplan, and Eshel), neurosensory deficits (Lew, Tanaka, Hall, and Pogoda), and fatigue (Lewis). Important subpopulations of individuals who are at high risk for one or more concussions are then addressed in sections on sports-related injury (Dec, Kelly, and Gilman), pediatric mTBI (Master), military and veteran populations (Shura and Eapen), and women (Tapia). Lastly, a provocative chapter on cutting-edge and next-generation research is authored by Dr. Goldberg to bring the text into the 21st century of precision medicine. In summary, this handbook offers readers of all knowledge and experience levels useful and evidence-influenced information that can be used to enhance one's knowledge base and to assist in the management of an individual who has sustained a concussion. It provides an important contribution to the healthcare literature and is a vital resource to any clinical library.

Blessen Eapen, MD
Chief, Physical Medicine and Rehabilitation Service
VA Greater Los Angeles Health Care System

David X. Cifu, MD
Associate Dean of Innovation and System Integration
Herman J. Flax, MD Professor and Chair
Department of Physical Medicine and Rehabilitation
Virginia Commonwealth University School of
Medicine

Senior TBI Specialist
U.S. Department of Veterans Affairs

Principal Investigator
Chronic Effects of Neurotrauma Consortium -
Long-term Effects of Mild Brain Injury program
(CENC-LIMBIC 2013-2024), U.S. Departments of
Defense and Veterans Affairs

Contents

CHAPTER 1

Acute Management of Concussion and Diagnostic Criteria

AMY MATHEWS, MD • AIWANE IBOAYA, MD • JASON A.D. SMITH, PHD •
KATHLEEN R. BELL, MD

INTRODUCTION

Concussion, or mild traumatic brain injury (mTBI), is a common, yet complex clinical entity. As concussion gains more attention within the medical, sport, military, and civilian populations, there has been a drive toward producing a common definition, diagnosis, and management approach. Currently, the diagnosis of concussion is clinical—based on history, symptoms, and examination. Early treatment centers on symptom management and reassurance is key as most concussions are self-limiting. This chapter provides a high-level overview of mTBI including the current working definitions, relevant epidemiology, and pathophysiology, as well as an evidence-based approach to acute diagnosis and management. Early mTBI will be covered over time, delineating the evaluation and management of mTBI in the minutes, hours, days, and weeks following concussion.

DIAGNOSTIC CRITERIA

Currently, there is no singular and universal definition for concussion. The terms mTBI, minor head trauma, minor head injury, and concussion have all been used to describe the same entity. For purposes of this chapter, these terms will be used interchangeably.

Several medical, governmental, and professional associations have created individual definitions of TBI within the framework of each institution's purpose. Although these definitions vary, there has been some progress toward a consensus definition with many definitions of concussion sharing commonalities in criteria including force to the head and an alteration in consciousness or cognition. Delineations between mild, moderate, and severe brain injury are typically based on duration of unconsciousness, length of post-traumatic amnesia, and/or level of responsiveness (i.e., Glasgow Coma Scale [GCS] score). Select

consensus definitions of TBI are included in Table 1.1.[1-5] Even within the category of mTBI, further stratification into complicated and uncomplicated mTBI may occur based on imaging. "Complicated mTBI" is defined by intracranial abnormality on day-of-injury CT or on other imaging, such as an MRI during follow-up examination.[6] Ultimately, the utility of diagnostic criteria in the initial diagnosis of concussion is maximized within the context of a systematic and comprehensive clinical evaluation as covered within this chapter. ·

EPIDEMIOLOGY

Any discussion of the prevalence and incidence of mTBI must be framed by an understanding of the current limitations in concussion reporting. An unknown quantity of concussions goes undiagnosed and, therefore, unreported for a number of reasons. First, as noted previously, there remains great variability in the diagnosis of concussion, which impacts identification of concussion. This inconsistent identification of mTBI ultimately impacts reporting for incidence and prevalence measures. Second, mTBI that is accompanied by more severe or distracting injuries may go unidentified as providers attend to concomitant injuries. Third, commonly occurring comorbid factors such as alcohol consumption, psychotropic medications, or hospital-administered narcotics may complicate the identification of mTBI in the trauma setting.[7] Lastly, there is no surveillance method to determine the number of individuals who may have had TBI but did not seek any medical care.

Despite these limitations in reporting, the substantial public health burden of TBI cannot be disputed. The Centers for Disease Control and Prevention (CDC) reported that TBI accounted for nearly 2.5 million emergency department (ED) visits, hospitalizations, and deaths in the United States in

Concussion. https://doi.org/10.1016/B978-0-323-65384-8.00001-8
Copyright © 2020 Elsevier Inc. All rights reserved.

TABLE 1.1
Professional Organizational Definitions of TBI and mTBI/Concussion.

Organization	Definition	Mental Status Change	LOC	Amnesia	GCS	Last Update
CDC[1]	Disruption in normal brain function, causes: Bump, blow, or jolt to the head, or penetrating head injury	"Brief"	"Brief"			2018
DoD[2]	Structural injury and/or physiological disruption of brain function from external force with at least one of the following: LOC, PTA, altered mental state, neurologic deficits, intracranial lesion	0–24 h	0–30 min	0–1 day	13–15	2013
ACRM[3]	Physiological disruption of brain function with one of the following: LOC, PTA, altered mental status, focal neurologic deficits	Alteration at time of injury	0–30 min	<1 day	13–15	1993
CISG[4]	Biomechanical forces from direct blow to the head, face, neck or body with an impulsive force transmitted to the head					2017
DSM-5 (APA)[5]	Impact to the head or other rapid displacement of the brain within the skull with at least one of the following: LOC, PTA, altered mental state, focal neurologic signs, intracranial lesion on imaging, seizure, visual field cuts					2013

ACRM, American Congress of Rehabilitation Medicine; *CDC*, Centers for Disease Control and Prevention; *CISG*, Concussion in Sport Group; *DoD*, United States Department of Defense; *DSM 5 (APA)*, Diagnostic and Statistical Manual of Mental Disorders, Fifth Edition (American Psychiatric Association); *GCS*, Glasgow Coma Scale; *LOC*, Loss of Consciousness; *PTA*, post-traumatic amnesia.

2010.[8] Approximately 80% of these patients are seen and discharged from the ED within the same day, which is commonly considered an indirect indicator of mTBI.[9] The CDC report did not account for US military or veterans' services. The Department of Defense reported that between the year 2000 and the first quarter of the year 2018, the total TBI incidence was 383,947, with mTBI making up 82.3% of that total.[10] Work-related and industrial injuries constitute a sizable proportion of civilian, nonsport concussions. The US Bureau of Labor Statistics reported 94,360 nonfatal head injuries for the year 2015, across private, state, and local government settings.[11]

Age, gender, and prior history of concussion are important risk factors. Between 2007 and 2013, the highest rates of TBI-related ED visits, hospitalizations, and deaths were in individuals >75 years, 0–4 years, and 15–24 years.[12] Within these groups, the most common etiology for nonfatal TBI in children 0–14 years old and adults >45 years old was falls.[12,13] Motor vehicle accidents were the most frequent cause for nonfatal TBI in the age group between 15 and 44 years old. History of concussion is a risk factor for another concussion.[14] An important and emerging area of study is the role of sex and gender in risk of TBI, prevalence, incidence, symptom presentation, and recovery. It has been demonstrated that females have a 1.5 times greater incidence of sustaining mTBI compared to males playing the same sport.[15] Gender, as a factor in social roles is being increasingly recognized as a necessary and underappreciated aspect of concussion research in areas beyond sports, such as in vocational settings.[16] Gender-specific issues in females with mTBI are discussed later in chapter 14.

PATHOANATOMY AND PATHOPHYSIOLOGY

Understanding of the mechanisms underlying concussion and associated symptoms is evolving rapidly with new means of imaging and genetic characterization. Displacement of the brain in response to perturbation results in stretching and torsion of neuronal and especially axonal tissue. Immediately after concussion, ionic fluxes result from this stretch with an efflux of potassium and influx of calcium and sodium via mechanoporation of lipid membranes; see Fig. 1.1. These ionic fluxes cause further depolarization of the axonal membrane, resulting in a "spreading depression-like" state that may be the basis for acute symptoms of loss of consciousness and confusion.[17]

In an effort to restore balance between the sudden increases in metabolic demand, there is a rapid increase in glutamate and glucose concentrations. Ionic pumps at the membranes become hyperactive, depleting stores of ATP and requiring increased mitochondrial activity. This quickly results in an exhaustion of energy availability. However, there is an accompanying decrement in cerebral blood flow as well, resulting in a mismatch in metabolic demand and glucose availability which lasts for at least a week after concussion.[18]

At this point, the high levels of intracellular calcium begin to cause mitochondrial failure, which further interfere with the production of ATP necessary for membrane pump function and other processes.[19] Due to the persisting metabolic shifts, the redox state of the cell is disturbed, which results in the production of free radicals and excitatory compounds. These continued disturbances of energy and pH balance set the stage for cellular and axonal vulnerability for a potential second injury.[17]

During this metabolic crisis, gene expression is altered and enzymatic and transporter moieties are affected, diminishing cellular function. The upregulation of inflammatory genes and cytokine production will then cause microglial activation with potential subsequent cell damage.[20] High levels of intracellular calcium are transported to the axons where calcium enhances the phosphorylation of the axonal neurofilaments, leading to structural weakening of the axon and disruption of the microtubule, interfering with axonal transport of neurotransmitters.[21] Disruption of neurovascular coupling may last for weeks and potentially longer, continuing to affect the oxidative capacity of the neuron.[22] Protein degradation and toxin clearing require energy; it is postulated that the slowed clearance may impact deposition of proteins (amyloid, tau) which may form abnormal complexes over time with repeated injury.[23]

The Clinical Concussion Clock

Effective diagnosis and management of concussion requires serial evaluations. Management goals and approaches change as time from injury progresses (Fig. 1.2). Providers should aim to provide systematic and effective care for any particular point in recovery.

Minutes

The goals within the first few minutes after a suspected concussion are to assess medical stability and to determine, in a timely manner, if the individual requires escalated medical evaluation. The initial assessment of the concussed individual can be challenging, especially in the setting of sporting events or in-theater military injuries where the need for expeditious evaluation, the individual's desire to return to activity, and uncontrolled testing environments require a systematic and efficient approach. First, the provider should evaluate the airway,

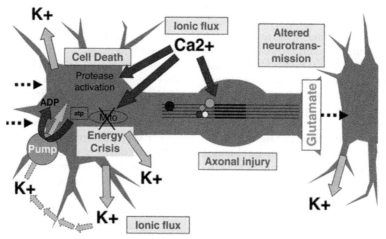

Neurometabolic Cascade of mTBI

FIG. 1.1 Neurometabolic cascade of mTBI.

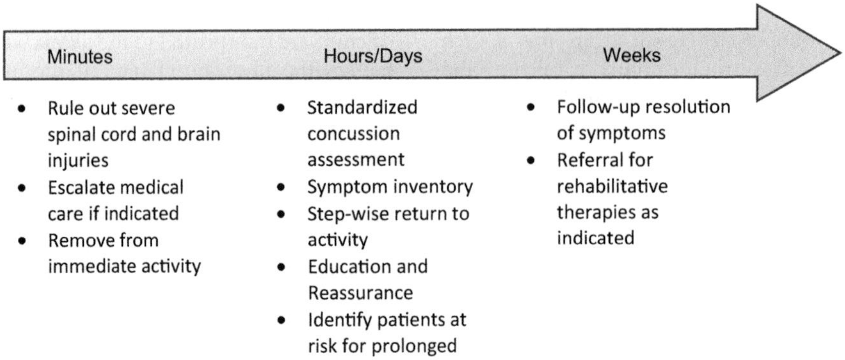

Minutes	Hours/Days	Weeks
• Rule out severe spinal cord and brain injuries • Escalate medical care if indicated • Remove from immediate activity	• Standardized concussion assessment • Symptom inventory • Step-wise return to activity • Education and Reassurance • Identify patients at risk for prolonged	• Follow-up resolution of symptoms • Referral for rehabilitative therapies as indicated

FIG. 1.2 Clinical concussion clock.

breathing, and circulatory functions of the patient. If any of these are compromised, the provider should escalate care using the appropriate Advanced Cardiac Life Support/Basic Life Support (ACLS/BLS) protocols. If none of these elements are affected, the provider should then proceed to evaluate for more serious cervical spine and/or brain injuries. Further cervical stabilization and evaluation is needed for patients exhibiting midline tenderness, focal neurologic deficits, distracting injuries, altered level of consciousness, or intoxication.[24] More serious brain injury may be suspected in patients who exhibit focal neurologic deficits, prolonged or deteriorating loss of consciousness, seizures, escalating headaches, persistent emesis, agitation, or signs of skull fracture. Skull fracture may be suspected with hemotympanum, otorrhea, rhinorrhea, or palpable skull deformity. Other signs and symptoms that may prompt further evaluation include an individual who appears dazed, "sees stars", or exhibits labored or uncoordinated movements after a direct or indirect force to the head.[4,25–27] A GCS score should be obtained initially and can be repeated serially to monitor for improvement or deterioration. A brief orientation screen such as Maddocks questions for sport-related concussion or the orientation section of the Standardized Assessment of Concussion (SAC) should be obtained.[28,29] Individuals who are suspected of having a concussion should immediately be removed from activity for further evaluation and to avoid immediate second impact. Serial assessments are necessary in the early phase after injury to monitor for progression of symptoms or signs.[4,27]

Although a more thorough history may be obtained in the hours and days following a concussion, the first-response provider should note a few elements within the immediate minutes after an injury. A history of the inciting injury should be obtained including method of injury (fall, blunt object, car accident, blast, etc.), degree and direction of force, and presence of protective headgear. History of a high-risk mechanism, such as high-speed impact, fall from significant height, or rotational component, is sufficient to warrant further evaluation in a higher level of care.[4] Loss of consciousness, which was once considered a requisite for diagnosis of concussion, is now known to occur in less than 10% of concussions and may not reflect injury severity.[30] Loss of consciousness, when present, should be documented as self-reported or witnessed.[25] The presence and duration of retrograde and post-traumatic amnesia should also be elicited, but may also need corroboration from witnesses. In the setting of suspected concussion, individuals should be immediately removed from activity in which they are at risk for subsequent injury until further evaluation can be completed.

Hours to days
The goals within the first few hours to days following a concussion are to evaluate for suspected concussion, identify concomitant injuries, and assess plan of care (immediate acute medical attention, observation at home, or outpatient evaluation). Patients may report a spectrum of nonspecific postconcussive symptoms ranging from transiently mild to prolonged disabling impairments (Table 1.2). To date, there is no pathognomonic symptom(s) or direct measurements for concussion diagnosis. The American Academy of Neurology (AAN) recommends utilizing assessment tools along with a focused history and physical examination (H&P) to evaluate and diagnose concussion.[31]

For sports-related concussions, the goal of the on-field assessment is to quickly determine if the athlete should be removed from play for a more thorough sideline evaluation. Sideline evaluations are then used to elucidate degree of suspicion of concussion which, if moderate or high, should prompt removal from the remainder of the game. Any player with concussion should not be returned to play within the same game.

TABLE 1.2
Symptoms of Concussion.

SOMATIC OR PHYSICAL

- Headache
- Dizziness
- Balance difficulties
- Fatigue
- Sleep disturbance (insomnia or excessive sleepiness)
- Visual changes
- Nausea
- Photophobia
- Phonophobia

COGNITIVE

- Difficulty paying attention
- Memory deficits
- Difficulty multitasking
- Cognitive "fog"
- Disorientation/confusion

BEHAVIORAL OR AFFECTIVE

- Emotional lability
- Agitation
- Personality changes
- Anxiety

Sideline assessment tools are useful in the evaluation of a concussed athlete and will be discussed in greater detail elsewhere in this book. Notably, the Sport Concussion Assessment Tool-5 (SCAT5), revised in 2017, is endorsed by a consensus statement on concussion in sport for use in individuals ages 13 years and older. The evaluation takes approximately 10 minutes to administer and includes a symptom checklist, cognitive screen, neurologic screen, and Modified Balance Error Scoring System (mBESS) balance test. Cutoff scores that are diagnostic of concussion have not been elucidated, rather the SCAT5 and other tools should be used as a tool within clinical evaluation.[4] Other useful tools include the SAC, Maddocks's questions, sensory organization test, and King-Devick (K-D) test.[28,29]

In the military realm, the Military Acute Concussion Evaluation (MACE) test is a standardized instrument that evaluates concussion in a combat or deployed setting. This screening tool was designed by the Defense and Veterans Brain Injury Center (DVBIC) in cooperation with leading civilian and military brain injury experts for the purpose of evaluating a person with a suspected concussion within the first 24–48 hours after military-related injury.[32] MACE is comprised of two parts: a focused history section and the neurocognitive examination which includes the SAC to assess acute cognitive effects. Utilizing the MACE assists in

determining if the duty member needs to seek further medical attention or if they can return to duty.

Goals at the initial clinical encounter, which are likely to occur either in the ED or outpatient setting, are to obtain a thorough history, perform a systematic physical examination, order additional testing as indicated, identify symptoms requiring early intervention, and educate the patient on concussion diagnosis and prognosis.

History. A concise but complete history of injury should include mechanism of injury, presence and duration of loss of consciousness, duration of anterograde and retrograde amnesia, and symptom evolution. A medical history including current medical diagnosis with medications, prior surgical interventions, family history, functional and occupational history should be obtained. It is useful in the first clinical encounter to identify risk factors for prolonged recovery. A history of prior concussions as well as details on the severity, duration, and resolution of subsequent symptoms may help with the evaluation and management of the concussion that is currently being evaluated. Comorbid diagnosis of attention-deficit hyperactivity disorder or learning disability, migraines, mental health disorder, and substance abuse has been identified as predictors of protracted recovery following concussion.[33–37]

When determining recommendations for follow-up care, providers should consider these risk factors for association with prolonged symptoms.

Concussion checklists may be useful in identifying the variety, duration, and severity of postconcussive symptoms, as well as for monitoring resolution or progression over subsequent encounters in order to create an individualized treatment plan. The Rivermead Post-Concussion Symptoms Questionnaire (RPQ) and the Post-Concussion Symptom Checklist (PCSC) are two commonly used tools. The RPQ compares premorbid and postconcussive symptoms 24 hours following the injury. The PCSC categorizes symptoms into physical/somatic, cognitive, affective, and sleep disturbances and is measured 2 days post concussion. Self-report checklists are potentially easy and quick measures of progression and/or recovery of symptoms; however, interpretation of these checklists requires an understanding of their limitations. Reliability and sensitivity may be impacted by the patient's impaired ability to provide accurate responses, misunderstanding of the directions, variable interpretations of the rating scales, response bias based on subjective interpretation of symptoms, and presence of overlapping symptoms and/or diagnoses such as chronic pain and/or malingering.[38] Screening for comorbid mood and sleep conditions that may produce symptom overlap with concussion is also valuable. Screens such as the Patient Health Questionnaire-9 (PHQ-9) for depression, PTSD Checklist (PCL-5) for post-traumatic stress disorder, Generalized Anxiety Disorder-7 (GAD-7) for anxiety, CAGE-AID for substance misuse, and STOP-BANG for obstructive sleep apnea may be helpful in assessing patients.

Computerized tools can be used to provide a baseline assessment and track cognitive recovery. Some examples are the Automated Neuropsychological Assessment Metrics (ANAM), ImPACT, CogSport, and Concussion Resolution Index (CRI).[39]

Physical examination. Concussion is a physiologic disruption to the brain that can affect somatic, cognitive, vestibular, affective, and sleep domains.[40] A thorough and systematic neurological and functional physical examination should be performed to assess these multiple domains. Evaluating with a top-down approach allows one to efficiently consider the spectrum of symptoms that may or may not be actively present. The recommended domains to assess including neurologic, mental status, psychiatric, somatic, vestibular, ocular, and balance as well as respective examination maneuvers are listed in Table 1.3.

Laboratory investigations. In the acute setting the role for laboratory examinations are limited. For patients with complicated mTBI, who require in-hospital monitoring, serum sodium levels should be checked within the first 24 hours.[41] There has been an increasing interest from concussion providers for early diagnostic and prognostic tools, such as serum, salivary, and cerebrospinal fluid biomarkers. Currently, there is no laboratory test that can diagnose concussion. Ongoing studies are investigating the use of a number of biomarkers including, but not limited to, S100β, Ubiquitin C-Terminal Hydrolase L1 (UCH-L1), glial fibrillary acidic protein (GFAP), brain-derived neurotrophic factor (BDNF), tau, neurofilament light protein (NFL), neuron specific enolase (NSE), amyloid protein, creatinine kinase (CK), and heart-type fatty acid binding protein (h-FABP). As of February 2018, the Food and Drug Administration has approved the first serum biomarkers, UCH-L1 and GFAP, to help predict which patients will have intracranial lesions visible by CT scan. Serum levels must be drawn within 12 hours of injury and results are typically available within 3—4 hours. Results from these tests can help clinicians decide whether to obtain cranial imaging, ideally leading to more efficient use of healthcare resources and minimizing unnecessary exposure to radiation.[42,43] Biomarkers to detect presence of concussion, stratify patients based on prognosis, and monitor for recovery are still in development.

Imaging. A total of 6%—10% of patients with mTBI demonstrate acute intracranial changes on head CT such as hemorrhage in the epidural, subdural, subarachnoid, or parenchymal spaces. These mTBIs with objective changes on imaging are referred to as complicated mTBIs.[44,45] The New Orleans Criteria and Canadian Head CT guidelines are tools to aid in the decision to obtain cranial imaging acutely after concussion. New Orleans Criteria recommends obtaining head CT in patients with GCS of 15 if they are older than 60 years, display drug or alcohol intoxication, headache, vomiting, seizures, visible trauma above the clavicle, or lasting anterograde amnesia.[46,47] The Canadian Head CT rule limits use of CT after an mTBI to patients if any of the following are present: GCS less than 15 in the first 2 hours after injury, dangerous mechanism (i.e., motor-pedestrian accident, motor vehicle accident with ejection, fall from >3 feet or >5 stairs), age greater than 65 years, retrograde amnesia longer than 30 minutes prior to impact, greater than two episodes of vomiting, or suspicion for open or depressed skull fracture, including basilar skull fracture, or suspected

TABLE 1.3
Appoach to Physical Examination of Concussed Individuals.

Domain	Examination
Neurologic	Cranial nerves Manual muscle strength testing Sensory assessment Coordination Proprioception Deep tendon reflexes Gait
Cognitive	Level of arousal Orientation Language Attention Memory Executive function
Behavior	Affect Comportment
Somatic/ musculoskeletal	Temporomandibular joint Cervical and thoracic ROM Spurling's test Sharp purser test: ligamentous instability Pain: Myofascial, cervicalgia, vertebral, tender points, etc.
Vestibular	Otoscopic evaluation Modified VOMS Halmagyi head thrust: peripheral vestibulopathy Dix–Hallpike test: BPPV
Ophthalmologic	Fundoscopic evaluation Confrontation, visual field evaluation Extraocular movements Smooth pursuit, saccades, near point vergence Horizontal and vertical nystagmus Accommodation
Balance	M-BESS Tandem gait Static and dynamic balance assessment

BPPV, Benign Paroxysmal Positional Vertigo; *M-BESS*, Modified-Balance Error Scoring System; *ROM*, range of motion; *VOMS*, Vestibular Ocular Motor Screening.

cerebrospinal fluid leak.[48] Patients with coagulopathy also warrant special consideration for early imaging. MRI is not indicated in the evaluation of acute concussion.[47] Transcranial doppler ultrasound holds promise in the detection of acute changes in cerebral blood flow and cerebral autoregulation after mTBI which may have diagnostic and prognostic significance.[49,50] fMRI, PET, magnetic resonance spectroscopy (MRS), SPECT, and DTI are not indicated in the acute clinical setting, but may have a role in research.

Initial treatment approach. Education is a vital component in the initial treatment of individuals who have sustained a concussion. Patients should be provided information on the natural history of concussion. In sports-related concussion, most individuals demonstrate complete recovery of somatic, cognitive, postural, and affective symptoms in the first 3 weeks after injury.[50a] Estimates in nonsport concussion are slightly longer, but complete symptom resolution occurs for the vast majority of patients within the first 3 months.[51] Positive prognostic factors should be highlighted to the patient. It has been demonstrated that education on expected symptoms and natural progression of concussion has been associated with reduced mean symptom duration, number of symptoms, and level of distress following concussion.[52,53]

Though rare, due to its potentially fatal condition, patients should be counseled regarding second-impact syndrome (SIS). SIS occurs when an individual experiences a second head injury while still recovering from a prior concussion. The vulnerable, acutely dysregulated brain diffusely and rapidly swells which leads to herniation of the brain. Providers should counsel patients to avoid activities that pose a high risk of obtaining a second head injury during the recovery phase as these may lead to worsening morbidity or mortality.[54]

Recommendations for physical and cognitive rest should be discussed with the patient. Activities should be "modulated" rather than completely ceased. Prolonged cognitive and physical restrictions may adversely contribute to harmful effects such as physiological deconditioning and psychological complications such as fatigue, depression, and anxiety, which lead to prolonged recovery.[53,55,56] Concussed individuals should be encouraged to continue with essential daily activities while staying cognizant of symptom provocation. In short, patients may work "to the point" of symptoms but not "through" symptoms. Activities that require high cognitive or physical load, such as school, work, or physical labor, may need accommodations. Cognitive modulation may be challenging to guide because a universal protocol has yet to be standardized. Generally, endurance and dedicated time should be slowly increased for tasks that involve high levels of concentration such as school or work attendance, sports participation, and mental activities such as technology use (television, mobile device, and computer/laptop). Once resolution of symptoms at rest occurs, return to activities in a stepwise fashion is advised. Exercise has been shown to attenuate cognitive impairment after concussion.[57] Exercise, specifically aerobic exercise, has been shown to promote neurocognitive recovery, reduce symptoms, and improve depressive symptoms. After establishing a symptom-free exercise capacity, testing a preliminary trial of aerobic exercise training has been shown in postconcussed athletes and nonathletes to substantially improve recovery of symptoms and return to normal physical activities.[58] The approach to return to school, work, and physical activity will be discussed later in this book.

Although many symptoms are self-limited and will spontaneously resolve, select symptoms may benefit from early intervention. Post-traumatic headaches (PTHs) and sleep disturbances following concussion should be addressed in initial clinical encounters due to their potential to exacerbate comorbidities and sequelae following injury.

PTHs are the most commonly reported symptom after concussion. PTHs are classified as secondary headaches due to head injury, typically starting within 7 days of injury.[59] They are most commonly characterized based on primary headache phenotype: migraine, tension-type, cluster, cervicogenic, etc. PTH may occur in people with and without premorbid primary headaches. If requiring pharmacologic intervention, simple analgesics (aspirin, acetaminophen or paracetamol, and nonsteroidal anti-inflammatory drugs) are the first-line treatment. Care must be made to avoid the production of medication overuse/rebound headaches that occur when analgesics are used more than 2−3 days per week or on average 10 days per month. If simple analgesics are ineffective, acute or abortive agents such as triptans or ergotamine derivatives can be used for headaches with migrainous features on an as-needed basis. These abortive agents are contraindicated in people with central, coronary, or peripheral vascular disease due to their vasoconstrictive properties. Preventive therapy or prophylaxis for chronic daily headaches will be addressed in Chapter 6. Recommendation of narcotic use should be avoided if possible due to its cognitive and sedative effects, risk of rebound headaches, and threat for dependency.[60]

Sleep disorders following concussion are associated with long-term sequelae and morbidity following TBI. Providing techniques to ensure proper sleep is necessary to combat potential consequences such as anxiety, depression, PTSD, chronic pain, functional impairments, and diminished health-related quality of life.[61] Formulation of proper sleep hygiene is a mainstay of recovery. Sleep hygiene includes following a regular consistent sleep schedule; avoiding heavy exercise during the evening; limiting late and prolonged naps; eliminating caffeine, heavy meals, or alcohol shortly before sleeping; and avoiding bright lights from computers, television, tablets, and video games before and during bedtime.[62] Evaluation for premorbid sleep issues or conditions that may have been exacerbated after concussion, such as obstructive sleep apnea or circadian dysregulation may help guide treatment. Pharmacotherapy, such as off-label use of melatonin or trazodone, in sleep disorders following concussion may be considered in refractory cases. A more in-depth discussion of sleep management after mTBI can be found in Chapter 7.

Complementary and alternative medicine (CAM) has increased in popularity throughout the years as a potential primary and/or adjunctive form of treatment. These therapies warrant further investigation as most lack well-designed and appropriately powered studies. Some popular treatments include acupuncture; Ayurveda; craniosacral therapy, meditation, and mindfulness practices; neurobiofeedback; t'ai chi; and yoga.[63,64] Hyperbaric oxygen therapy (HBOT) has gained publicity as a potential nonpharmacologic intervention after TBI. A Cochrane review and meta-analysis which is the most rigorous review published regarding HBOT in TBI demonstrated that there was no evidence of improvement in overall long-term functional outcome or performance of activities of daily living in those who received HBOT, and there was in fact evidence of some increased risk of significant pulmonary impairment in those receiving HBOT.[65]

Currently, there lacks strong evidence to support the use of supplements for acute concussion management. However, there are animal-based studies along with limited human studies showing promise of supplementation use in severe TBI. Clinical trials evaluating supplement use in concussion management have yet to be completed.[66] Animal studies following concussion show that omega-3-fatty acids (O3FAs) can help maintain genomic and cellular homeostasis, as well as decrease the extent of injury the brain sustains. Curcumin, one of the phytochemicals in turmeric, also reduces neural inflammation. *Scutellaria baicalensis*, a herb used frequently in Chinese herbal medicine, is shown to decrease brain edema, inflammatory mediators, and cell death and increase overall neurologic function. Vitamins C, D, and E have been studied more than other vitamins in severe TBI. Use of vitamins E and C together have shown to significantly decrease the amount of brain injury due to oxidative stress than supplementation of either alone. Vitamin D in combination with progesterone has shown reduced neuronal loss and decreased oxidative damage.[66]

Weeks to Months

Follow-up encounters should include serial monitoring of postconcussive symptoms as well as monitoring of changes to functional parameters or computer-based assessments. Progressive or persistent symptoms may warrant further diagnostic studies and/or referral for specialized rehabilitative services, such as vestibular therapy, oculomotor therapy, and/or cognitive therapy.

Persistent symptoms after concussion may be termed postconcussion syndrome (PCS). PCS encompasses a multitude of nonspecific physical, psychological, and cognitive symptoms seen in concussion that are linked to several possible causes; however, the symptoms do not necessarily reflect ongoing, active, physiologic brain injury. Diagnosis and management of these projected symptoms will be addressed in a future chapter.

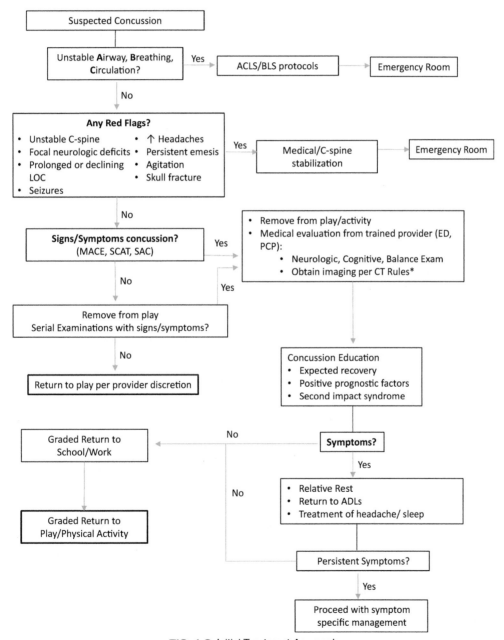

FIG. 1.3 Initial Treatment Approach.

CONCLUSION

Concussion, or mTBI, is a major public health concern. Timely identification, evaluation, and management of mTBI are essential. The pathophysiology of mTBI is typically self-limited and usually temporary. In the acute phase of concussion, education regarding the likelihood of recovery is key. Treatment of symptoms with significant functional impact, such as PTH and sleep disturbance, may be useful in the prevention of long-term sequelae. Future progress is needed toward standardized diagnostic criteria and stratification methods to identify patients who would benefit from further aggressive and early interventions.

REFERENCES

1. CDC-National Center for Health Statistics - Homepage. http://www.cdc.gov/nchs/. December 8, 2018.
2. Department of Veterans Affairs D of D. *VA/DoD Clinical Practice Guideline for the Management of Concussion-Mild Traumatic Brain Injury.* 2016. Version 2.0.
3. Kay T, Harrington DE, Adams R, et al. American congress of rehabilitation medicine mild traumatic brain injury committee of the head injury interdisciplinary special interest group. Definition of mild traumatic brain injury. *J Head Trauma Rehabil.* 1993. https://doi.org/10.1097/00001199-199309000-00010.
4. McCrory P, Meeuwisse W, Dvořák J, et al. Consensus statement on concussion in sport—the 5thinternational conference on concussion in sport held in Berlin, October 2016. *Br J Sports Med.* 2017. https://doi.org/10.1136/bjsports-2017-097699.
5. American Psychiatric Association. *Diagnostic and Statistical Manual of Mental Disorders DMS V.* 2013. https://doi.org/10.1176/appi.books.978089042596.744053.
6. Iverson GL, Lange RT, W M. Outcome from complicated versus uncomplicated mild traumatic brain injury. *Rehabil Res Pr.* 2012:415740.
7. Furger RE, Nelson LD, Lerner EB, McCrea MA. Frequency of factors that complicate the identification of mild traumatic brain injury in level I trauma center patients. *Concussion.* 2016. https://doi.org/10.1016/j.scitotenv.2013.03.021.
8. Frieden TR, Houry D, Baldwin G. Report to congress on traumatic brain injury in the United States: epidemiology and rehabilitation. *CDC NIH Rep to Congr.* 2015. https://doi.org/10.3171/2009.10.JNS091500.
9. Laker SR. Epidemiology of concussion and mild traumatic brain injury. *Pharm Manag PM R.* 2011. https://doi.org/10.1016/j.pmrj.2011.07.017.
10. Defense and Veterans Brain Injury Center. DoD Worldwide Numbers for TBI. https://dvbic.dcoe.mil/dod-worldwide-numbers-tbi. December 8, 2018.
11. Department of Labor B of LS. News Release: Nonfatal Occupational Injuries and Illnesses Requiring Days Away From Work, 2015 [online].
12. Taylor CA, Bell JM, Breiding MJ, Xu L. Traumatic brain injury—related emergency department visits, hospitalizations, and deaths — United States, 2007 and 2013. *MMWR Surveill Summ.* 2017. https://doi.org/10.15585/mmwr.ss6609a1.
13. Frieden TR, Houry D, Baldwin G. Traumatic brain injury in the United States: epidemiology and rehabilitation. *CDC NIH Rep to Congr.* 2015:1—74. https://doi.org/10.3171/2009.10.JNS091500.
14. Harmon KG, Drezner JA, Gammons M, et al. American Medical Society for Sports Medicine position statement: concussion in sport. *Br J Sports Med.* 2013. https://doi.org/10.1136/bjsports-2012-091941.
15. Covassin T, Moran R, Elbin RJ. Sex differences in reported concussion injury rates and time loss from participation: an update of the national collegiate athletic association injury surveillance program from 2004-2005 through 2008-2009. *J Athl Train.* 2016. https://doi.org/10.4085/1062-6050-51.3.05.
16. Mollayeva T, El-Khechen-Richandi G, Colantonio A. Sex & gender considerations in concussion research. *Int Spec Conf Probabilistic Saf Struct.* 1980. https://doi.org/10.2217/cnc-2017-0015.
17. Giza CC, Hovda DA. The new metabolic cascade of concussion. *Neurosurgery.* 2014;75(suppl_4):S24—S33. https://doi.org/:10.1227/NEU.0000000000000505.
18. Barlow KM, Marcil LD, Dewey D, et al. Cerebral perfusion changes in post-concussion syndrome: a prospective controlled cohort study. *J Neurotrauma.* 2017. https://doi.org/10.1089/neu.2016.4634.
19. Kim S, Han SC, Gallan AJ, Hayes JP. Neurometabolic indicators of mitochondrial dysfunction in repetitive mild traumatic brain injury. *Concussion.* 2017. https://doi.org/10.2217/cnc-2017-0013.
20. Chiu CC, Liao YE, Yang LY, et al. Neuroinflammation in animal models of traumatic brain injury. *J Neurosci Methods.* 2016. https://doi.org/10.1016/j.jneumeth.2016.06.018.
21. Johnson VE, Stewart W, Smith DH. Axonal pathology in traumatic brain injury. *Exp Neurol.* 2013. https://doi.org/10.1016/j.expneurol.2012.01.013.
22. Purkayastha S, Sorond FA, Lyng S, Frantz J, Murphy MN, Hynan LS, Sabo T, Bell KR. Impaired cerebral vasoreactivity despite symptom resolution in sports-related concussion. *J Neurotrauma.* Publ online 23 Apr 2019. https://doi.org/10.1089/neu.2018.5861.
23. Ling H, Hardy J, Zetterberg H. Neurological consequences of traumatic brain injuries in sports. *Mol Cell Neurosci.* 2015. https://doi.org/10.1016/j.mcn.2015.03.012.
24. Stiell IG, Clement CM, McKnight RD, et al. The Canadian C-spine rule versus the NEXUS low-risk criteria in patients with trauma. *N Engl J Med.* 2003. https://doi.org/10.1056/NEJMoa031375.
25. McCrea M, Jafee M, Helmick K, Guskiewicz S. *Validation of the Military Acute Concussion Evaluation (MACE) for In-Theater Evaluation of Combat-Related Traumatic Brain Injury.* 2009.
26. Coldren RL, Kellly MP, Parish RV, Dretsch M, Russell ML. Evaluation of the Military Acute Concussion Evaluation

for use in combat operations more than 12 hours after injury. *Mil Med.* 2010. https://doi.org/10.7205/MILMED-D-09-00258.

27. By D, Concussion THE, Sport IN, et al. Sport concussion assessment tool - 5th edition. *Br J Sports Med.* 2017. https://doi.org/10.1136/bjsports-2017-097506SCAT5.

28. Maddocks D. The assessment of orientation following concussion in athletes. *Clin J Sport.* 1995. https://doi.org/10.1097/00042752-199501000-00006.

29. McCrea M, Kelly JP, Randolph C, et al. Standardized assessment of concussion (SAC): on-site mental status evaluation of the athlete. *J Head Trauma Rehabil.* 1998. https://doi.org/10.1097/00001199-199804000-00005.

30. Cantu RC. Return to play guidelines after a head injury. *Clin Sports Med.* 1998. https://doi.org/10.1016/S0278-5919(05)70060-0.

31. Giza CC, Kutcher JS, Ashwal S, et al. Summary of evidence-based guideline update: evaluation and management of concussion in sports. *Neurology.* 2013. https://doi.org/10.1212/WNL.0b013e31828d57dd.

32. McCrea M, Guskiewicz K, Doncevic S, et al. Day of injury cognitive performance on the military acute concussion evaluation (MACE) by U.S. Military service members in OEF/OIF. *Mil Med.* 2014. https://doi.org/10.7205/MILMED-D-13-00349.

33. Mautner K, Sussman WI, Axtman M, Al-Farsi Y, Al-Adawi S. Relationship of attention deficit hyperactivity disorder and postconcussion recovery in youth athletes. *Clin J Sport Med.* 2015. https://doi.org/10.1097/JSM.0000000000000151.

34. Zemek R, Barrowman N, Freedman SB, et al. Clinical risk score for persistent postconcussion symptomsamong children with acute concussion in the ED. *JAMA, J Am Med Assoc.* 2016. https://doi.org/10.1001/jama.2016.1203.

35. Morgan CD, Zuckerman SL, Lee YM, et al. Predictors of postconcussion syndrome after sports-related concussion in young athletes: a matched case-control study. *J Neurosurg Pediatr.* 2015. https://doi.org/10.3171/2014.10.PEDS14356.

36. Iverson GL. Misdiagnosis of the persistent postconcussion syndrome in patients with depression. *Arch Clin Neuropsychol.* 2006. https://doi.org/10.1016/j.acn.2005.12.008.

37. Iverson GL, Lange RT, Franzen MD. Effects of mild traumatic brain injury cannot be differentiated from substance abuse. *Brain Inj.* 2005. https://doi.org/10.1080/02699050410001720068.

38. Register-Mihalik JK, Guskiewicz KM, Mihalik JP, Schmidt JD, Kerr ZY, McCrea MA. Reliable change, sensitivity, and specificity of a multidimensional concussion assessment battery: implications for caution in clinical practice. *J Head Trauma Rehabil.* 2013. https://doi.org/10.1097/HTR.0b013e3182585d37.

39. Grindel SH. The use, abuse, and future of neuropsychologic testing in mild traumatic brain injury. *Curr Sports Med Rep.* 2006. https://doi.org/10.1097/01.CSMR.0000306513.79430.03.

40. Scorza KA, Raleigh MF, O'connor FG. Current concepts in concussion: evaluation and management. *Am Fam Physician.* 2012. d10181 [pii].

41. Tanriverdi F, Schneider HJ, Aimaretti G, Masel BE, Casanueva FF, Kelestimur F. Pituitary dysfunction after traumatic brain injury: a clinical and pathophysiological approach. *Endocr Rev.* 2015. https://doi.org/10.1210/er.2014-1065.

42. Papa L, Brophy GM, Welch RD, et al. Time course and diagnostic accuracy of glial and neuronal blood biomarkers GFAP and UCH-L1 in a large cohort of trauma patients with and without mild traumatic brain injury. *JAMA Neurol.* 2016. https://doi.org/10.1001/jamaneurol.2016.0039.

43. Bazarian JJ, Biberthaler P, Welch RD, et al. Serum GFAP and UCH-L1 for prediction of absence of intracranial injuries on head CT (ALERT-TBI): a multicentre observational study. *Lancet Neurol.* 2018. https://doi.org/10.1016/S1474-4422(18)30231-X.

44. Kisat M, Zafar SN, Latif A, et al. Predictors of positive head CT scan and neurosurgical procedures after minor head trauma. *J Surg Res.* 2012. https://doi.org/10.1016/j.jss.2011.04.059.

45. Kreitzer N, Hart K, Lindsell CJ, et al. Factors associated with adverse outcomes in patients with traumatic intracranial hemorrhage and Glasgow Coma Scale of 15. *Am J Emerg Med.* 2017. https://doi.org/10.1016/j.ajem.2017.01.051.

46. Haydel MJ, Preston CA, Mills TJ, Luber S, Blaudeau EBA, Deblieux PMC. Indications for computed tomography in patients. *N Engl J Med.* 2000. https://doi.org/10.1056/NEJM200007133430204.

47. Jagoda AS, Bazarian JJ, Bruns JJ, et al. Clinical policy: neuroimaging and decisionmaking in adult mild traumatic brain injury in the acute setting. *Ann Emerg Med.* 2008. https://doi.org/10.1016/j.annemergmed.2008.08.021.

48. Stiell IG, Wells GA, Vandemheen K, et al. The Canadian CT Head Rule for patients with minor head injury. *Lancet.* 2001. https://doi.org/10.1016/S0140-6736(00)04561-X.

49. Meier TB, Bellgowan PSF, Singh R, Kuplicki R, Polanski DW, Mayer AR. Recovery of cerebral blood flow following sports-related concussion. *JAMA Neurol.* 2015. https://doi.org/10.1001/jamaneurol.2014.4778.

50. Tan CO, Meehan WP, Iverson GL, Taylor JA. Cerebrovascular regulation, exercise, and mild traumatic brain injury. *Neurology.* 2014. https://doi.org/10.1212/WNL.0000000000000944.

50a. Belanger HG, Vanderploeg RD. The neuropsychological impact of sports-related concussion: a meta-analysis. *J Int Neuropsychol Soc.* 2005 Jul;11(4):345−357. PubMed PMID: 16209414.

51. Binder LM, Rohling ML, Larrabee GJ. A review of mild head trauma. Part I: meta-analytic review of neuropsychological studies. *J Clin Exp Neuropsychol.* 1997. https://doi.org/10.1080/01688639708403870.

52. Miller LJ, Mittenberg W. Brief cognitive behavioral interventions in mild traumatic brain injury. *Appl Neuropsychol.* 1998. https://doi.org/10.1207/s15324826an0504_2.

53. Ponsford J, Willmott C, Rothwell A, et al. Impact of early intervention on outcome after mild traumatic brain injury in children. *Pediatrics.* 2001. https://doi.org/10.1542/peds.108.6.1297.

54. McLendon LA, Kralik SF, Grayson PA, Golomb MR. The controversial second impact syndrome: a review of the literature. *Pediatr Neurol.* 2016. https://doi.org/10.1016/j.pediatrneurol.2016.03.009.

55. Grool AM, Aglipay M, Momoli F, et al. Association between early participation in physical activity following acute concussion and persistent postconcussive symptoms in children and adolescents. *JAMA, J Am Med Assoc.* 2016. https://doi.org/10.1001/jama.2016.17396.

56. DiFazio M, Silverberg ND, Kirkwood MW, Bernier R, Iverson GL. Prolonged activity restriction after concussion: are we worsening outcomes? *Clin Pediatr (Phila).* 2015. https://doi.org/10.1177/0009922815589914.

57. Leddy JJ, Haider MN, Ellis M, Willer BS. Exercise is medicine for concussion. *Curr Sports Med Rep.* 2018. https://doi.org/10.1249/JSR.0000000000000505.

58. Leddy JJ, Kozlowski K, Donnelly JP, Pendergast DR, Epstein LH, Willer B. A preliminary study of subsymptom threshold exercise training for refractory post-concussion syndrome. *Clin J Sport Med.* 2010. https://doi.org/10.1097/JSM.0b013e3181c6c22c.

59. Society HCS of the IH. *The International Classification of Headache Disorders.* 2nd ed. 2008. https://doi.org/10.1177/0333102413485658. Headache.

60. Lucas S. Characterization and management of headache after mild traumatic brain injury. In: *Brain Neurotrauma: Molecular, Neuropsychological, and Rehabilitation Aspects.* 2015. https://doi.org/10.1201/b18126.

61. Wickwire EM, Williams SG, Roth T, et al. Sleep, sleep disorders, and mild traumatic brain injury. What we know and what we need to know: findings from a national working group. *Neurotherapeutics.* 2016. https://doi.org/10.1007/s13311-016-0429-3.

62. Katz DI, Cohen SI, Alexander MP. Chapter 9 — mild traumatic brain injury. In: *Handbook of Clinical Neurology.* 2015. https://doi.org/10.1016/B978-0-444-52892-6.00009-X.

63. Richer AC. Functional medicine approach to traumatic brain injury. *Med Acupunct.* 2017. https://doi.org/10.1089/acu.2017.1217.

64. Cantor JB, Gumber S. Use of complementary and alternative medicine in treating individuals with traumatic brain injury. *Curr Phys Med Rehabil Reports.* 2013. https://doi.org/10.1007/s40141-013-0019-9.

65. Bennett MH, Trytko B, Jonker B. Hyperbaric oxygen therapy for the adjunctive treatment of traumatic brain injury. *Cochrane Database Syst Rev.* 2009. https://doi.org/10.1002/14651858.CD004609.pub2.

66. Ashbaugh A, McGrew C. The role of nutritional supplements in sports concussion treatment. *Curr Sports Med Rep.* 2016. https://doi.org/10.1249/JSR.0000000000000219.

CHAPTER 2

Neuropsychological Assessment

NANCY H. HSU, PSYD, ABPP-RP • PAUL DUKARM, PHD, ABPP-CN

Following a concussion, patients can present with cognitive, personality, and emotional changes. The affected neurocognitive domains may include learning and memory, language, executive functioning, working memory, and processing speed.[1–3] Examples of specific subjective complaints consist of short-term memory loss, difficulty focusing and concentrating, word-finding difficulty, inability to multitask, distractibility, and slowed thinking. In addition, patients commonly complain of mood lability, depressed mood, anxiousness, irritability, frustration, impulsivity, anger, and impatience.[3] While symptoms of concussion typically resolve within 3 months post injury, there is a small percentage of patients who continue to experience persistent post-concussion syndrome.[2] Regardless of time post injury, neuropsychological assessment can objectively quantify neurocognitive functioning and detect other biopsychosocial factors that may be contributing to persistent symptoms. It is an integral part of concussion care, guiding treatment planning, and assisting in making decision in regards to return to work, play, or duty.

NEUROPSYCHOLOGICAL METHODS

Evidence-based Neuropsychological Practice

Neuropsychological assessment can ascertain a large body of information associated with diagnostic and treatment-related concerns and questions. There are typically six broad categories that neuropsychological assessment referral questions generally fall under. These include (1) diagnosis, (2) describing neuropsychological status, (3) treatment planning or facility placement, (4) identifying effects of treatment response or change in functioning over time, (5) as a research evaluation tool, and (6) in forensic applications.[4] Shoenberg and Scott[5] discuss how evidence-based neuropsychological practice seeks "to provide guidelines for neuropsychologists to integrate outcomes of research, clinical expertise, the unique aspects of the patient, referral questions, and available costs and resources to the provision of neuropsychology services. Neuropsychology is uniquely positioned to answer concussion-related referral questions as well as provide a depth of information pertaining to the diagnosis and management of concussion. When neuropsychological assessment is requested due to a suspected concussion or persistent postconcussion complaints, there are a variety of methods currently being utilized for evaluating these types of referral questions. Neuropsychology is uniquely positioned to answer concussion-related referral questions as well as provide a depth of information pertaining to the diagnosis and management of concussion.

The Physical Examination

The initial evaluation of a concussion often begins in the setting for which it occurred. This is the most reliable temporal assessment since concussive symptoms do not have a "late onset" period and retrospective patient report can be unreliable. Most often, however, individuals experience a concussion outside of these settings or do not present to emergency department personnel. Acute physical examination procedures are generally conducted by healthcare providers who have been trained in neurological screening, such as emergency first responders, sports team physicians, or combat medics. Concussion providers are generally physicians trained in neurology, orthopedics, or physiatry. Acute manifestation of concussive sequelae can result in disorientation, confusion, as well as a host of other neurological symptoms. The physical examination generally tests for gait and coordination, oculomotor functioning and smooth pursuit eye movements, and general mental status.[6]

The determination of brain injury severity is often assessed using a standardized protocol for evaluating conscious states. These protocols and measurement instruments include the Glasgow Coma Scale,[7] Rancho Los Amigos Levels of Cognitive Functioning Scale,[8] and the Confusion Assessment Protocol.[9] These instruments

Concussion. https://doi.org/10.1016/B978-0-323-65384-8.00002-X
Copyright © 2020 Elsevier Inc. All rights reserved.

can be completed in the field by trained personnel to determine the level of consciousness or post-traumatic amnesia acutely after brain injury.

The utilization of standardized cognitive screening instruments to determine the presence of concussion initially began with the Standardized Assessment of Concussion (SAC).[10] This screening tool contains tasks that challenge orientation, concentration, and memory. The tool was subsequently introduced into combat military settings where a history section is completed in addition to the SAC. The Military Acute Concussion Evaluation (MACE) yields a score, which is essentially the SAC score. The MACE has been extended for use in the community settings.[11]

Questionnaires and Interviews

One method of rapidly and efficiently collecting a summary of subjective cognitive complaints ostensibly related to concussion is to administer a symptom checklist. These tools are widely used both in clinical and research settings. However, symptom checklists are notorious for being susceptible to overreporting. Clinicians need to be aware of the nonspecificity of symptoms associated with concussion, as well as several facets of social neuropsychological phenomena that could potentially influence the degree of concussion symptom endorsement. These include motivational and contextual factors such as the presence of litigation for monetary reward or other incentives to appear functionally disabled, expectancy bias, and iatrogenic factors.[12]

The preferred method of conducting a clinical interview in the context of postconcussion syndrome is an open-ended approach. Interviews are similarly vulnerable to such symptom validity issues. For example, as opposed to severe injuries where anosognosia may be present, symptom salience is high in individuals with persistent complaints with a history of mild head injury.[13] In an effort to enhance sensitivity and specificity of clinical traumatic brain injury (TBI) diagnosis, a hybrid interview application was developed for special populations in the Veterans Health Administration for the purpose of determining the likely presence of a remote brain injury.[14] This method has clinical utility with nonmilitary and veteran populations as well.

Computerized Neuropsychological Screening

Computerized cognitive screening has also been utilized in multiple settings. Used contemporarily by professions other than neuropsychology that include neurology, speech and language pathology, and occupational therapy, computerized cognitive testing has become a rather ubiquitous method in the evaluation of cognitive difficulties. Initially developed to obtain baseline and follow-up assessment for military personnel suffering from concussion, the Automated Neuropsychological Assessment Metrics (ANAM) has been used for operational military service branches to study the effects of concussion. Other commercially available computerized assessment devices (e.g., CogSport/Axon,[15] King-Devick[16]) have been marketed specifically for sports-related concussion evaluation.[15,17]

The Immediate Postconcussion Assessment and Cognitive Testing (ImPACT)[15] battery contains seven test modules that assess neurocognitive functioning. These include memory, reaction time, nonverbal problem-solving, response variability, sustained and selective attention time, and attention span. The battery contains six alternative forms to mitigate practice effects. For pediatric populations, the ImPACT Pediatric is an examiner-administered iOS-based battery of neuropsychological tests designed to measure cognitive functioning in children ages 5–11 years.[18]

Serial neuropsychological testing can potentially take place across various time periods, e.g., days, weeks, months, and even years. Clinicians should become familiar with test-retest reliability since those coefficients have been shown to vary across time period and task. For example, significant changes have been found in memory composite scores across testing, while motor speed and reaction time composites showed no significant growth.[16a]

The Fixed and Flexible Battery

The fixed battery approach to neuropsychological assessment offers some relative consistency for the examiner as well as the ability to derive an overall deficiency score. The fixed battery is common in settings where research data are concurrently being collected. The claim of many forensic specialists that the fixed battery is superior to the flexible approaches has been determined to be inaccurate.[19] The Meyers Neuropsychological Battery was validated in a mild traumatic brain injury population.[20] The battery consists of the Ward Seven Subtest version of the Wechsler Adult Intelligence Scale-III and a collection 15 independent neuropsychological tests presented in standard order.[20]

The flexible approach to neuropsychological assessment involves the hypothesis testing and deductive decision-making process that stem from qualitative observation of the patient. Differences of the flexible approach from the fixed approach include three general areas. These are (1) the timing of test selection, (2) reliance on neurological concepts about behavioral data versus psychometric (i.e., impairment score) data, and (3) reliance on qualitative versus quantitative data.[21] Decisions about test selection and which areas of cognition to concentrate resources on are made during the examination, not a priori such as in a fixed battery approach. These decisions are based on how the patient behaved (testing) as the information is integrated into a cognitive neurology framework about brain-behavior relationships. Finally, the qualitative aspects of testing tend to be weighted more than purely psychometric data points, such as in a binary impaired versus not impaired determination.[21]

The majority of neuropsychological assessment involves one-on-one paper and pencil testing. Testing session entails a patient completing a battery of tests that is administered by a trained psychometrician or a neuropsychologist. The selected tests assess neurocognitive functions that allow the clinician to address the referral questions and provide treatment recommendations. A comprehensive neuropsychological evaluation for concussion examines learning, memory, attention, language, executive functioning, visuospatial processing, motor skills, and neurobehavioral functioning (see Table 2.1). Depending on the context for testing, performance and symptoms validity measures could be included in the battery as well.

REASON AND TEMPORAL IMPACT OF REFERRAL

Treating physicians should consider referring their patients for neuropsychological assessment when there is question about cognitive and emotional functioning following concussion. When patients complain about changes to their cognition, personality, and emotional regulation, a neuropsychological assessment could validate their concerns or provide them with assurance that the symptoms would likely resolve over time. Treating physicians should also consider requesting a neuropsychological assessment when there is question about the impact of pain, trauma reactions, psychological sequela, sleep disturbance, other medical comorbidities, or preexisting mood disorders on their patients' recovery process.

The referring source should articulate the reason for testing by identifying questions they would like the neuropsychologist to address; "What do I want to know from testing?" Being specific with the referral question instead of making a generic request will yield better results and allow the neuropsychologist to tailor their battery to better respond to the referral question.

Documenting reason for referral will also support the need for the patients to undergo a neuropsychological assessment to their insurers. Furthermore, the treating physician should explain the reason for referral to their patients in order to increase follow-through with the evaluation.

Timing of the referral can influence the interpretation of test results. Acutely, cognitive status will be fluid as the brain is still healing from the injury. Test results would only capture a snapshot of cognitive functioning for that time period, and not allow for an accurate trajectory. However, test results could assist the treating physician to make referrals to appropriate rehabilitation services (e.g., occupational therapy, speech-language pathology, cognitive rehabilitation) and guide acute rehabilitation goals. When testing is conducted a year or more post injury, clinical judgment could be made regarding prognosis, as well as permanency of impairments and disability. Test results could provide nonphysician providers, including vocational rehabilitation counselors, case managers/social workers, and therapists, valuable information about their patients' cognitive strengths and weaknesses that could impact treatment. Finally, serial testing should be considered to help track progress in recovery, thereby assisting in making decisions regarding return to play/work/school.

NEUROPSYCHOLOGICAL OUTCOME OF CONCUSSION
Misconceptions

Misconceptions about brain injury recovery continue to persist despite educational and rehabilitation programs designed to enhance identification and management. Gouvier et al.[56] highlighted this in their seminal study on public knowledge and perceptions of brain injury. For example, more than 80% of those polled said that survivors of a brain injury can forget who they are and not recognize others, but be normal in every other way. Over half of the responses by the general public regarding recovery were considered to be incorrect. Over 70% were not aware that having one head injury increased probability for having a second. Despite over 60% believing that rest and inactivity was good advice for a recovering person to follow, over 70% incorrectly believed that it is the effort one puts into recovery that determines their outcome. Other surprising findings were noted and subsequent studies have replicated their findings. In order to define and address such misconceptions about brain injury, Block[57] developed the Traumatic Brain Injury

TABLE 2.1
Neuropsychological Tests and Associated Functions.

Domain	Functions Assessed	Tests
Performance validity	Task engagement	Test of Memory Malingering,[22] Word Memory Test,[23] Dot Counting Test,[24] Victoria Symptom Validity Test[25]
Symptom validity	Credibility of subjective symptom complaints	Structured Inventory of Malingered Symptoms,[26] Validity Scales of Minnesota Multiphasic Personality Test-2 Restructured Form (MMPI-2; RF)[27]
Psychological status	Psychological and emotional status	MMPI-2 (RF),[27] Personality Assessment Inventory,[28] Patient Health Questionnaire (PHQ-9),[29] Generalized Anxiety Disorder 7 (GAD-7)[30]
Intellectual ability	Premorbid functioning, estimation of intellectual abilities.	Wechsler Adult Intelligence Scale-Fourth Edition,[31] Shipley-2[32]
Language	Reading ability, auditory comprehension, word and object naming, academic skills proficiency.	Boston Diagnostic Aphasia Examination,[33] Neuropsychological Assessment Battery Language Module,[34] Academic Achievement Battery[35]
Complex attention	Attention capacity, serial digit sequencing and immediate memory, information transformation, calculation and updating; cognitive control, selective and sustained attention, speed of information processing	WAIS-IV Cognitive Proficiency Subtests,[a] Ruff 2 and 7 Selective Attention Test,[36] Brief Test of Attention,[37] Paced Auditory Serial Addition Test,[38] Trail Making Test[39]
Learning and memory	Single exposure and serial/rote immediate recall; aassociative learning and memory; rate of learning efficiency; delayed recall, recognition discrimination, proactive and retroactive interference, types and quality of memory errors.	Hopkins Verbal Learning Test-Revised,[40] California Verbal Learning Test-2,[41] Rey Auditory Verbal Learning Test,[42] Wechsler Memory Scale-Fourth Edition,[43] Brief Visuospatial Memory Test,[44] Continuous Visual Memory Test[45]
Executive control	Cognitive flexibility, inhibitory control, fluid reasoning (deductive and inductive logic), divergent thinking, initiative, planning, cognitive organization, self-monitoring, practical judgment.	Stroop Test,[46] Tower of London-2,[47] Wisconsin Card Sorting Test,[48] Controlled Oral word Association Test, Booklet Category Test,[49] Copy Trial of Rey-Osterrieth Complex Figure Test,[50] Copy Trial of Rey Complex Figure Test,[51] Delis-Kaplan Executive Functioning Battery[52]
Visuospatial processing	Analysis and integration, mental rotation, organization, spatial orientation, construction, visuomotor integration	WAIS-IV Perceptual Reasoning Subtests, Shipley-2 (Block Patterns)
Sensory/Motor	Near-point visual acuity, auditory acuity, tactile sensation, gait and station, fine motor dexterity, coordination, strength of grip, motor speed, lateralization dominance	Grooved Pegboard Test,[53] Finger Oscillation Test,[54] Dean-Woodcock Sensory Motor Battery[55]

[a] WAIS-IV Cognitive Proficiency Subtests: Digit Span, Arithmetic, Symbol Search, Coding.

Misconceptions/Misattribution Model (TBI-MM) in which the goal is to uncover and delineate the bases for the creation and maintenance of TBI misconceptions.

Rate of Cognitive Recovery

Immediate disruption of cognitive functioning is common in the acute phase. In the initial weeks after a concussion, individuals tend to perform about one-half of a standard deviation below peers on neuropsychological tasks matched on demographic variables. Overwhelming evidence has shown that for the vast majority of individuals, complete cognitive recovery happens over the course of several days to no more than a few months.[58,59] Moreover, inclusion of a nonconcussed orthopedic trauma control group is considered by many in the field of clinical neuropsychology to be a gold standard when researching neuropsychological outcome in mild TBI patients outside of sports. This is because studies have long demonstrated that in terms of neuropsychological performance, mild TBI patients and nonconcussed orthopedic trauma control participants have disparate neuropsychological performance profiles at 1 month post injury, but at 1 year those between group neuropsychological differences become similar in both cognitive performance and subjective post-traumatic complaint profiles.[59,60] Long-term outcome studies show average functioning and no cognitive decline in persons evaluated some 20–30 years post concussion.[61,62]

Myth of the "Miserable Minority"

A rather perpetual belief in the mild TBI literature is that there have been a percentage of people (roughly 15%) who do not recover within the expected trajectory and go on to experience permanent cognitive and functional disability as a consequence of concussion.[63] This myth is traceable to an influential review article written in 1995 on mild TBI.[64] Further reviews of additional source evidence found that in two source articles, one of the study's findings showed that cognitive dysfunction was based on self-report, and that of the 15% that reported continuing symptoms, over half were in litigation or judged to be malingering. In the second study, the only deficits detected in a subset of the study that included moderate-severe head injured persons were again based on self-report, and not objective testing.[1] To summarize, the 10%–15% "miserable minority" *complain* of cognitive dysfunction, but their subjective symptom reporting correlates less with actual brain impairment and more with contextual and other biopsychosocial factors.

Base Rate of Postconcussive Symptoms

In healthy samples, concussion symptoms occur rather frequently. Failure to account for this base rate information is common in large group studies on concussion symptoms.[65] These studies show that people are prone toward underestimating the presence and degree of pre-injury post concussive-like symptoms, a phenomena referred to as the good old days bias.[66,67] For example, in one seminal study, over 75% endorsed mild fatigue, over 70% endorsed mild irritability, and over 50% endorsed mild memory problems, feeling down or nervousness and headaches. Furthermore, over 15% of the healthy sample endorsed moderate-severe concentration problems, over 13% with memory problems and fatigue, 12% with poor sleep, and over 10% with moderate-severe temper problems and irritability.[67]

PERFORMANCE AND SYMPTOM VALIDITY

Symptom validity testing in traumatic brain injury has become a widely discussed topic in the field of neuropsychology.[68] Validity of test findings is considered a critical issue in assessment (see Table 2.1). Many tests have been developed for the main purpose of detecting magnification of deficits during a neuropsychological assessment. The most common approach involves forced-choice testing that is based on using validated cut-off scores to suggest suboptimal effort. However, relying solely on these measures has been criticized given the complexity of psychosocial, psychiatric, and medical symptoms typically presented by patients with concussion that might account for the underlying cause of insufficient effort. Iverson and Binder recommended the following steps for a comprehensive approach to assess for symptom exaggeration and/or suboptimal effort: (1) consider inconsistency between severity of cognitive deficits and injury severity, (2) thoroughly review medical records for discrepancies, (3) test for response bias as part of neurocognitive testing, and (4) identify potential bias that might interfere with the clinician's clinical judgment.[69]

Once validity of test performance is confirmed, neuropsychological assessment could objectively characterize cognitive deficits instead of relying on patients' self-report of symptoms. Depending on context and setting, patients with concussion could present with magnification or minimization of their symptoms. Patients might exaggerate/fabricate symptoms for secondary gains, such as disability eligibility or compensation in medicolegal cases. Exaggeration of symptoms might also reflect someone's need to be validated. Brain injury has been referred to as an "invisible injury" given that neurocognitive impairments are not visible; patients present outwardly as uninjured in the absence of orthopedic injuries. To validate the legitimacy of their injury, patients may magnify the severity of their symptoms. On the other hand, minimization of symptoms could occur in the context of desire to return to work/duty/play. Athletes who are motivated to return to play or active military servicemen who desire to return to duty may minimize their symptoms in order to be medically cleared by their treating physician.[70,71] There is also the avoidance of stigma that lead to minimization of symptoms.

INFLUENCE OF EXPECTATIONS ON TEST PERFORMANCE

Important mediating factors that can drive poor performance in some individuals in neuropsychological testing include expectation biases. People who expect that they should perform in a certain way, or have preconceived notions about how a person with particular brain injury would perform on neuropsychological testing, are prone to fulfill those expectations. Several specific biases have been identified in the field of social psychology and applied to neuropsychological assessment in the context of persistent postconcussive complaints.

Mittenberg's[72] groundbreaking study shed light on how automatic expectancies about the consequences of a mild brain injury shape persistent postconcussive complaints in some people. They postulated that without a readily available and alternative explanation, people will attribute the saliency of their symptoms to a concussion due to the automatic activation of the symptom expectancies associated with perceived concussion sequelae. Expectancies work to automatically bias selective attention, forcing the person to focus even more on their symptoms that further increases physiological arousal.

The expectation-as-etiology concept describes individuals who have persistent postconcussive complaints and are prone to fulfilling a predetermined expectation of a cluster of symptoms associated with a concussion. Furthermore, a second finding from their study indicated that individuals will report common concussion symptoms less frequently than normal, non–head injured controls. This phenomenon, termed the *good old days* bias, is illustrated by the finding that individuals who imagine they have had a concussion will attribute less symptoms as being present at preinjury baseline than even non–head injured control persons. These findings were extended and confirmed in athletes who

sustained sports-related concussions. Yet, the expectation-as-etiology bias may be overly narrow in its explanatory power.[73] Regardless of *any* negative event, people will underestimate their preinjury baseline and report less frequent and less magnitude of symptoms perceived prior to a negative event.

Stereotype threat is a situational phenomenon where activations of negative performance expectancies are generated and subsequently lead to worse performance. When confronted with tasks that one thinks are performed poorly, the threat of that group stereotype is believed to interfere and lead to worse performance. This finding also applies to individuals of that group who do not believe the stereotype. Moreover, people of any group can be made to perform inferiorly on a given task, if a stereotype threat is activated. The stereotype threat was applied to neuropsychological test performance in individuals with a history of concussion.[74] Their findings indicated that when people with a history of concussion are primed about neuropsychological effects with an emphasis to potential poor performance prior to testing, those individuals performed worse than people who received neutral instructions. Moreover, people in the diagnostic threat group rated the tasks more difficult, put forth less effort, and had less confidence in their performance. Subsequently, effort, anxiety, and depression were not contributing factors in test performance in diagnostic threat conditions.[75]

Diagnosis threat may not carry over into all groups. For reasons not fully understood, athletes who have sustained sports-related concussion do not produce the same lower performance in experimental conditions as their nonthreat counterparts. Moreover, athletes who were placed under diagnostic threat about a previous concussion injury did not perform worse on neuropsychological tasks than athletes who were given neutral threat instructions.[76] Potential reasons for these findings suggested that athletes as a group may be somewhat inoculated against poor outcome beliefs due to the a priori knowledge that concussions are an "occupational hazard." The athletes in the diagnosis threat condition may not have adopted the stereotype, as possible beliefs about recovery or positive outcome may have prevented such a low-performance expectation to take hold.

Another expectation-based phenomenon that can affect neuropsychiatric outcome is the power of suggestion.[77] The coin of suggestibility has two sides, the placebo effect and the nocebo effect. Placebo effects are well documented and are seen when individuals are primed to expect certain positive results from an innocuous treatment. Studies involving psychotherapy, pharmacological agents, and even surgical (sham) procedures have demonstrated the powerful effect that positive expectations can have on treatment effectiveness. On the other hand, expectations about negative outcome can be just as powerful. Individuals who have negative effects from an innocuous treatment suggested to them indeed tend to manifest and report such negative effects.[78] These nocebo effects become increasingly important when engaged in assessment and management of concussion. It is important to recognize that the inadvertent suggestibility of persistent concussion sequelae by treatment providers can potentially produce iatrogenesis in some patients.[79]

COMORBIDITIES AND DIFFERENTIAL DIAGNOSIS

PCS, which overlap with symptoms of a number of psychiatric/mood disorders and create a challenge in diagnosis as mood disorders, are common comorbidities of concussion.[80,81] Specifically, development of postinjury depression and post-traumatic stress disorder (PTSD) is well documented and researched.[82,83] Overlapping symptoms of PCS and depression include difficulty concentrating and focusing, memory problems, fatigue, sleep disturbance, and reduced motivation. Similarly, there is also significant overlap between PCS and PTSD, such as anxiety, insomnia, difficulty concentrating, fatigue, hyperarousal, avoidance, amnesia, negative emotions (i.e., anger, fear, guilt), loss of interest in previously enjoyable activities, and irritability/anger outbursts.[84,85] Part of the neuropsychological assessment is to consider these caveats when making diagnoses. Furthermore, interpretation of test results require the knowledge of how depression and PTSD impact neurocognitive functioning.

Alcohol use is another comorbid condition that needs to be screened as part of neurocognitive testing.[86] Prevalence rate for alcohol intoxication at time of injury ranges between 36% and 51%.[87] Although alcohol use initially decline in the first year post injury, it has shown to increase 2 years post.[88] Thorough assessment of patients' alcohol use history is therefore essential in concussive care. Chronic alcohol use has shown to impact learning, memory, attention, and aspects of executive control,[89] a similar presentation as patients who are affected from concussion.[90] demonstrated that neurocognitive profile of patients with substance problems could not be differentiated from patients with mild TBIs.

Multiple factors, such as chronic pain, sleep deprivation, and medication side-effects, could influence performance on neurocognitive testing.[91,92] Chronic pain can impact someone's ability to focus, concentrate, and remember.[91] Pain also impacts someone's ability to fall and stay asleep, although insomnia is a common symptom post injury regardless of presence of pain. As a consequence of these symptoms, patients are frequently prescribed a myriad of medications (benzodiazepines, analgesics) that impact cognitive functioning, particularly memory.[93] Patients are also often prescribed an antiepileptic drug for prophylactic purpose, which has been shown to cause cognitive dysfunction.[94] When interpreting test results, these factors need to be taken into consideration as not to misattribute impairments solely to concussion itself.

SPECIAL POPULATIONS
Pediatrics

Working with the pediatric population requires specialized training. Neuropsychological assessment should be conducted by a child neuropsychologist. One of the factors to consider when conducting testing with this population is age at the time of injury as it influences test interpretation and recommendations. The neuropsychologist needs to consider the child's developmental stage in creating an impression and drawing conclusions. For adolescents, presenting symptoms could be related to concussion and/or age-appropriate behaviors (e.g., irritability, impulsivity). Academic functioning is a major issue in working with this population. Neuropsychological assessment needs to address the issue of returning to school, determining whether the child will need accommodations in order to achieve academic success. The treatment team also needs to work closely with parents and the school systems to ensure smooth transition back to the classrooms.

Geriatrics

Assessing concussion in the geriatric population poses challenges as well. Many older adults have a greater number of chronic health conditions pre-injury compared to younger persons. Moreover, estimating pre-injury baseline may be just as susceptible as other groups in terms of cognitive biases, as well as the presence of unidentified cognitive decline. Anticoagulant therapy may create added risk for bleeding associated with accidents, making seemingly minor events more dangerous. Concussion in geriatric populations may have intuitive validity that outcome is worse and postconcussive sequelae are probably associated with a prior concussion. However, the research in this area points to a flaw in this reasoning. Elderly persons who sustain an uncomplicated concussion, usually as a result of fall, tend to have similar outcome trajectories as their younger counterparts.[95]

Military/Veterans

Concussions in the military are as ubiquitous as they are in the general population. Falls, motor vehicle accidents, and blunt trauma accidents are the most frequent etiology. However, assessing concussion in the combat theater is a special challenge. Injuries from blast-related events are common and span the range of polytrauma injuries to concussion. Similar to sports-related contexts, military personnel who may sustain an altered mental status without additional injury may, as a result of training and culture, underreport their initial symptoms in order to return to duty as soon as possible. In-field assessment may be dangerous and unreliable since the environment may be full of potential distractions. Delayed assessment may thus miss acute sequelae. Screening measures have been adapted and applied to aid medics and other personnel to identify cognitively based acute concussion.[11] Despite these challenges to accurate assessment, persistent postconcussive complaints from combat personnel follow similar PCS complaint explanations. Studies show that when psychological factors are accounted for, there is essentially no significant contribution of the actual concussion to PCS complaints. Thus, PCS has been attributed to psychological factors and not neurological sequelae.[11,96] Concussion assessment in military veterans presents its own challenges. Many active duty military service personnel are referred for neuropsychological assessment over a self-reported history of concussion during deployment, often without any corroborating medical documentation. Similarly, when veterans are routinely screened for a personal history of TBI, and if the screen is positive, they are referred for a TBI second-level examination where clinicians are asked to determine if there has been a likely TBI incurred, often only based on self-report.[97] These second-level examinations are usually clinical in nature and involve an interview and possibly the completion of self-report checklists covering neurobehavioral symptoms. If the second-level examination is positive, or if the patient continues to report neurobehavioral complaints, they are often referred for formal neuropsychological assessment.[98] Another pathway that veterans receive neuropsychological assessment for a reported concussion history is through a referral to compensation and pension through the veteran's benefits administration (VBA).[99]

Forensics

It is not uncommon for patients who have sustained a concussion to be involved in litigation. Patients could have been involved in a vehicular accident or sustained their injury at work, resulting in worker's compensation status. Patients who become disabled from working post injury also often apply for disability benefits. In these cases, it is necessary to incorporate effort testing as part of the neuropsychological battery. Secondary gain in these cases is a motivating factor in symptom exaggeration and/or inadequate effort on test performance. When testing is requested as part of litigation or disability determination, our client becomes the referring source, whether that is the attorney representing the case, worker's compensation company, or social security administration. The reason for referral and the question at hand is different than for clinical purpose. The focus of the assessment is then to determine disability status, support evidence of direct relationship between injury and impairments, and address ability to return to work. The clinician should clearly explain the purpose of the evaluation to these patients up front to avoid misunderstandings, and encourage full effort.

CONCLUSION

Neuropsychological assessment can provide the patient, family, and the healthcare team with valuable information pertaining to the management of postconcussion recovery. Keen understanding of concussion outcome trajectories, utilization of valid and reliable measures, and familiarity with biopsychosocial factors that can impede recovery are essential for determining appropriate consultative recommendations and interventional strategies. The context in which the concussion occurred, as well as premorbid adjustment also play a vital role in understanding patient presentation and the recovery profile. It is therefore essential to incorporate neuropsychological assessment as part of postconcussion treatment protocol in order to delineate these important issues and provide neurobehavioral information pertinent for managing and decision-making regarding returning to work, school, or play.

REFERENCES

1. Iverson GL. Outcome from mild traumatic brain injury. Curr Opin Psychiatr. 2005;18(3):301. http://www.lww.com/giverson@interchange.ubc.ca http://search.epnet.com/login.aspx?direct=true&AuthType=ip,url,cookie,uid&db=psyh&an=2005-05821-012.

2. McInnes K, Friesen CL, MacKenzie DE, Westwood DA, Boe SG. Mild Traumatic Brain Injury (mTBI) and chronic cognitive impairment: a scoping review. *PLoS One.* 2017; 12(4):e0174847. https://doi.org/10.1371/journal.pone. 0174847.

3. Rabinowitz AR, Levin HS. Cognitive sequelae of traumatic brain injury. *Psychiatr Clin.* 2014;37(1):1—11. https://doi.org/10.1016/j.psc.2013.11.004.

4. Lezak MD, Howieson DB, Bigler ED, Tranel D. *Neuropsychological Assessment.* 5th ed. New York, NY: Oxford University Press; 2012.

5. Shoenberg M, Scott J. The neuropsychology referral and answering the referral question. In: Shoenberg M, Scott J, eds. *The Little Black Book of Neuropsychology: A Syndrome-Based Approach.* New York: Springer; 2011:3.

6. Matuszak JM, McVige J, McPherson J, Willer B, Leddy J. A practical concussion physical examination toolbox. *Sport Health.* 2016;8(3):260—269. https://doi.org/ 10.1177/1941738116641394.

7. Teasdale G, Jennett B. Assessment of coma and impaired consciousness. A practical scale. *Lancet.* 1974;2(7872): 81—84. http://www.ncbi.nlm.nih.gov/entrez/query. fcgi?cmd=Retrieve&db=PubMed&dopt=Citation&list_ uids=4136544.

8. Hagen C, Malkmus D, Durham P. *Levels of Cognitive Functioning.* Downey, CA: Ranchos Los Amigos Hospital; 1972.

9. Sherer M, Nakase-Thompson R, Yablon SA, Gontkovsky ST. Multidimensional assessment of acute confusion after traumatic brain injury. *Arch Phys Med Rehabil.* 2005;86(5):896—904. https://doi.org/10.1016/ j.apmr.2004.09.029.

10. McCrea M. Standardized mental status assessment of sports concussion. *Clin J Sport Med Off J Can Acad Sport Med.* 2001;11(3):176—181.

11. Kelly MP, Coldren RL, Parish RV, Dretsch MN, Russell ML. Assessment of acute concussion in the combat environment. *Arch Clin Neuropsychol.* 2012;27(4): 375—388. https://doi.org/10.1093/arclin/acs036.

12. Iverson G, Lange R. Post-concussion syndrome. In: Shoenberg M, Scott JL, eds. *The Little Black Book of Neuropsychology: A Syndrome-Based Approach.* New York: Springer; 2011.

13. Larrabee GJ, Rohling ML. Neuropsychological differential diagnosis of mild traumatic brain injury. *Behav Sci Law.* 2013;31(6):686—701. https://doi.org/10.1002/bsl.2087.

14. Vanderploeg RD, Groer S, Belanger HG. Initial developmental process of a VA semistructured clinical interview for TBI identification. *J Rehabil Res Dev.* 2012;49(4): 545—556.

15. Louey AG, Cromer JA, Schembri AJ, et al. Detecting cognitive impairment after concussion: sensitivity of change from baseline and normative data methods using the CogSport/Axon cognitive test battery. *Arch Clin Neuropsychol.* 2014;29(5):432—441. https://doi.org/10.1093/ arclin/acu020.

16. Galetta KM, Brandes LE, Maki K, et al. The King-Devick test and sports-related concussion: study of a rapid visual screening tool in a collegiate cohort. *J Neurol Sci.* 2011;309(1—2):34—39. https://doi.org/ 10.1016/j.jns.2011.07.039.

16a. Maerlender AC, Masterson CJ, James TD, et al. Test-retest, retest, and retest: growth curve models of repeat testing with immediate post-concussion assessment and cognitive testing (ImPACT). *J Clin Exp Neuropsychol.* 2016;38(8):869—874. https://doi.org/10.1080/138033 95.2016.1168781.

17. Lovell MR, Collins MW. New developments in the evaluation of sports-related concussion. *Curr Sports Med Rep.* 2002;1(5):287—292.

18. Iverson GL, Schatz P. Brief ipad-based assessment of cognitive functioning with ImPACT(R) pediatric. *Dev Neuropsychol.* November 2018:1—6. https://doi.org/ 10.1080/87565641.2018.1545844.

19. Larrabee GJ. Flexible vs. fixed batteries in forensic neuropsychological assessment: reply to Bigler and Hom. *Arch Clin Neuropsychol.* 2008;23(7—8):763—776. https:// doi.org/10.1016/j.acn.2008.09.004.

20. Meyers JE, Rohling ML. Validation of the Meyers short battery on mild TBI patients. *Arch Clin Neuropsychol.* 2004;19(5):637—651. https://doi.org/10.1016/j.acn. 2003.08.007.

21. Bauer R. The flexible battery approach to neuropsychological assessment. In: Vanderploeg RD, ed. *Clinician's Guide to Neuropsychological Assessment.* Hillsdale, NJ: Lawrence Erlbaum Associates, Inc; 1994:259—290.

22. Tombaugh TN. *The Test of Memory Malingering (TOMM).* North Tonawanda, NY: Multi-Health Systems; 1996.

23. Green P. *Word Memory Test.* Edmonton, AB: Green's Publishing Inc.; 2005.

24. Boone K, Lu P, Herzberg D. *The Dot Counting Test. Manual.* Los Angeles, CA: Western Psychological Services; 2002.

25. Slick D, Hopp G, Strauss E, Thompson G. *Victoria Symptom Validity Test. Professional Manual.* Lutz, FL: Psychological Assessment Resources, Inc.; 2005.

26. Widows MR, Smith GP. *Structured Inventory of Malingered Symptomatology Professional Manual.* Odessa, FL: Psychological Assessment Resources; 2005.

27. Ben-Porath YS, Tellegen A. *The Minnesota Multiphasic Personality Inventory-2 Restructured Form: Manual for Administration, Scoring, and Interpretation.* Minneapolis, MN: University of Minnesota; 2008.

28. Morey LC. *The Personality Assessment Inventory Manual.* Odessa, FL: Psychological Assessment Resources; 1991.

29. Spitzer RL, Kroenke K, Williams JB. Validation and utility of a self-report version of PRIME-MD:the PHQ primary care study. Primary care evaluation of mental disorders. Patient Health Questionnaire. *J Am Med Assoc.* 1999; 282(18):1737—1744.

30. Spitzer RL, Kroenke K, Williams JB, Lowe B. A brief measure for assessing generalized anxiety disorder: the GAD-7. *Arch Intern Med.* 2006;166(10):1092—1097, 166/10/1092 [pii].

31. Wechsler D. Wechsler Adult Intelligence Scale-4th ed. San Antonio, TX: Pearson.

32. Shipley W, Gruber C, Martin T, Klein A. *Shipley-2. Manual.* Los Angeles, CA: Western Psychological Services; 2009.

33. Goodglass H, Kaplan E, Barresi B. *Boston Diagnostic Aphasia Exam.* 3rd ed. San Antonio, TX: Pearson Assessment; 2000.

34. Stern R, White T. *Neuropsychological Assessment Battery: Administration, Scoring, and Interpretation Manual.* Lutz, FL: Psychological Assessment Resources, Inc.; 2005.

35. Messer M. *Academic Achievement Battery. Professional Manual.* Lutz, FL: Psychological Assessment Resources, Inc.; 2014.

36. Ruff R, Allen C. *Ruff 2 & 7 Selective Attention Test. Professional Manual.* Lutz, FL: Psychological Assessment Resources, Inc.; 1995.

37. Schretlen D. *Brief Test of Attention Professional Manual.* Odessa, FL: Psychological Assessment Resources; 1997.

38. Tombaugh TN. A comprehensive review of the paced auditory serial addition test (PASAT). *Arch Clin Neuropsychol.* 2006;21(1):53–76. https://doi.org/10.1016/j.acn.2005.07.006.

39. Reitan RM. *Trail Making Test: Manual for Administration and Scoring.* Tucson, AZ: Reitan Neuropsychology Laboratory; 1992.

40. Brandt J, Benedict R. *Hopkins Verbal Learning Test-Revised. Professional Manual.* Lutz, FL: Psychological Assessment Resources, Inc.; 2001.

41. Delis DC, Kremer JH, Kaplan E, Ober BA. *California Verbal Learning Test Second Edition-Adult Version Manual.* San Antonio, TX: The Psychological Corporation; 2000.

42. Schmidt M. *Rey Auditory-Verbal Learning Test.* Los Angeles: Western Psychological Services; 1996.

43. Wechsler D. *Wechsler Memory Scale—Fourth Edition (WMS-IV).* San Antonio, TX: Pearson Assessment; 2009.

44. Benedict R. *Brief Visuospatial Memory Test-Revised. Professional Manual.* Lutz, FL: Psychological Assessment Resources, Inc.; 1997.

45. Trahan D, Larrabee G. *Continuous Visual Memory.* Lutz, FL: Psychological Assessment Resources, Inc.; 1999.

46. Golden C, Freshwater S. *Stroop Color and Word Test Adult Version. A Manual for Clinical and Experimental Uses.* Wood Dale, IL: Stoelting; 1998.

47. Culbertson W, Zillmer E. *Tower of London-Drexal University (TOLDX™).* 2nd ed. North Tonawanda, NY: Multi-Health Systems, Inc.; 2005. Technical Manual.

48. Heaton R, Chelune G, Talley J, Kay G, Curtiss G. *Wisconsin Card Sorting Test Manual. Revised and Expanded.* Lutz, FL: Psychological Assessment Resources, Inc.; 1993.

49. DeFilippis NA, Campbell E. *The Booklet Category Test Professional Manual.* 2nd ed. Odessa, FL: Psychological Assessment Resources; 1997.

50. Mitrushina MN, Boone KB, D'Elia LF. Rey-osterrieth complex figure. In: Mitrushina MN, Boone KB, D'Elia LF, eds. *Handbook of Normative Data for Neuropsychological Assessment.* New York: Oxford University Press; 1999: 157–185.

51. Meyers JE, Meyers KR. *Rey Complex Figure Test and Recognition Trial- Professional Manual.* Odessa, FL: Psychological Assessment Resources, Inc.; 1995.

52. Delis D, Kaplan E, Kramer J. *Delis-Kaplan Executive Function System:Technical Manual.* San Antonio, TX: Harcourt Assessment Company; 2001.

53. Matthews CG, Klove K. *Instruction Manual for the Adult Neuropsychology Test Battery.* Madison, WI: University of Wisconsin Medical School; 1964.

54. Heaton RK, Miller W, Taylor MJ, Grant I. *Revised Comprehensive Norms for an Expanded Halstead-Reitan Battery: Demographically Adjusted Neuropsychological Norms for African American and Caucasian Adults.* Odessa, FL: Psychological Assessment Resources; 2004.

55. Dean R, Woodcock R. *Dean-Woodcock Neuropsychological Battery.* Rolling Meadows, IL: Riverside; 2003.

56. Gouvier WD, Prestholdt PH, Warner MS. A survey of common misconceptions about head injury and recovery. *Arch Clin Neuropsychol.* 1988;3(4):331–343.

57. Block CK, West SE, Goldin Y. Misconceptions and misattributions about traumatic brain injury: an integrated conceptual framework. *Pharm Manag PM R.* 2016;8(1): 58–68 e4. https://doi.org/10.1016/j.pmrj.2015.05.022.

58. Belanger HG, Curtiss G, Demery JA, Lebowitz BK, Vanderploeg RD. Factors moderating neuropsychological outcomes following mild traumatic brain injury: a meta-analysis. *J Int Neuropsychol Soc.* 2005;11(03): 215–227.

59. Dikmen S, Machamer JE, Winn HR, Temkin NR. Neuropsychological outcome at 1-year post head injury. *Neuropsychology.* 1995;9:80–90.

60. Dikmen S, Machamer J, Temkin N. Mild traumatic brain injury: longitudinal study of cognition, functional status, and post-traumatic symptoms. *J Neurotrauma.* 2017; 34(8):1524–1530. https://doi.org/10.1089/neu.2016.4618.

61. Himanen L, Portin R, Isoniemi H, Helenius H, Kurki T, Tenovuo O. Cognitive functions in relation to MRI findings 30 years after traumatic brain injury. *Brain Inj.* 2005; 19(2):93–100.

62. Hessen E, Nestvold K, Anderson V. Neuropsychological function 23 years after mild traumatic brain injury: a comparison of outcome after paediatric and adult head injuries. *Brain Inj.* 2007;21(9):963–979. https://doi.org/10.1080/02699050701528454.

63. Greiffenstein MF. Clinical myths of forensic neuropsychology. *Clin Neuropsychol.* 2009;23(2): 286–296. https://doi.org/10.1080/13854040802104873.

64. Alexander MP. Mild traumatic brain injury: Pathophysiology, natural history, and clinical management. *Neurology.* 1995;45(7):1253. http://www.lww.com/http://search.epnet.com/login.aspx?direct=true&AuthType=ip,url,cookie,uid&db=psyh&an=1996-92438-001.

65. Gouvier WD, Uddo-Crane M, Brown LM. Base rates of postconcussional symptoms. *Arch Clin Neuropsychol.* 1988;3:273–278.

66. Lange RT, Iverson GL, Rose A. Post-concussion symptom reporting and the "good-old-days" bias following mild traumatic brain injury. *Arch Clin Neuropsychol.* 2010;25(5):442–450. https://doi.org/10.1093/arclin/acq031.

67. Iverson GL, Lange RT. Examination of "postconcussion-like" symptoms in a healthy sample. *Appl Neuropsychol.* 2003;10(3):137−144. https://doi.org/10.1207/S15324826AN1003_02.

68. Bigler ED. Effort, symptom validity testing, performance validity testing and traumatic brain injury. *Brain Inj.* 2014;28(13−14):1623−1638. https://doi.org/10.3109/02699052.2014.947627.

69. Iverson GL, Binder LM. Detecting exaggeration and malingering in neuropsychological assessment. *J Head Trauma Rehabil.* 2000;15(2):829−858.

70. Lovell M,W, Collins M, Maroon J, et al. *Inaccuracy of Symptom Reporting Following Concussion in Athletes.* Vol. 34. 2002. https://doi.org/10.1097/00005768-200205001-01680.

71. Rigg JL, Mooney SR. Concussions and the military: issues specific to service members. *Pharm Manag PM R.* 2011; 3(10 Suppl 2):S380−S386. https://doi.org/10.1016/j.pmrj.2011.08.005.

72. Mittenberg W, DiGiulio DV, Perrin S, Bass AE. Symptoms following mild head injury: expectation as aetiology. *J Neurol Neurosurg Psychiatry.* 1992;55(3):200−204.

73. Gunstad J, Suhr JA. "Expectation as etiology" versus "the good old days": postconcussion syndrome symptom reporting in athletes, headache sufferers, and depressed individuals. *J Int Neuropsychol Soc.* 2001;7(3): 323−333.

74. Gunstad J, Suhr JA. Perception of illness: nonspecificity of postconcussion syndrome symptom expectation. *J Int Neuropsychol Soc.* 2002;8(1):37−47.

75. Suhr JA, Gunstad J. Further exploration of the effect of "diagnosis threat" on cognitive performance in individuals with mild head injury. *J Int Neuropsychol Soc.* 2005;11(1):23−29. https://doi.org/10.1017/S1355617705050010.

76. Carter-Allison SN, Potter S, Rimes K. Diagnosis threat and injury beliefs after mild traumatic brain injury. *Arch Clin Neuropsychol.* August 2016. https://doi.org/10.1093/arclin/acw062.

77. Murray D, Stoessl AJ. Mechanisms and therapeutic implications of the placebo effect in neurological and psychiatric conditions. *Pharmacol Ther.* 2013;140(3):306−318. https://doi.org/10.1016/j.pharmthera.2013.07.009.

78. Kennedy WP. The nocebo reaction. *Med World.* 1961;95: 203−205.

79. Alexander MP. Minor traumatic brain injury: A review of physiogenesis and psychogenesis. *Semin Clin Neuropsychiatry.* 1997;2(3):177−187.

80. Jorge RE, Arciniegas DB. Mood disorders after TBI. *Psychiatr Clin North Am.* 2014;37(1):13−29. https://doi.org/10.1016/j.psc.2013.11.005.

81. Jorge R, Robinson RG. Mood disorders following traumatic brain injury. *NeuroRehabilitation.* 2002;17(4): 311−324.

82. Jorge RE, Robinson RG, Moser D, Tateno A, Crespo-Facorro B, Arndt S. Major depression following traumatic brain injury. *Arch Gen Psychiatry.* 2004;61(1):42−50.

83. Dikmen SS, Bombardier CH, Machamer JE, Fann JR, Temkin NR. Natural history of depression in traumatic brain injury. *Arch Phys Med Rehabil.* 2004;85(9): 1457−1464.

84. Hendrickson RC, Schindler AG, Pagulayan KF. Untangling PTSD and TBI: challenges and strategies in clinical care and research. *Curr Neurol Neurosci Rep.* 2018;18(12):106. https://doi.org/10.1007/s11910-018-0908-5.

85. Bryant R. Post-traumatic stress disorder vs traumatic brain injury. *Dialogues Clin Neurosci.* 2011;13(3): 251−262.

86. Ashman TA, Schwartz ME, Cantor JB, Hibbard MR, Gordon WA. Screening for substance abuse in individuals with traumatic brain injury. *Brain Inj.* 2004;18(2): 191−202.

87. Parry-Jones BL, Vaughan FL, Miles Cox W. Traumatic brain injury and substance misuse: a systematic review of prevalence and outcomes research (1994-2004). *Neuropsychol Rehabil.* 2006;16(5):537−560. https://doi.org/10.1080/09602010500231875.

88. Ponsford J, Whelan-Goodinson R, Bahar-Fuchs A. Alcohol and drug use following traumatic brain injury: a prospective study. *Brain Inj.* 2007;21(13−14): 1385−1392. https://doi.org/10.1080/02699050701796960.

89. Gould TJ. Addiction and cognition. *Addict Sci Clin Pract.* 2010;5(2):4−14.

90. Lange RT, Iverson GL, Franzen MD. Comparability of neuropsychological test profiles in patients with chronic substance abuse and mild traumatic brain injury. *Clin Neuropsychol.* 2008;22(2):209−227. https://doi.org/10.1080/13854040701290062.

91. Hart RP, Wade JB, Martelli MF. Cognitive impairment in patients with chronic pain: the significance of stress. *Curr Pain Headache Rep.* 2003;7(2):116−126.

92. Killgore WDS. Effects of sleep deprivation on cognition. *Prog Brain Res.* 2010;185:105−129. https://doi.org/10.1016/B978-0-444-53702-7.00007-5.

93. Crowe SF, Stranks EK. The residual medium and long-term cognitive effects of benzodiazepine use: an updated meta-analysis. *Arch Clin Neuropsychol.* 2018;33(7): 901−911. https://doi.org/10.1093/arclin/acx120.

94. Beltramini GC, Cendes F, Yasuda CL. The effects of anti-epileptic drugs on cognitive functional magnetic resonance imaging. *Quant Imag Med Surg.* 2015;5(2): 238−246. https://doi.org/10.3978/j.issn.2223-4292.2015.01.04.

95. Goldstein FC, Levin HS. Cognitive outcome after mild and moderate traumatic brain injury in older adults. *J Clin Exp Neuropsychol.* 2001;23(6):739−753. https://doi.org/10.1076/jcen.23.6.739.1028.

96. Silverberg ND, Iverson GL. Etiology of the post-concussion syndrome: physiogenesis and Psychogenesis revisited. *NeuroRehabilitation.* 2011;29(4):317−329. https://doi.org/10.3233/NRE-2011-0708.

97. Broshek DK, De Marco AP, Freeman JR. A review of postconcussion syndrome and psychological factors associated

with concussion. *Brain Inj.* 2015;29(2):228–237. https://doi.org/10.3109/02699052.2014.974674.

98. Belanger HG, Vanderploeg RD, Sayer N. Screening for remote history of mild traumatic brain injury in vha: a critical literature review. *J Head Trauma Rehabil.* 2016; 31(3):204–214.   https://doi.org/10.1097/HTR.0000 000000000168.

99. Belanger HG, Uomoto JM, Vanderploeg RD. The Veterans Health Administration's (VHA's) Polytrauma System of Care for mild traumatic brain injury: costs, benefits, and controversies. *J Head Trauma Rehabil.* 2009;24(1):4–13. https://doi.org/10.1097/HTR.0b013e3181957032.

CHAPTER 3

Neuroimaging in Traumatic Brain Injury Rehabilitation

DAVID F. TATE, PHD • ELISABETH A. WILDE, PHD • GERALD E. YORK, MD • ERIN D. BIGLER, PHD, ABPP

INTRODUCTION

The number of published treatment studies in traumatic brain injury (TBI) has grown considerably in the past several years. Unfortunately, treatments vary widely across studies and typically demonstrate equivocal results. Furthermore, these studies often omit any biological explanations that might explain the response to or outcomes following treatment. This makes it difficult to identify any biological factors that might inform treatment and any therapeutic "active ingredients" that might be common to those studies where a positive response to treatment is evident. Thus, there is still much to be learned about rehabilitation following TBI, especially with regards to what makes a biological potent treatment.

Though not without criticism, one of the promising methods for studying the biological underpinnings of treatment-related change in brain tissue is magnetic resonance imaging (MRI). Part of the interest in MRI stems from its ability to visualize tissue in vivo, to localize potential abnormalities, and to monitor evolution and progression of change in tissue. However, one of the main criticisms is that imaging has often produced equivocal results in TBI patient groups, especially in the cross-sectional group analyses common to the literature. Given the disparate findings across studies, one could go so far as suggesting that imaging has been unable to provide any meaningful consistent biomarker/s that could be used to track/plan treatment interventions. However, there are a number of important caveats to this literature that likely contribute to these disparate findings, including the use of inconsistent postinjury intervals, cross-sectional exploration of only a single time point, the use of analytic methods that fail to capture the complexity and spatially heterogenous distribution of injury, and the inclusion of patients with varying mechanisms of injury.[1] Thus,

imaging should not be discounted yet, especially as many new improved acquisitions, postprocessing, and/or statistical methods promise to improve sensitivity and accuracy in this unique patient population.

In particular, prospective studies that examine within-subject changes in structure or function have additional potential to shape our clinical, biological, and functional understanding of rehabilitation in TBI in new ways. However, to date, there are only a limited number of studies that have used MRI prospectively to determine what changes take place during treatment. The purpose of this chapter is to briefly describe common imaging findings in both animal and human TBI studies that might have important clinical implications for rehabilitation, review recent studies that have used imaging to monitor rehabilitation in TBI patients, and briefly describe methods that might improve our ability to utilize imaging to guide therapeutic efforts in the individual patient. Given the multiple ways that MRI can characterize both structural and functional aspects of the brain following TBI, more objective information about the various neural structures and systems involved in rehabilitation could improve treatment planning in the individual patient following TBI.[2]

REHABILITATION RELEVANT CROSS-SECTIONAL MRI FINDING

MRI findings among TBI cohorts have been reviewed extensively elsewhere.[3-5] This literature can be difficult to accurately summarize without first acknowledging the significant methodological (i.e., diffusion MRI [dMRI] processing methods) and sample (i.e., TBI severity, military vs. civilian, age, time since injury, sample size, etc.) differences between the studies. However, the following few representative studies that focus on the connection between significant MRI

Concussion. https://doi.org/10.1016/B978-0-323-65384-8.00003-1
Copyright © 2020 Elsevier Inc. All rights reserved.

findings and outcomes (cognitive, mood, or symptoms) highlight findings that improved our diagnostic and prognostic understanding and perhaps even may be used to inform rehabilitation.

Structural Imaging Findings

The primary clinical and research application of MRI has traditionally been used to assess structural integrity of tissue and to quantify the size and shape of lesions, various regions of interest (ROI; i.e., subcortical nuclei), or cortical thickness. Across the spectrum of TBI severity, MRI consistently demonstrates global and regional atrophy of gray and white matter volumes. However, these global imaging abnormalities are likely too general in nature and as such often lack clear relationships with important functional outcomes that might inform rehabilitation.[6]

Regardless, there are a few important conclusions that can be gleaned from structural MRI. First, it is clear from studies that include the full range of severity that several regions of the brain tend to be more vulnerable to the effects of TBI, including the frontal and temporal poles, the medial temporal lobes, inferior frontal gyri, and deep white matter structures.[7,8] In addition, volumetric findings have been noted in subcortical structures such as the thalamus, hippocampus, putamen, and pallidum.[9–13] These more specific findings may have potential implications for rehabilitation as the size of these structures has often been shown to be related to important cognitive and behavioral functions, including memory, motor function, processing speed, and executive function.[14–16] Interestingly, these functions are often part of the symptom constellation typical to patients following TBI (see Fig. 3.1). However, cautious interpretation of these findings is often warranted as the associations between the size of these ROIs and cognitive function following TBI are typically observed in cross-sectional samples. This makes it difficult to understand the temporal relationships between these measures and limits the information that might be needed in order to translate simple brain behavior relationships to treatments that might impact these relationships in predictable ways. As such, additional research is yet required to fully understand the implications of the observed brain-behavior relationships.

More sophisticated postprocessing methods of structural MRI appear to demonstrate additional abnormalities following TBI. For example, using shape features of subcortical structures, differences for several subcortical gray matter structures including the thalamus and the nucleus accumbens are noted following TBI.[17,18] Shape features may ultimately be more sensitive to subtler changes in cellular features within subcortical

structures. These findings may be important as cell types may play therapeutic roles not yet understood. For example, a recent study from the animal literature demonstrates the importance of cholinergic cell populations in rehabilitation.[19] After undergoing 2 weeks of motor skills training, a subset of rats first underwent cholinergic ablations (chemical lesion in the nucleus basalis). One week later, each rat received a brain injury to the motor cortex which resulted in significant loss of the motor skill (85% loss in skilled grasping). Rats then underwent 5 weeks of intensive training on the same motor skill task. Rehabilitation resulted in the gradual recovery of the prelesion performance (60% recovery) in animals with intact cholinergic systems while those with the cholinergic ablations showed significantly less functional recovery. In addition, the neuronal structure of the cholinergic depleted rats showed less complexity and fewer dendritic spines. Combined, these functional and cellular changes suggest that cholinergic cell populations are important in promoting recovery through rehabilitation following injury.

Diffusion MRI Findings

dMRI has been shown to be sensitive to the microstructural changes in white matter following TBI by quantifying the movement of water within brain parenchyma,[20,21] and local changes in dMRI measurements can provide important quantifiable information regarding the integrity of the underlying tissue. Given dMRI's sensitivity in imaging white matter, it has garnered much interest in investigating TBI.

Using simple ROIs and/or voxel-based methods across TBI severity and patient populations (i.e., sports, military/veterans, civilian), studies have demonstrated significant differences in various scalar metrics (predominately fractional anisotropy [FA]) for several ROIs including the corpus callosum, cingulate gyrus, cerebellar peduncles, superior longitudinal fasciculus, and orbitofrontal white matter.[22–26] Significant findings were consistently worse with increasing TBI severity,[27] with multiple TBI exposures,[28] and with the presence of additional common comorbid conditions (i.e., PTSD[29,30]; major depressive disorder [MDD][24,31]; alcohol use disorder.)[32] In addition, significant relationships have been shown between many of these scalar metrics and poorer outcomes including worse symptom reporting and mood problems, including suicidality.[25,26] Worsening cognitive performance across several domains including processing speed, executive function, and memory are also commonly associated with worse dMRI measures.

Recently, prospective studies have improved our understanding of the evolution and progression of the

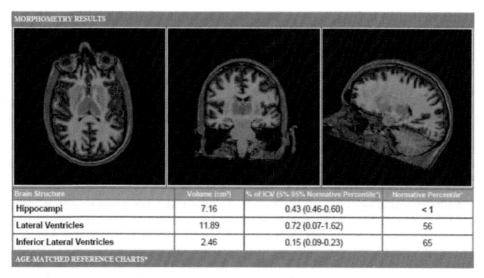

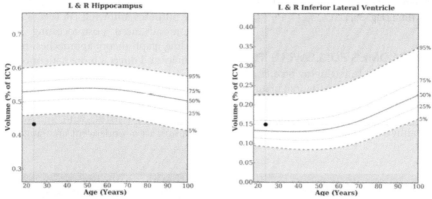

Brain Structure	Volume (cm³)	% of ICV (5%-95% Normative Percentile*)	Normative Percentile*
Hippocampi	7.16	0.43 (0.46-0.60)	< 1
Lateral Ventricles	11.89	0.72 (0.07-1.62)	56
Inferior Lateral Ventricles	2.46	0.15 (0.09-0.23)	65

*Charts and normative values are provided for reference purposes only. The FDA has not approved their use for diagnostic purposes.

FIG. 3.1 Quantitative radiology report (NeuroQuant) showing reduced hippocampal volume in a 24-year-old patient with a blast-related injury, headaches, post-traumatic stress disorder (PTSD), hearing loss, and memory lapse/loss.

dMRI metrics following TBI. In the Ljungqvist et al., study, dMRI measures in the corpus callosum continue to show change 6 and 12 months post injury when compared to controls (continued reductions in FA).[33] In the Edlow et al. study, changes (reductions in FA) over time were correlated with outcomes including dementia rating scale (DRS) scores.[34] In the Dennis et al., study differences in dMRI measures were not noted until in the chronic phase with TBI patients having reduced FA that is related to cognitive performance including memory and executive function.[35] In a study examining dMRI-derived metrics as predictors of functional outcome following rehabilitation in children with TBI, FA in the ipsilesional corticospinal tract provided relatively high predictive accuracy (sensitivity = 95%, specificity = 78%), which exceeded the predictive ability of lesion volume or other clinical variables. Mean FA of the ipsilesional corticospinal tract also correlated positively with the pediatric functional independence measures (WeeFIM) discharge motor scores.[36,37] Future studies that focus on rehabilitation more specifically will help clinicians identify the structural connectivity patterns most likely to result in successful response to treatment or at the very least identify patterns that may more accurately predict the heterogeneous outcomes common in TBI patient populations.

MRI Summary

Global, regional, and more specific MRI abnormalities are related to TBI severity, making MRI a potentially important diagnostic, prognostic, and scientific tool. Importantly, it is possible that MRI sensitivity and specificity could be dramatically improved by finding ways to combine the pathological features from various imaging sequences. It is clear that unique information from each of the MRI sequences provides distinctive information about the extent and distribution of injury pathology in the individual patient (see Fig 3.2), and one might reasonably conclude that together this information might improve the ability of the clinician to predict outcome or recovery. Furthermore, the commonness of post-TBI symptoms that relate to mood regulation, drive, fatigability, and motivation, which are often major hindrances to rehabilitation, may relate to subcortical pathology that can be observed in medical imaging. For the rehabilitation clinician, recognizing these types of quantitative image analysis findings may allow prediction of impaired processing speed, provide objective information to help guide therapies, and track improvement over time (Fig. 3.4).

PREDICTING OUTCOMES FOLLOWING TBI

Recent studies have also used imaging to predict outcomes following TBI that may be important in planning more effective rehabilitation treatments. For example, when a sample of 75 mild TBI (mTBI) patients was compared to 47 healthy control participants, functional networks observed using resting state fMRI (rsfMRI) were noted to be significantly different independent of whether or not the TBI patients were positive for day-of-injury (DOI) CT/MRI findings.[38] Even when DOI imaging in TBI patients is negative for the presence of lesions, alterations in functional networks have been demonstrated in the semi-acute stages (within 2 weeks) following injury. More importantly, the observed alterations that were temporally close to the injury were predictive of functional outcomes (i.e., neuropsychological performance) at 6 months post injury. More specifically, patients with more significant alterations in rsfMRI networks (default mode, executive control, frontoparietal, and dorsal attentional networks) had worse neuropsychological performance (processing speed, memory) and greater symptom reporting as measured by the Rivermead Post Concussion Questionnaire. Thus, rsfMRI may be viewed as a more sensitive biomarker for both diagnostic and functional prognostic purposes following TBI (Fig. 3.3).

More advanced postprocessing of rsfMRI data, including graph theory approaches, may also improve sensitivity and direct a more patient-centered approach following TBI. These types of metrics and analyses are expertly summarized elsewhere,[39] though the following study typifies this form of data analysis. In a study of 38 individuals with mTBI, with and without persistent symptoms who underwent imaging at 3 weeks and

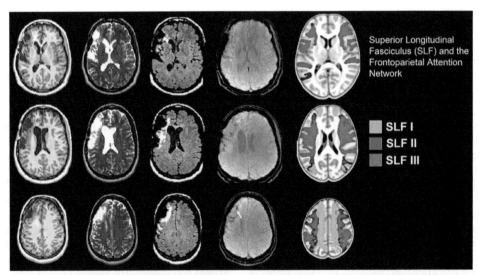

Superior Longitudinal Fasciculus (SLF) and the Frontoparietal Attention Network

■ SLF I
■ SLF II
■ SLF III

FIG. 3.2 Structural MRI using different sequences (columns; T1, T2, FLAIR, SWI) in severe TBI patient at different levels in the brain (rows). Using information from the different sequences can improve the characterization of the extent and pathological nature of the injury. By combining this information with known functional networks (column 5), behavioral profiles can emerge that can then be used to inform treatment planning and aid clinicians in making more accurate prognostic conclusions.

Day of Injury   **4 Years Post**

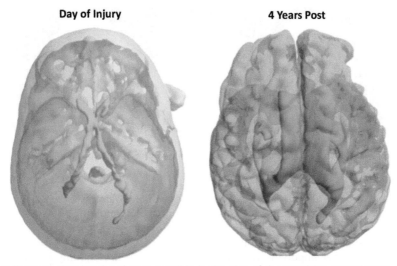

FIG. 3.3 3-D image showing the change possible in the size of the ventricles several years post injury. Understanding the clinical features that impact these kinds of changes in the brain following a TBI will be critical when trying to predict outcomes and response to treatment.

6 months post injury, investigators demonstrated unique graph metric results in the different phases (subacute or chronic) of injury recovery, especially in the thalamic and temporal brain regions.[40] The alterations were positively correlated with increased symptom reporting, especially for patients with persistent symptoms following TBI, suggesting that networks involving these regions may be of particular interest when explaining symptom presentation or planning treatments.

IMAGING FINDINGS TRACKING MORE TRADITIONAL REHABILITATION APPROACHES

The current literature includes a growing number of studies that examine the effects of treatment on the brain after a TBI.[41] As summarized in a review by Galetto and Sacco,[41] there are just a handful of functional neuroimaging studies than have monitored change over time. Nonetheless, the use of integrated, multimodality methodology to assess both the functional and structural integrity of neural systems and ROIs in response to rehabilitation therapies holds great promise. These studies demonstrate potential treatment-related change as manifest in imaging findings and objective cognitive improvement that suggest the capacity for significant neuroplasticity following TBI, even in the chronic stages of recovery (Fig. 3.4).[39]

Functional MRI (fMRI), including both task-based and rsfMRI have been particularly useful in documenting cerebral blood flow changes from pre- to posttreatment. Changes in the blood oxygen level dependent (BOLD) contrast are thought to be linked to neuronal activity, and as such, functional connectivity can be quantified and visualized. For example, Han and colleagues (2016) used both structural (cortical thickness) and functional imaging sequences to examine the effects of training strategies in adults following mild and moderate TBI.[42] Their sample of 60 patients was randomized to one of two groups for 8 weeks. Participants were assessed at baseline, then received 12 sessions of either strategy or knowledge-based training, and were then reassessed. Results demonstrated significant improvements in cognitive functioning and changes in both the cortical thickness maps and the functional imaging between the two time points. The active therapy group showed an increase in the complex structural and functional connectivity patterns between pre- and posttreatment time points that were shown to be associated with improvements in cognitive performance on a test of simple attention and processing speed (i.e., Trails A). In this same cohort, additional positive improvements were noted in depressive symptoms following cognitive rehabilitation treatment (i.e., reduction in Beck Depression Scores and PTSD Checklist).[43] These improved mood scores were associated with increased cortical thickness in four separate ROIs

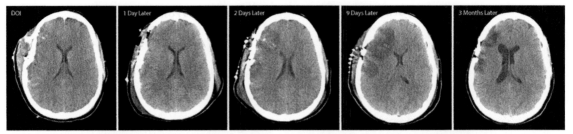

FIG. 3.4 Repeated computed tomography study in an individual patient should the significant change possible in time. This illustrates how important it is to monitor change as this likely influences outcomes in this patient group.

in the right prefrontal cortex as well as a decrease in BOLD signal activation in the same frontal regions. Importantly, these findings suggest that cognitive rehabilitation may have important effects in patients with TBI that can generalize to other important aspects of function.

In a follow-on study, Han and colleagues investigated the effects of strategy-based cognitive training in a sample of 56 chronic mTBI patients following 8 weeks of training.[44] Participants were evaluated at baseline, immediately following treatment, and 3 months post treatment. Across the three time points, the participants undergoing the strategy-based training showed significant monotonic increases in connectivity measures in the cingulo-opercular and frontoparietal networks, two known cognitive control networks. The improvements in these networks were then positively related to Trail Making Test scores.

In a study of story memory rehabilitation techniques in TBI, Chiaravalloti and colleagues examined the effects of memory training following TBI in a cohort of 18 individual patients.[45] Baseline and posttreatment MRI were collected while patients participated in a memory task while in the scanner (task-related fMRI). Analysis of these scans demonstrated significant changes in the functional imaging activation between the baseline and posttreatment scanning in the default mode and executive control networks. More specifically, there was an interaction between groups (treatment vs. control) for BOLD signal changes within the anterior cingulate, posterior insula, and cerebellum, with the treatment group demonstrating significant relative improvements compared to the placebo control condition. The activation differences were interpreted as being associated with increased use of memory strategies taught to each patient during the treatment phase.

In a larger sample of 60 patients with mild but persistent functional problems following TBI, Vas and colleagues examined the effects of another memory training protocol (Strategic Memory Advanced

Reasoning Training [SMART]) immediately post training and 3 months post training.[46] Compared to a control training paradigm (psychoeducation-based treatment), TBI patients trained using SMART showed significant behavioral improvements in cognitive control, executive function, memory, and daily function, as well as reductions in symptoms associated with mood disturbance (i.e., depressive symptoms). The improvement in scores was associated with improvements in cerebral blood flow bilaterally in the precuneus, inferior frontal lobes, left insula, and the bilateral anterior cingulate cortex as measured by pseudocontinuous arterial spin-labeled (pCASL) MRI. Importantly, localized increases in blood flow may indicate increased use of these regions when patients are engaged in these types of cognitive tasks; these increases may be ultimately associated with neuroplasticity following training or rehabilitation.

In a study of attention and executive control training following TBI, Chen et al. (2011) examined 12 patients who underwent 5 weeks of intensive training (ten 2-hour group trainings, three 1-hour individual trainings, and 20 hours at home practice).[47] Following treatment, significant improvements in behavioral measures of attention and executive control were demonstrated. fMRI demonstrated improvements in the extrastriate cortex independent of baseline fMRI that was observed in the group undergoing attention regulation training. Improvement of functional signal in the prefrontal regions was shown to be dependent on baseline functional signal and preintervention scores on attention measures in the treatment group. These results suggest that functional changes in these regions may underlie improvement in attention and executive control in patients following TBI.

Neuroimaging has also been applied in persons with chronic TBI to guide and tailor rehabilitation strategies, as well as to select patients which may benefit most from therapies. Strangman and colleagues collected fMRI measures while participants performed a verbal memory task.[48] Magnitude of the fMRI activation predicted rehabilitation success following a 12-week cognitive rehabilitation intervention; extreme under- or overactivation of the ventrolateral prefrontal cortex was associated with less successful learning after rehabilitation.

In more complicated TBI patient groups (i.e., those with comorbid PTSD), treatment focused on PTSD also demonstrates significant changes post treatment that may help improve outcomes.[49] The results from this study demonstrated significant improvement in functional imaging measures (i.e., amygdala, subcallosal gyrus, anterior cingulate gyrus, and lateral prefrontal gyrus) following virtual exposure therapy to treat PTSD symptoms in service members with TBI. Changes in the imaging signal associated positively with improvements in the clinicians' Clinical Global Impression (CGI) scores. However, only modest associations were noted between the imaging signal changes and the Clinician-Administered PTSD Scale (CAPS) scores.

Though additional research is needed to fully appreciate the effects of rehabilitation following TBI, these studies suggest the utility of imaging in understanding of the biological effects and general efficacy of traditional cognitive rehabilitation in TBI.[41] In addition, these findings identify several important ROIs that appear to be associated with unique rehabilitation efforts following TBI and other comorbid conditions. Combined, these findings are encouraging in that they demonstrate probable functional and biological biomarkers that are associated with rehabilitation even in the chronic stages of TBI recovery. Confirmation of these findings could lead to the development of more detailed and specific rehabilitation procedures targeting activation in ROIs identified in these studies.

IMAGING FINDINGS TRACKING MORE EXPERIMENTAL REHABILITATION APPROACHES

In addition to the investigation of more traditional cognitive rehabilitation interventions, others have begun to examine the potential benefits of techniques that are meant to augment more traditional therapeutic treatments. For example, in a small randomized clinical trial, Yuan and colleagues[50] studied the effects of aerobic training in 22 children with persistent symptoms following TBI. Each child underwent aerobic and stretching exercise training and demonstrated imaging-detectable effects in structural connectivity measures including dMRI and rsMRI network and graph theory results. These findings were also associated with

reductions in symptom burden in the TBI group, suggesting that improved structural and functional connectivity can be improved using simple aerobic exercises.

Transcranial direct current stimulation (tDCS) has also begun to garner some interest in TBI rehabilitation. In this treatment paradigm, traditional cognitive therapies are combined with electrical stimulation, where the electrical stimulation appears to create a preparatory brain state that allows the patient to benefit more directly or efficiently from traditional cognitive rehabilitation. For example, in 32 adult TBI patients with TBI (across the spectrum of TBI severity), improvements in attention and communicative functional measures are demonstrated when using tDCS to augment computer-assisted attention training paradigms.[51] Importantly, rsfMRI results showed a "renormalization" of the BOLD response (reduction in hyperactivation) in the middle temporal gyrus, superior temporal gyrus, cingulate gyrus, and precentral gyrus that were associated with improvements in cognitive measures. In addition, 3-month follow-up testing continued to demonstrate stable cognitive performance and improved EEG measures (amplitude of low frequency fluctuation [ALFF]). This augmentation approach to rehabilitation in TBI may yet prove to be a required feature of future rehabilitation efforts that can be used to supplement and improve rehabilitation outcomes regardless of treatment choice.

Similar findings have been noted by other groups when using tDCS. In fact, single session, frontal, anodal tDCS has been shown to improve attention immediately after administration in patients with mTBI, although the persistence of treatment effects has not been systematically proven.[52] Improved immediate auditory memory is also facilitated in mTBI using tDCS.[53] In another study, 10 sessions of tDCS were shown to improve cognitive function across a broad neuropsychological test battery and to improve abnormal EEG in patients with mTBI.[54] Similarly, mTBI subjects stimulated by tDCS, but not control groups, improved in terms of reaction time and misses in a divided attention task with concomitant changes in fMRI activation during the divided attention task.[51] Interestingly, and of particular interest to personalized rehabilitation, Sacco et al. varied the placements of electrodes based on the specific pattern of injury in each mTBI patient in order to achieve a more individualized approach to treatment. The possibility of establishing an individual profile of brain injury, derived from MRI, for each patient to design subject-specific treatment approaches is consistent with the goal of more personalized rehabilitation approached desired by clinicians and patients.

Though there is a limited literature at this point directly investigating imaging changes over the course of treatment following TBI, the few studies that exist clearly demonstrate effects that may be specific to the types of therapy conducted. However, it is clear that additional research is required, but these types of research could ultimately be extremely useful in planning treatments for patients following TBI.

CLINICAL RECOMMENDATIONS

Clinical recommendations for the use of imaging following TBI have long been established and are described in detail elsewhere.[55–58] However, these recommendations are generally limited to the identification of life-threatening complications in the acute and subacute post injury intervals (i.e., hemorrhages) or to visualization of the extent of the structural damage in the more chronic timeframes (i.e., lesions, atrophy, encephalomalacia). Thus, the clinical indications for the use of imaging following TBI remains limited to the characterization of the severity and extent of injury. Furthermore, when imaging is indicated, the type of imaging or the MRI sequences recommended for clinical purposes is typically limited to computed tomography (CT) imaging and/or basic structural MRI sequences (T1-weighted, FLAIR, SWI), while more advanced imaging modalities and sequences (i.e., dMRI, rsfMRI) are almost exclusively reserved for research purposes. Important improvements in quality and the speed with which postprocessing quantification of clinical relevant brain changes appear on imaging will likely lead to additional revisions for future recommendations as these more experimental imaging methods appear to be more sensitive to common pathological and functional changes following TBI.

Clinical guidelines or recommendations for the use of imaging specific to the rehabilitation setting do not currently exist, except for the recommendation to image in situations of unanticipated functional decline or persistent symptoms. However, it is becoming increasingly clear from discussions like the one above, that imaging could play additional roles in predicting response to treatments, planning treatments, and/or establishing or monitoring treatment efficacy. At present, the role of neuroimaging in clinical rehabilitation following TBI is often limited to the identification of lesions in regions of the brain that are ascribed to specific functional domains that may affect the focus of and ability to participate in rehabilitation. Additionally, clinical imaging

may be used to monitor tissue for evidence of focal injury resolution or diffuse degenerative change, though the connection between brain changes and relevant functional benefits of these changes remains to be determined. Though the role of imaging in rehabilitation research is expanding dramatically, technological and conceptual advances used in acquisition and analysis of neuroimaging data will continue to provide a foundation for an ever-expanding role in the clinical setting. However, additional research discoveries may yet be required before effective clinical recommendations can be made in the rehabilitation realm.

FUTURE DIRECTIONS AND CONCLUSIONS

Though specific clinical recommendations for the use of imaging in rehabilitation settings are premature at this point, advanced applications of MRI have become increasingly quantitative. This is expected to allow for a more refined characterization of tissue change for diagnostic and prognostic purposes as well as for more personalized treatment planning and evaluation of treatment response. Although differences in quantitative values derived across scanner hardware and software have historically presented obstacles for the development of normative data and clinical utilization of some kinds of MRI-based data obtained across sites or across time, consensus guidelines and methods are being developed both to monitor and reduce variability at the time of acquisition[59] and also to address differences or "harmonize" data retrospectively[60,61] utilizing advanced statistical approaches.

One criticism and potential limitation in neuroimaging studies to date is the reliance upon group-level analyses. Group results can be sample dependent and lack ready translation to clinical practice since the spatial distribution of injury and the specific nature of functional outcomes in TBI patients is often heterogeneous.[62] This heterogeneity limits the utility of imaging when attempting to integrate findings to determine a more personalized approach to the rehabilitation process. Thus, for imaging to better inform rehabilitation, new patient-centric or individualized medicine methods in neuroradiology will need to be applied. Various analytic approaches are being tested that might improve our ability to generate very specific treatments for the individual patient following TBI.

Another limitation to this literature is that many of our assumptions about what imaging variables are associated with important clinical outcomes is dependent on cross-sectional analyses. This is quickly evolving, but caution is warranted in attributing causal relationships to any significant associations between variables, particularly in smaller sample sizes. Debate persists around the optimal time to acquire imaging for use in diagnosis and prognosis as the expected pattern of quantitative results may change from the acute to subacute to chronic phases of injury. An additional criticism is that many studies rely on sample sizes that are insufficient. The studies that examined treatment outcomes directly relied on sample sizes between 8 and 31 participants. In fact, most published studies to date include less than 10 participants in the treatment arm. Conclusions from these smaller sample sizes require additional validation, though important preliminary hypotheses can be tested and developed.

While the potential role of neuroimaging has not yet been fully realized in clinical rehabilitation in TBI, recent studies have highlighted innovative future applications of quantitative neuroimaging, not only in diagnosis and prognosis but also in treatment planning and evaluation of treatment response. Neuroimaging may allow clinicians to better identify areas of the brain requiring specific or targeted intervention and to direct treatment resources for maximal benefit within a given patient. Additionally, imaging may have a future role in evaluating efficacy of novel interventions and in more objectively monitoring treatment response.

REFERENCES

1. Rosenbaum SB, Lipton ML. Embracing chaos: the scope and importance of clinical and pathological heterogeneity in mTBI. *Brain Imaging Behav.* 2012;6(2):255–282.
2. Konigs M, Pouwels PJ, Ernest van Heurn LW, et al. Relevance of neuroimaging for neurocognitive and behavioral outcome after pediatric traumatic brain injury. *Brain Imaging Behav.* 2018, Feb;12(1):29–43.
3. Asken BM, DeKosky ST, Clugston JR, Jaffee MS, Bauer RM. Diffusion tensor imaging (DTI) findings in adult civilian, military, and sport-related mild traumatic brain injury (mTBI): a systematic critical review. *Brain Imaging Behav.* 2017.
4. Koerte IK, Lin AP, Willems A, et al. A review of neuroimaging findings in repetitive brain trauma. *Brain Pathol.* 2015; 25(3):318–349.
5. Wilde EA, Bouix S, Tate DF, et al. Advanced neuroimaging applied to veterans and service personnel with traumatic brain injury: state of the art and potential benefits. *Brain Imaging Behav.* 2015;9(3):367–402.
6. Slobounov S, Gay M, Johnson B, Zhang K. Concussion in athletics: ongoing clinical and brain imaging research controversies. *Brain Imaging Behav.* 2012;6(2): 224–243.
7. Bigler ED, Tate DF. Brain volume, intracranial volume, and dementia. *Invest Radiol.* 2001;36(9):539–546.
8. Levin HS, Zhang L, Dennis M, et al. Psychosocial outcome of TBI in children with unilateral frontal lesions. *J Int Neuropsychol Soc.* 2004;10(3):305–316.
9. Beauchamp MH, Ditchfield M, Maller JJ, et al. Hippocampus, amygdala and global brain changes 10 years after childhood traumatic brain injury. *Int J Dev Neurosci.* 2011;29(2):137–143.
10. Gooijers J, Chalavi S, Beeckmans K, et al. Subcortical volume loss in the thalamus, putamen, and pallidum, induced by traumatic brain injury, is associated with motor performance deficits. *Neurorehabil Neural Repair.* 2016;30(7):603–614.
11. Isoniemi H, Kurki T, Tenovuo O, Kairisto V, Portin R. Hippocampal volume, brain atrophy, and APOE genotype after traumatic brain injury. *Neurology.* 2006;67(5): 756–760.
12. Spanos GK, Wilde EA, Bigler ED, et al. Cerebellar atrophy after moderate-to-severe pediatric traumatic brain injury. *AJNR Am J Neuroradiol.* 2007;28(3):537–542.
13. Takayanagi Y, Gerner G, Takayanagi M, et al. Hippocampal volume reduction correlates with apathy in traumatic brain injury, but not schizophrenia. *J Neuropsychiatry Clin Neurosci.* 2013;25(4):292–301.
14. Irimia A, Van Horn JD. Functional neuroimaging of traumatic brain injury: advances and clinical utility. *Neuropsychiatric Dis Treat.* 2015;11:2355–2365.
15. Shenton ME, Hamoda HM, Schneiderman JS, et al. A review of magnetic resonance imaging and diffusion tensor imaging findings in mild traumatic brain injury. *Brain Imaging Behav.* 2012;6(2):137–192.
16. Voelbel GT, Genova HM, Chiaravalotti ND, Hoptman MJ. Diffusion tensor imaging of traumatic brain injury review: implications for neurorehabilitation. *Neuro Rehab.* 2012; 31(3):281–293.
17. Tate DF, Wade BS, Velez CS, et al. Volumetric and shape analyses of subcortical structures in United States service members with mild traumatic brain injury. *J Neurol.* 2016;263(10):2065–2079.
18. Tate DF, Wade BSC, Velez CS, et al. Subcortical shape and neuropsychological function among U.S. service members with mild traumatic brain injury. *Brain Imaging Behav.* 2018.
19. Wang L, Conner JM, Nagahara AH, Tuszynski MH. Rehabilitation drives enhancement of neuronal structure in functionally relevant neuronal subsets. *Proc Natl Acad Sci U S A.* 2016;113(10):2750–2755.
20. Basser PJ, Mattiello J, LeBihan D. MR diffusion tensor spectroscopy and imaging. *Biophys J.* 1994;66(1):259–267.
21. Pierpaoli C, Basser PJ. Toward a quantitative assessment of diffusion anisotropy. *Magn Reson Med.* 1996;36(6): 893–906.
22. Little DM, Kraus MF, Joseph J, et al. Thalamic integrity underlies executive dysfunction in traumatic brain injury. *Neurology.* 2010;74(7):558–564.
23. Matsushita M, Hosoda K, Naitoh Y, Yamashita H, Kohmura E. Utility of diffusion tensor imaging in the acute stage of mild to moderate traumatic brain injury for detecting white matter lesions and predicting long-term cognitive function in adults. *J Neurosurg.* 2011;115(1):130–139.

24. Matthews SC, Strigo IA, Simmons AN, O'Connell RM, Reinhardt LE, Moseley SA. A multimodal imaging study in U.S. veterans of Operations Iraqi and Enduring Freedom with and without major depression after blast-related concussion. *Neuroimage*. 2011;54(suppl 1):S69–S75.

25. Messe A, Caplain S, Paradot G, et al. Diffusion tensor imaging and white matter lesions at the subacute stage in mild traumatic brain injury with persistent neurobehavioral impairment. *Hum Brain Mapp*. 2011;32(6):999–1011.

26. Yurgelun-Todd DA, Bueler CE, McGlade EC, Churchwell JC, Brenner LA, Lopez-Larson MP. Neuroimaging correlates of traumatic brain injury and suicidal behavior. *J Head Trauma Rehabil*. 2011;26(4):276–289.

27. Kraus MF, Susmaras T, Caughlin BP, Walker CJ, Sweeney JA, Little DM. White matter integrity and cognition in chronic traumatic brain injury: a diffusion tensor imaging study. *Brain*. 2007;130(Pt 10):2508–2519.

28. Davenport ND, Lim KO, Armstrong MT, Sponheim SR. Diffuse and spatially variable white matter disruptions are associated with blast-related mild traumatic brain injury. *Neuroimage*. 2012;59(3):2017–2024.

29. Davenport ND, Lamberty GJ, Nelson NW, Lim KO, Armstrong MT, Sponheim SR. PTSD confounds detection of compromised cerebral white matter integrity in military veterans reporting a history of mild traumatic brain injury. *Brain Inj*. 2016;30(12):1491–1500.

30. Waltzman D, Soman S, Hantke NC, et al. Altered microstructural caudate integrity in posttraumatic stress disorder but not traumatic brain injury. *PLoS One*. 2017;12(1):e0170564.

31. Spitz G, Alway Y, Gould KR, Ponsford JL. Disrupted white matter microstructure and mood disorders after traumatic brain injury. *J Neurotrauma*. 2017;34(4):807–815.

32. Lange RT, Shewchuk JR, Rauscher A, et al. A prospective study of the influence of acute alcohol intoxication versus chronic alcohol consumption on outcome following traumatic brain injury. *Arch Clin Neuropsychol*. 2014;29(5):478–495.

33. Ljungqvist J, Nilsson D, Ljungberg M, Esbjornsson E, Eriksson-Ritzen C, Skoglund T. Longitudinal changes in diffusion tensor imaging parameters of the corpus callosum between 6 and 12 months after diffuse axonal injury. *Brain Inj*. 2017;31(3):344–350.

34. Edlow BL, Copen WA, Izzy S, et al. Diffusion tensor imaging in acute-to-subacute traumatic brain injury: a longitudinal analysis. *BMC Neurol*. 2016;16:2.

35. Dennis EL, Jin Y, Villalon-Reina JE, et al. White matter disruption in moderate/severe pediatric traumatic brain injury: advanced tract-based analyses. *Neuroimage Clin*. 2015;7:493–505.

36. Ressel V, O'Gorman Tuura R, Scheer I, van Hedel HJ. Diffusion tensor imaging predicts motor outcome in children with acquired brain injury. *Brain Imaging Behav*. 2016.

37. Strauss S, Hulkower M, Gulko E, et al. Current clinical applications and future potential of diffusion tensor imaging in traumatic brain injury. *Top Magn Reson Imag*. 2015;24(6):353–362.

38. Palacios EM, Yuh EL, Chang YS, et al. Resting-state functional connectivity alterations associated with six-month outcomes in mild traumatic brain injury. *J Neurotrauma*. 2017;34(8):1546–1557.

39. Caeyenberghs K, Verhelst H, Clemente A, Wilson PH. Mapping the functional connectome in traumatic brain injury: what can graph metrics tell us? *Neuroimage*. 2017;160:113–123.

40. Messe A, Caplain S, Pelegrini-Issac M, et al. Specific and evolving resting-state network alterations in post-concussion syndrome following mild traumatic brain injury. *PLoS One*. 2013;8(6):e65470.

41. Galetto V, Sacco K. Neuroplastic changes induced by cognitive rehabilitation in traumatic brain injury: a review. *Neurorehabil Neural Repair*. 2017, 1545968317723748.

42. Han K, Davis RA, Chapman SB, Krawczyk DC. Strategy-based reasoning training modulates cortical thickness and resting-state functional connectivity in adults with chronic traumatic brain injury. *Brain Behav*. 2017;7(5):e00687.

43. Han K, Martinez D, Chapman SB, Krawczyk DC. Neural correlates of reduced depressive symptoms following cognitive training for chronic traumatic brain injury. *Hum Brain Mapp*. 2018;39(7):2955–2971.

44. Han K, Chapman SB, Krawczyk DC. Neuroplasticity of cognitive control networks following cognitive training for chronic traumatic brain injury. *Neuroimage Clin*. 2018;18:262–278.

45. Chiaravalloti ND, Dobryakova E, Wylie GR, DeLuca J. Examining the efficacy of the modified story memory technique (mSMT) in persons with TBI using functional magnetic resonance imaging (fMRI): the TBI-MEM trial. *J Head Trauma Rehabil*. 2015;30(4):261–269.

46. Vas A, Chapman S, Aslan S, et al. Reasoning training in veteran and civilian traumatic brain injury with persistent mild impairment. *Neuropsychol Rehabil*. 2016;26(4):502–531.

47. Chen AJ, Novakovic-Agopian T, Nycum TJ, et al. Training of goal-directed attention regulation enhances control over neural processing for individuals with brain injury. *Brain*. 2011;134(Pt 5):1541–1554.

48. Strangman GE, O'Neil-Pirozzi TM, Goldstein R, et al. Prediction of memory rehabilitation outcomes in traumatic brain injury by using functional magnetic resonance imaging. *Arch Phys Med Rehabil*. 2008;89(5):974–981.

49. Roy MJ, Francis J, Friedlander J, et al. Improvement in cerebral function with treatment of posttraumatic stress disorder. *Ann N Y Acad Sci*. 2010;1208:142–149.

50. Yuan W, Wade SL, Quatman-Yates C, Hugentobler JA, Gubanich PJ, Kurowski BG. Structural connectivity related to persistent symptoms after mild TBI in adolescents and response to aerobic training: preliminary investigation. *J Head Trauma Rehabil*. 2017.

51. Sacco K, Galetto V, Dimitri D, et al. Concomitant use of transcranial direct current stimulation and computer-assisted training for the rehabilitation of attention in

traumatic brain injured patients: behavioral and neuroimaging results. *Front Behav Neurosci.* 2016;10:57.

52. Kang EK, Kim DY, Paik NJ. Transcranial direct current stimulation of the left prefrontal cortex improves attention in patients with traumatic brain injury: a pilot study. *J Rehabil Med.* 2012;44(4):346—350.

53. O'Neil-Pirozzi TM, Doruk D, Thomson JM, Fregni F. Immediate memory and electrophysiologic effects of prefrontal cortex transcranial direct current stimulation on neurotypical individuals and individuals with chronic traumatic brain injury: a pilot study. *Int J Neurosci.* 2017; 127(7):592—600.

54. Ulam F, Shelton C, Richards L, et al. Cumulative effects of transcranial direct current stimulation on EEG oscillations and attention/working memory during subacute neurorehabilitation of traumatic brain injury. *Clin Neurophysiol.* 2015;126(3):486—496.

55. Centers DVBI. *Neuroimaging Following Mild TBI in the Nondeployed Setting;* 2013. https://dvbic.dcoe.mil/material/neuroimaging-following-mild-tbi-non-deployed-setting-clinical-recommendation.

56. Wintermark M, Sanelli PC, Anzai Y, Tsiouris AJ, Whitlow CT, Institute AHI. Imaging evidence and recommendations for traumatic brain injury: conventional neuroimaging techniques. *J Am Coll Radiol.* 2015;12(2):e1—e14.

57. Beauchamp MH, Ditchfield M, Babl FE, et al. Detecting traumatic brain lesions in children: CT versus MRI versus susceptibility weighted imaging (SWI). *J Neurotrauma.* 2011;28(6):915—927.

58. Wintermark M, Sanelli PC, Anzai Y, Tsiouris AJ, Whitlow CT, Radiolgy ACo. Imaging evidence and recommendations for traumatic brain injury: advanced neuro- and neurovascular imaging techniques. *Am J Neuroradiol.* 2015;36(2):E1—E11.

59. Wilde EA, Provenzale JM, Taylor BA, et al. Assessment of quantitative magnetic resonance imaging metrics in the brain through the use of a novel phantom. *Brain Inj.* 2018;32(10):1266—1276.

60. Cetin Karayumak S, Bouix S, Ning L, et al. Retrospective harmonization of multi-site diffusion MRI data acquired with different acquisition parameters. *Neuroimage.* 2019; 184:180—200.

61. Mirzaalian H, Ning L, Savadjiev P, et al. Multi-site harmonization of diffusion MRI data in a registration framework. *Brain Imaging Behav.* 2018;12(1):284—295.

62. Ware JB, Hart T, Whyte J, Rabinowitz A, Detre JA, Kim J. Inter-subject variability of axonal injury in diffuse traumatic brain injury. *J Neurotrauma.* 2017;34(14): 2243—2253.

CHAPTER 4

Postconcussive Syndrome (PCS)

WILLIAM C. WALKER, MD • RUSSELL W. LACEY, MD

PART 1. DIAGNOSIS, RISK FACTORS AND EVALUATION OF POSTCONCUSSIVE SYNDROME

Definition and Diagnosis

The physiologic effects of a mild traumatic brain injury (mTBI), or concussion, may provoke any number of immediate brain injury type symptoms. The term postconcussive (or postconcussion) syndrome (PCS) is applied when several or more of these early symptoms persist beyond the expected time frame for resolution of the physiologic effects of the mTBI. Using common symptom measures such as the Rivermead Post-Concussion Symptoms Questionnaire (RPQ)[1] or Neurobehavioral Symptom Inventory (NSI),[2] factor analysis studies have generally grouped PCS symptoms into three or four domains as shown in Table 4.1.

Unfortunately, the literature contains varying definitions and criteria for meeting a PCS diagnosis, with a lack of consensus among experts. The two most commonly used definitions for both clinical use and research purposes are put forth in the International Classification of Diseases (ICD) by the World Health Organization[3] and the Diagnostic and Statistical Manual of Mental Disorders (DSM) from the American Psychiatric Association.[4] However, the criteria differ, and both have changed over time across subsequent editions.

In the current ICD edition, ICD-10, criteria for "postconcussional syndrome" require the occurrence of head trauma "usually sufficiently severe to result in loss of consciousness" that occurred within 4 weeks of symptom onset and that the patient must have at least three of the following eight symptoms: headaches, dizziness, fatigue, irritability, insomnia, memory problems, concentration issues, and reduced tolerance to stress, emotional excitement, or alcohol. This definition is problematic in that there is no required duration of symptoms and the definition of mTBI (described in Chapter 1) is not applied, i.e., immediate alteration of consciousness, as was the case for ICD-9.

In the previous version of DSM, DSM-IV, the criteria for "postconcussional disorder" required the following: (1) history of head trauma that has caused "significant cerebral concussion"; (2) evidence of difficulty in attention or memory on neuropsychological testing or quantified cognitive assessment; (3) at least three of the following eight symptoms: easily fatigued, disordered sleep, headache, vertigo or dizziness, irritability or aggression on little or no provocation, anxiety, depression or affective lability, changes in personality (e.g., social or sexual inappropriateness), and apathy or lack of spontaneity; (4) symptoms must last at least 3 months with onset either following the concussion or significant worsening of a premorbid symptom; (5) symptoms cannot be accounted for by other mental diagnosis; and (6) a demonstrated significant decline in previous level of functioning, such as in social, occupational, or academic settings. Compared to ICD-9, fewer individuals met these criteria because of the requirement for neuropsychologic testing abnormalities and minimum symptom of 3 months. But when the DSM-5 was published in 2013, postconcussional disorder was removed altogether. Instead there are diagnoses for mild (and major) neurocognitive disorder due to TBI, which potentially could be applied if the first two criteria under DSM IV were met.

One commonality across all definitions is the requirement for at least three new (or worsening of preexisting) TBI-like symptoms beginning shortly after head injury in which TBI severity was not greater than mild. Thus, the term PCS does not apply if TBI severity was moderate or severe or if only one or two persistent symptoms follow mTBI (e.g., isolated post-traumatic headaches). A common cutoff used by experts for duration of symptoms to be classified as PCS is 3 months as per DSM-IV. There is empirical support for this in the neuropsychological testing literature where group differences in cognitive performance are rarely found after 3 months when patients with mTBI are compared to controls.[5] Additionally, it is useful clinically to

Concussion. https://doi.org/10.1016/B978-0-323-65384-8.00004-3
Copyright © 2020 Elsevier Inc. All rights reserved.

TABLE 4.1 Postconcussive Syndrome Symptom Domains.			
SOMATIC			
Somatosensory	**Vestibular-motor**	**Affective**	**Cognitive**
Headache, nausea, vomiting, visual disturbance, phonophobia, photophobia, change in taste or smell	Dizziness, imbalance, incoordination	Depression, anxiety, irritability, easily angered or frustrated, fatigue[a], insomnia[a]	Poor concentration, forgetful, slow thinking, problems with decision-making, multitasking, or word finding

[a] Sometimes grouped with somatosensory or cognitive.

differentiate when the persistence of these symptoms is associated with a disruption of life as described in the DSM-IV criteria. Regardless, the controversy in the operational definition of PCS highlights the importance of an individualized symptom and function-oriented approach to treatment that will be presented in Part 2 of this chapter.

Epidemiology

Given the divergent diagnostic criteria, it is unsurprising that prevalence rates for PCS vary widely across the literature. Easier to measure is the incidence of TBI cases of all severities presenting acutely for medical attention. In the United States, an estimated 2.8 million TBI-related emergency department visits, hospitalizations, and deaths occur annually and 80%–90% are classified as mTBI.[6] This is likely an underestimate given that many individuals do not present to a hospital after an mTBI. Regardless, the reported proportion of mTBI cases that develop PCS ranges widely from 5% to 43%.[7] This reflects not only differing diagnostic criteria but also differences in patient recruitment settings and sample selection. The most widely accepted range is 10%–20% of people that will develop PCS following mTBI, but this remains controversial due to the overlapping nature of PCS symptoms with common comorbidities such as PTSD, depression, and chronic pain. Additionally, some believe that many cases of PCS simply represent preinjury symptoms that are later misattributed to mTB in what has been termed the "good old days" bias.[8] Nevertheless, a constellation of persistent and even worsening nonspecific TBI-like symptoms many months after mTBI is a common clinical presentation such that practitioners in related fields must have strategies to evaluate and treat these patients.

Pathophysiology

A clear pathological link between the initial metabolic changes of diffuse axonal injury from mTBI described in Chapter 1 to the persistence of PCS symptoms and

life dysfunction has not been demonstrated. If the link exists, it remains unclear why the effects of mTBI are transient and reversible in most individuals but not in others. One of the more prominent theories is that of increased vulnerability due to reduced brain reserves and/or preexisting neuropsychiatric disorders. Empirical evidence for this comes from the literature on risk factors for developing PCS after TBI, namely increased age and comorbid psychiatric diagnoses (see below). Many other confounding factors have been identified in the harboring of PCS including chronic pain disorders, personality traits, medication side effects, and secondary gain.

Risk Factors

The most commonly identified risk factors for developing PCS after mTBI are increased age and female gender.[7,9] Their preeminence may in part stem from their universal inclusion as variables of interest in observational studies owing to their ease of collection in both prospective and retrospective designs. Other commonly identified risk factors are premorbid mental health conditions, lower education, and secondary gain factors (litigation, workers compensation). There is also growing evidence that a history of multiple prior concussions may confer a greater risk for developing PCS after the next mTBI.[10,11] Lastly, there is evidence that the presence of post-traumatic amnesia with mTBI signifies slower recovery after athletic concussions and thus higher grade mTBI,[12,13] but whether this translates into greater risk for PCS has not been well examined. It is worth noting that many patients with PCS after mTBI have much greater symptoms and life dysfunction than many survivors of severe TBI which again raises the specter of nonorganic components to PCS.

Evaluation

The first step in evaluating a patient with possible PCS is obtaining a thorough history of the traumatic event and immediate aftermath to determine that the patient did indeed have an mTBI; refer to the Chapter 1 for details on this aspect. Many patients present with PCS-type symptoms after a head or neck injury without having sustained a clinical mTBI. The symptoms may instead arise from PTSD, whiplash-associated disorder, and/or other causes. If it is determined an mTBI did occur, it is still important to probe through interview for comorbid whiplash disorders, PTSD, or other mental health disorders. Although not diagnostic, the PTSD Checklist for DSM-5 (PCL-5),[14] the two-item version of the Patient Health Questionnaire (PHQ-2), the two-item version of the Generalized Anxiety Disorder scale (GAD-2) are excellent screening tools for PTSD, depression, and anxiety, respectively. Positive screens require follow-up interview to determine if clinical PTSD, depression, or anxiety disorder is present.

During interview, each individual symptom should be queried including time of onset and course. This can be overwhelming in patients with full-blown PCS, who may endorse every or almost every symptom. In these cases, each symptom should be acknowledged, but is useful to redirect the patient toward what the worse one to three symptoms are for the purpose of prioritizing the treatment plan. For such patients, screening for symptom aggrandizement with the Mild Brain Injury Atypical Symptom (mBIAS) questionnaire can also help to alert the need to address nonorganic factors.[15]

The focus of physical examination is to assess for evidence of comorbidities given that neurologic examination in PCS is likely to be normal. Based on evidence from acute mTBI literature, the most likely abnormalities will be postural instability or eye convergence insufficiency. Heel to toe gait, also termed tandem gait, is more sensitive than the Romberg maneuver or its variants as an office test for postural instability. In patients with dizziness or vertigo symptoms, the Dix–Hallpike maneuver should be included to evaluate for possible benign paroxysmal positional vertigo (BPPV). Consideration for ENT referral should be given for dizziness that does not respond to vestibular rehabilitation therapy (see treatment section below). In patients with headaches, the neck should be ranged and palpated and the skull should be palpated for areas of tenderness or neuralgia.

During examination, the clinician should stay alert for evidence of a "functional" PCS. Previously termed psychosomatic disorders, functional neurologic disorders are quite common.[16] Evidence of functional PCS can be seen in overt nonphysiolgic exaggerations of eye and eyelid movements on cranial nerve testing (i.e., excessive fluttering or darting), nonphysiologic

swaying or loss of balance on tandem gait, or excessive jerking on finger-nose-finger testing. Further evidence can come from observing a mismatch of poorer motor function during formal testing compared to stealth observation of gait, gaze, and coordination when the patient is unaware of being observed.

There is little role for imaging in PCS. Rarely, subdural hematoma can present postacutely, in which case conventional head CT could rule it in or out. Warning signs for this include advanced age, worsening headache over time, frank mental status abnormalities, or focal neurologic deficit. If transient ischemic attack–like symptoms exist and there was significant neck trauma, then CTA (CT angiography) should be considered to assess for occult carotid dissection or other types of traumatic cervical artery injury. The only role for brain MRI in PCS is if other potential causes of the presenting symptoms or examination findings should be investigated (e.g., stroke, brain tumor, demyelinating disease).

Insomnia is a common symptom in PCS, and when present, sleep apnea or other sleep disorders should be considered as a contributing factor. Importantly, insomnia in of itself can cause or contribute to all the other symptoms of PCS. Symptoms or reports of witnessed loud snoring and/or pauses in breathing while asleep should prompt consideration for sleep apnea testing (see Chapter 7 for more detail). If fatigue is a prominent complaint, consideration should be given to neuroendocrine screening for which guidelines have recently been published by West et al.[17] (see Chapter 10 for more detail on fatigue).

Referral for neuropsychological testing is warranted when cognitive symptoms are prominent, especially if they are interfering with performance of vocational or avocational daily activities. Under the old DSM-IV criteria for PCS, deficits on neuropsychological testing were required along with the symptom complex in order to diagnose PCS. However, neuropsychological test results are not diagnostic for either mTBI or PCS. Although some areas of cognition are more vulnerable than others to mTBI, there is no signature pattern of test findings that are specific for TBI.[5] So before referral, it is important to maximize treatment of other aspects of PCS and comorbidities because insomnia, pain, depression, PTSD, and other factors can contribute to deficits found on neurocognitive testing. Regardless, findings can guide treatment recommendations, including the most appropriate compensatory strategies or potential pharmacology. Chapter 2 contains further detail on neuropsychological testing after mTBI.

Cognitive screening instruments designed for dementia (i.e., MMSE, MoCA) have limited utility in the evaluation of PCS because they are insensitive for mTBI-related cognitive impairment. Suspicion of dementia should prompt workup for reversible causes with lab work, at a minimum thyroid-stimulating hormone and vitamin B12 levels, and strong consideration for head CT.[18]

Prognosis

Once entrenched, the prognosis for complete resolution of full-blown PCS is very poor. Hence the clinical focus is on early education and intervention to prevent the persistence of symptoms as well as detection of and addressal of confounding factors and comorbidities. On the other hand, TBI is not a progressive disorder, and projecting pessimism of prognosis to the patient should be avoided. Using evidence from the moderate to severe TBI literature, the patient can be educated that gradual improvements in functional status can continue to occur for many years after TBI.[19] Nevertheless, the patient's expectations must be toned down toward a goal of symptom management rather than complete cure of symptoms (see more on this in treatment sections below).

PART 2 TREATMENT OF PCS
Introduction and General Principles of PCS Management

There is very little evidence from randomized controlled trials (RCTs) to guide treatment of PCS, but the literature reveals a general expert consensus on appropriate treatment principles. This chapter will review these principles along with author recommendations on specific interventions and strategies. Patients with persistent PCS are often suffering, distressed, and in need of guidance, education, support, and understanding. In general, the management approach should focus on promoting recovery and avoiding harm. Early on, an expectation of recovery should be counseled. Once firmly entrenched, education should shift toward promoting an expectation of controlling rather than curing symptoms and patient activation to overcome symptoms (i.e., promoting resiliency, self-help strategies, positive outlook). A patient-centered approach should be used to provide the needed reassurance and motivation.[20] Motivational interviewing is useful to foster the patient's participation in functional goal setting (e.g., increase in physical activity level, increase in life participation).[21]

Education

Education is the mainstay of PCS prevention and treatment. In one RCT, patients with mTBI showed significantly less PCS symptoms at 6 months post injury after receiving telephone-based counseling focused on education and symptom management compared to patients who received standard hospital discharge materials.[22] Points of emphasis in education are as follows:[23]

- Early on, assure the patient that symptoms are part of the normal recovery process.
- Throughout, assure the patient that symptoms are not a sign of permanent brain dysfunction (including no credible evidence of increased risk from chronic traumatic encephalopathy after one or a few concussions).
- Noncontact, aerobic, and recreational activities are safe and should be encouraged within the limits of the patient's symptoms; increased headache or irritability suggests that this level has been exceeded. (See Physical Exercise, below, for further details)
- Encourage resumption of occupational, educational, and social responsibilities in a graded fashion to minimize stress and avoid fatigue.
- Ascertain current sleep/wake cycle and provide counseling regarding appropriate sleep hygiene as needed.
- Provide printed and verbal education.

General Approach to Somatic Symptoms

Treatment for somatic complaints (e.g., insomnia, dizziness/incoordination, nausea, alterations of smell/taste, appetite problems, vision/hearing changes, numbness, headache, and fatigue) should be based on individual factors and symptom presentation. The somatic symptom most amenable to simple education and behavioral intervention is insomnia (see Table 4.2).[23]

In the subacute to early chronic phase, each symptom should be considered for possible diagnostic workup and treatable factors should be entertained and sought (refer to the other chapters in this textbook for more information on this). In the late chronic phase, if treatable factors have already been maximally addressed, the treatment focus should shift to a biopsychosocial model as indicated in the General Principles section above. A point of emphasis becomes teaching the patient to adopt a rehabilitation approach rather than an allopathic approach to recovery (i.e., active role of patient, functional goals, noncurative).

General Approach to Pharmacotherapy

Where evidence-based data exist to direct pharmacotherapeutic decision-making in PCS, it will be presented; where such data are not presented, the recommendations made represent the opinions of the authors. For the treatment of PCS as a whole, quality

TABLE 4.2
Education for Sleep Hygiene.
Avoid going to bed too early in the evening
Avoid stimulants, caffeinated beverages, power drinks, and nicotine during the evening
Avoid stimulating activities before bedtime (e.g., exercise, video games, TV)
Avoid alcohol
Restrict the nighttime sleep period to about 8 hour
Wake up and arise from bed at a consistent time in the morning (e.g., 7 a.m.)
Reduce (to less than 30 minute) or abolish daytime naps
Engage in daytime physical and mental activities (within the limits of the individual's functional capacity)
Use room darkening and noise protection methods (e.g., close blinds, eye shades, ear plugs, white noise)

evidence is lacking on the effectiveness of any medication, either for or against it. Despite a paucity of evidence from clinical trials in patients with mTBI, the prevailing standard of care is to base medication recommendations for PCS on individual symptom profiles. In many cases these recommendations are based on evidence in non-TBI populations. According to one survey, neurologists most commonly prescribe antidepressants for PCS[24] and secondly nonsteroidal anti-inflammatory agents (presumably for headache and/or accompanying musculoskeletal pain). Details on pharmacotherapy for common individual PCS symptoms and deficits including depression are provided in other chapters; this chapter will focus on general principles of pharmacotherapy in PCS.

Given the general lack of evidence, a ruling principle of pharmacotherapy in PCS is to minimize the number of medications in order to minimize side effects including potential drug-drug interactions. To do this, thorough medication reconciliation is crucial. The existing medication list should be reviewed for agents that can cause negative mental status or other neurologic effects (centrally acting medications, pain medications, sleep aids, anticholinergics, etc.). If a medication with neurologic side effects is identified, consider discontinuing or decreasing the dose and reevaluate after 1 week. Any medication added for symptom control must be carefully prescribed after consideration of sedating properties or other side effects. When adding medications, judicious choices that might target multiple

problematic symptoms via one medication are prudent. Some dual-role medications commonly used by the authors include low-dose amitriptyline (or nortriptyline) at bedtime to target insomnia and prevent headache; low-dose mirtazapine at bedtime to target the same as well as depression and decreased appetite; fluoxetine or other activating antidepressants to target depression and fatigue; valproic acid (Depakote) to target mood lability and prevent headache; propranolol to target headache prevention, anxiety, and dysautonomia. If there is compelling reason to use multiple medications for PCS, then medication start dates should be staggered such that the benefits and/or side effects of each's addition can be observed and potentially acted upon. The medication most closely targeting the symptom or deficit that is believed leading to the most widespread effects should be initiated first, which may account for the previously mentioned popularity of antidepressants by neurologists. Once a medication has been established to be giving greater benefit than harm for a patient, future drug holiday trials should be considered to determine continued need. In general, three consecutive months being free of the primary targeted symptom should trigger a trial of down-titration or discontinuation.

Overview of Pharmacotherapy for Some Common Individual PCS Symptoms

Emotional and mood symptoms including anxiety and depression can be treated with a variety of medications. The choice is usually dictated by comorbid symptoms and the side effect profile of the various agents. In general, selective serotonin reuptake inhibitors (e.g., sertraline, citalopram, fluoxetine, paroxetine) are preferred first-line agents because of their relatively benign side effect profiles and lower cost generic availability. Serotonin-norepinephrine reuptake inhibitors (e.g., duloxetine, venlafaxine) and atypical antidepressants (e.g., mirtazapine, bupropion) may also be considered. In the authors' experience, irritability and anger also often respond to the aforementioned antidepressants. The antiepileptic mood stabilizers (e.g., valproic acid and carbamazepine) may also be acceptable options, especially if neither depression nor anxiety is prominent. A recent RCT showed amantadine improved irritability and aggression in chronic TBI of mixed severity with the caveats that PCS (mTBI) was not specifically studied, and observer ratings did not improve relative to placebo.[25,26] The combination agent dextromethorphan/quinidine is being investigated for pseudobulbar affect in TBI populations including mTBI, but only level III evidence is available to support it (i.e., open label trial).[27] See Chapter 5 for more on treating mental health conditions.

Headache is the most common PCS symptom. Management should be tailored to the subtype of headache. See Chapter 6 for a detailed discussion of this subject.

Fatigue symptoms, both mental and physical, may be secondary to comorbid conditions such as depression, insomnia, sleep apnea, and endocrine dysfunction and/or side effects from current medications. Suboptimal physical activity and exercise levels may also contribute to both physical and mental fatigue symptoms. After suspect medications have been stopped or changed, comorbid conditions have been ruled out or maximally treated, and routine physical exercise has been established, then adding medication for any significant residual fatigue symptoms may be appropriate. An activating antidepressant (e.g., fluoxetine) is a reasonable agent to try initially, particularly with coexisting anhedonia or sadness symptoms. If the patient is already on an antidepressant medication, consider switching to one with a less sedating profile. Amphetamine-like stimulants (e.g., methylphenidate and dexedrine) may be beneficial, although careful monitoring is needed given their abuse potential. A recent small crossover trial showed efficacy of methylphenidate for mental fatigue and processing speed in mTBI patients.[28] Methylphenidate often elevates blood pressure and heart rate, so caution should be exercised with cardiac patients. Modafinil, a medication approved by the FDA for narcolepsy and shift work sleep syndrome, is a higher cost alternative. However, a study of 53 patients on an average of 6 years after TBI severe enough to require inpatient rehabilitation showed no consistent benefit for fatigue or excessive daytime sleepiness.[29] Amantadine has mixed evidence of efficacy for fatigue symptoms in multiple sclerosis, and is considered by some to be an option for PCS-related fatigue.[30] Refer to Chapter 10 for more information on fatigue after mTBI.

For sleep dysfunction, education and buy-in from patients on use of behavioral strategies are paramount (refer to Table 4.2 on education). Behavioral interventions, including meditation, relaxation training, and white noise devices, are preferred over pharmacotherapy. Primary sleep disorders should also be considered and ruled out with a sleep study as indicated. Melatonin is an excellent nutraceutical agent to try before resorting to prescription medication. The prescription drug of choice of insomnia after TBI is trazodone. Benzodiazepines and their derivatives including zolpidem and related agents should be avoided. Additional management recommendations can be found in Chapter 7.

For dizziness and disequilibrium, medication review and reconciliation are again crucial because numerous medications have dizziness as a potential side effect. Vestibular suppressants (e.g., meclizine) might be helpful during the acute period of several vestibular disorders but have not been shown to be effective in chronic dizziness after concussion.[31] The mainstays of treatment for persisting symptoms is vestibular therapy, ideally provided and taught by a physical therapist with neurologic expertise, which includes a combination of gaze stabilization, habituation, and balance exercises. Vestibular suppressants like meclizine should not be used concurrent with the habituation exercises as they will counter the goal of provoking symptoms and eliciting brain network reorganization. Regular performance of home exercises is an important piece of success of vestibular therapy. Other specific treatments may be indicated for some potential causes of dizziness (e.g., Eppley maneuvers for BPPV). See Chapter 9 for more information on treatment of vestibular and sensory disorders after mTBI.

Physical Exercise

Concussion is believed to cause autonomic nervous system dysfunction leading to elevated $PaCO_2$ which increases cerebral blood flow out of proportion to exercise intensity to incite symptoms that limit exercise performance (i.e., exercise intolerance).[32] There is also experimental evidence linking such higher cerebral vasoreactivity with greater PCS symptoms.[33] To restore autonomic nervous system and cerebral vasoreactivity homeostasis, some experts have advocated exercise as medicine for concussions, both early on and with persistent PCS.[32] The literature suggests that low-intensity graduated exercise programs can lead to several benefits for patients with persistent PCS besides better exercise tolerance including symptom reduction and ability (or time) to return to activity (e.g., work, sport).[34] A recent literature review concluded that there is moderate evidence to support subsymptomatic aerobic exercise as a treatment of PCS such that it should be considered a clinical "option" in evidence-based medicine hierarchy.[35] Specifically, the authors concluded there is level C evidence that the aerobic exercise protocol is more effective than the current standard of care in treating PCS, and recommended use of previously validated protocols, such as the Buffalo Concussion Treadmill test, Balke protocol, or rating of perceived exertion, to measure baseline values and treatment progression.[34] When access to such supervised programs is not feasible, the patient can be educated on a similar home program. Although the literature to date has primarily critically examined aerobic exercise, a general exercise program that includes strength training, core stability, aerobic activities, and range of motion is probably ideal. Note that physical (or cognitive) exertion can temporarily increase symptoms at any point in recovery and the long-term consequences from brief increases in symptoms are unknown.[36] Thus, the patient should be counseled to start with low exertion and gradually increase duration and intensity to avoid provoking major or prolonged symptom increases. Generally, the longer the PCS has been present, the slower the pace of progression should be and the longer it will take to overcome the exercise intolerance. If a person's normal activity involves significant physical activity, then exertional testing (i.e., stressing the body) should be conducted before permitting full resumption.

General Cognitive Treatment

Individuals with memory, attention, and/or executive function deficits that do not respond to treatment already described (e.g., reassurance, management of sleep dysfunction, mood disorders, and somatic complaints) may benefit from cognitive therapy delivered by speech and language pathology, neuropsychology, or occupational therapy. This can consist of functional training with compensatory strategies (e.g., use of external memory aids such as a smartphone or pocket notebook), which has the best evidence for efficacy, and/or cognitive remediation (e.g., memory or other basic cognitive skills training exercises).[37] As noted previously, neuropsychological assessment and consultation can help direct cognitive treatment and offer further targeted education. Cognitive rehabilitation and pharmacotherapy for cognitive symptoms and deficits are covered in more detail in Chapter 8.

General Psychological Treatment

Psychological treatment typically includes education, reassurance, teaching of anxiety reduction techniques, and cognitive-behavioral therapy to target and modify cognitive biases and misattribution. Psychotherapy can also be useful in identifying psychosocial factors contributing to symptom presentation and the teaching of specific coping skills for dealing with psychosocial pressure.[38] Early after mTBI, psychological treatment may help protect against developing PCS. One meta-analysis determined that patients who receive brief psychological treatment after mTBI have a significantly reduced incidence of persisting PCS compared to patients who receive standard acute care alone.[24] Efficacy data are lacking once PCS is established (i.e., if symptoms persist for >3 months), but physicians often

include psychologist referral in their treatment plan.[24] In these authors' opinion, referral to a neuropsychologist or psychologist with expertise in PCS is indicated when there is failure to respond to initial treatments, worsening stress, deterioration in function, or significant impairment in vocational or social function. More information on psychological treatment after mTBI can be found in Chapter 5.

Cognitive Behavioral Therapy

Beyond traditional psychotherapy approaches for mood disorders covered in Chapter 5, there is some evidence of efficacy for cognitive behavioral therapy (CBT) in PCS.[24] CBT in PCS is focused on techniques to encourage increased appropriate activation, including pacing of activities and the use of coping skills, relaxation strategies, sleep hygiene, cognitive restructuring, and positive thinking in the face of symptoms. Cognitive restructuring involves the reattribution of subjective symptoms to normal (nonbrain injury) causes and extensive empirical evidence supports its use in PCS treatment.[24] Patients with PCS often underestimate their premorbid experiences of headache, fatigue, inattention, memory difficulty, and dysphoria. These symptoms occur with regular frequency in the normal population, and their frequency of occurrence is increased by anxiety and stressful events. The effects of premorbid stress and anxiety may also be reattributed to the concussion, as may the effect of injury-related pain. Misattribution can foster a viscous cycle of feeling worse with belief that these symptoms are due to brain injury causing additional anxiety, stress, and depression.

Secondary Gain

Recognizing the presence and understanding the dynamics of secondary gain factors such as compensation, litigation, or sick role as a relief from stressors is important to help tailor the education and other treatments provided. It can be challenging to address them without tainting the clinician-patient therapeutic bond, so care must be taken in the style of interview and feedback. Factors that are not directly tied to financial outcomes may be amenable to education and or psychotherapy.

Interdisciplinary Programs

Interdisciplinary or collaborative models of care for PCS have demonstrated some efficacy in adults and adolescents in terms of symptom reduction and improved quality of life.[39,40] However, the durability of gains has not been demonstrated and because of difficulties implementing sham control, there remains questions about how much of the benefit is due to nonspecific effects of attention and care. Access to such programs is also quite limited because of restrictions on insurance coverage outside of the military/VA system.

Novel Interventions

Hyperbaric oxygenation (HBO) has been touted by many advocates as being effective in a multitude of brain disorders including PCS. However, a recent meta-analysis concluded that evidence from several RCTs demonstrates HBO therapy has no significant effect on PCS compared to sham.[41] Nutraceuticals have been advocated including prebiotics and probiotics based on purported central nervous system anti-inflammatory and immune regulation effects, but evidence is lacking.[42]

Monitoring Progress

One effective semiquantitative way to monitor the course of PCS and success of applied treatments is by quantifying the number and intensity of individual symptoms using one of the available standardized inventories such as the previously mentioned RPQ[1] or NSI,[2] or the Postconcussion Syndrome Checklist[43] or Concussion Symptom Checklist.[44] The authors of this chapter find this more useful early on in the course of PCS to help direct management toward the worst symptoms or combination of symptoms. Once entrenched, functional gains such as activity levels and participation outcomes (e.g., return to work, homemaking, or recreational activities) are better markers of rehabilitation success.

REFERENCES

1. King NS, Crawford S, Wenden FJ, Moss NE, Wade DT. The Rivermead Post Concussion Symptoms Questionnaire: a measure of symptoms commonly experienced after head injury and its reliability. *J Neurol*. 1995;242(9):587–592.
2. King PR, Donnelly KT, Donnelly JP, et al. Psychometric study of the neurobehavioral symptom inventory. *J Rehabil Res Dev*. 2012;49(6):879–888.
3. International Statistical Classification of Diseases and Related Health Problems 10th Revision. https://icd.who.int/browse10/2016/en. Accessed January 4, 2019.
4. *Diagnostic and Statistical Manual of Mental Disorders*. 5th ed. American Psychiatric Association; 2013.
5. Vanderploeg R, Curtiss G, Belanger H. Long-term neuropsychological outcomes following mild traumatic brain injury. *J Int Neuropsychol Soc*. 2005;11(3):228–236. https://doi.org/10.1017/S1355617705050289.
6. unknown. *Traumatic Brain Injury (TBI): Incidence & Distribution-National Center for Injury Prevention and Control*; 2005 (Journal Article). http://www.cdc.gov/ncipc/factsheets/tbi.htm
7. Voormolen DC, Cnossen MC, Polinder S, von Steinbuechel N, Vos PE, Haagsma JA. Divergent classification methods of post-concussion syndrome after mild traumatic brain injury: prevalence rates, risk factors, and functional outcome. *J Neurotrauma*. 2018;35(11):1233–1241. https://doi.org/10.1089/neu.2017.5257.
8. Sullivan K, Edmed S. The good-old-days bias and post-concussion syndrome symptom reporting in a non-clinical sample. *Brain Injury*. 2012;26(9):1098–1104. https://doi.org/10.3109/02699052.2012.666367.
9. Silverberg ND, Gardner AJ, Brubacher JR, Panenka WJ, Li JJ, Iverson GL. Systematic review of multivariable prognostic models for mild traumatic brain injury. *J Neurotrauma*. 2015;32(8):517–526. https://doi.org/10.1089/neu.2014.3600.
10. Dretsch MN, Silverberg ND, Iverson GL. Multiple past concussions are associated with ongoing post-concussive symptoms but not cognitive impairment in active-duty army soldiers. *J Neurotrauma*. 2015;32(17):1301–1306. https://doi.org/10.1089/neu.2014.3810.
11. Walker WC, Nowak KJ, Kenney K, et al. Is balance performance reduced after mild traumatic brain injury?: interim analysis from chronic effects of neurotrauma consortium (CENC) multi-centre study. *Brain Inj*. 2018;32(10):1156–1168. https://doi.org/10.1080/02699052.2018.1483529.
12. Collins MWP, Iverson GLP, Lovell MRP, McKeag DBMDMS, Norwig JMAATC, Maroon JMD. On-field predictors of neuropsychological and symptom deficit following sports-related concussion. *Clin J Sport Med*. 2003;13(4):222–229.
13. Teel EF, Marshall SW, Shankar V, McCrea M, Guskiewicz KM. Predicting recovery patterns after sport-related concussion. *J Athl Train*. 2017;52(3):288–298. https://doi.org/10.4085/1062-6050-52.1.12.
14. Blevins CA, Weathers FW, Davis MT, Witte TK, Domino JL. The posttraumatic stress disorder checklist for DSM-5 (PCL-5): development and initial psychometric evaluation. *J Trauma Stress*. 2015;28(6):489–498. https://doi.org/10.1002/jts.22059.
15. Cooper D, Nelson L, Armistead Jehle P, Bowles A. Utility of the mild brain injury atypical symptoms scale as a screening measure for symptom over-reporting in operation enduring freedom/operation iraqi freedom service members with post-concussive complaints. *Arch Clin Neuropsychol*. 2011;26(8):718–727. https://doi.org/10.1093/arclin/acr070.
16. Demartini B, D'Agostino A, Gambini O. From conversion disorder (DSM-IV-TR) to functional neurological symptom disorder (DSM-5): when a label changes the perspective for the neurologist, the psychiatrist and the patient. *J Neurol Sci*. 2016;360:55–56. https://doi.org/10.1016/j.jns.2015.11.026.
17. West TA, Sharp S. Neuroendocrine dysfunction following mild TBI: when to screen for it. *J Fam Pract*. 2014;63(1):11–16.

18. Adelman AM, Daly MP. Initial evaluation of the patient with suspected dementia. *Am Fam Physician.* 2005;71(9): 1745–1750.
19. Walker WC, Stromberg KA, Marwitz JH, et al. Predicting long-term global outcome after traumatic brain injury: development of a practical prognostic tool using the traumatic brain injury model systems national database. *J Neurotrauma.* 2018;35(14):1587–1595. https://doi.org/10.1089/neu.2017.5359.
20. Dwamena F, Holmes-Rovner M, Gaulden CM, et al. Interventions for providers to promote a patient-centred approach in clinical consultations. *Cochrane Database Syst Rev.* 2012;12(Journal Article):CD003267. https://doi.org/10.1002/14651858.CD003267.pub2.
21. Searight HR. Counseling patients in primary care: evidence-based strategies. *Am Fam Physician.* 2018; 98(12):719–728.
22. Bell KR, Hoffman JM, Temkin NR, et al. The effect of telephone counselling on reducing post-traumatic symptoms after mild traumatic brain injury: a randomised trial. *J Neurol Neuro surg Psychiatry.* 2008;79(11):1275–1281. https://doi.org/10.1136/jnnp.2007.141762.
23. The management of Concussion/mTBI Working Group. *Va/DoD Clinical Practice Guideline for Managment of Concussion/Mild Traumatic Brain Injury (mTBI)*; 2009. http://www.healthquality.va.gov/mtbi/concussion_mtbi_full.
24. Mittenberg W, Canyock EM, Condit D, Patton C. Treatment of post-concussion syndrome following mild head injury. *J Clin Exp Neuropsychol.* 2001;23(6):829.
25. Hammond FM, Bickett AK, Norton JH, Pershad R. Effectiveness of amantadine hydrochloride in the reduction of chronic traumatic brain injury irritability and aggression. *J Head Trauma Rehabil.* 2014;29(5):391–399. https://doi.org/10.1097/01.HTR.0000438116.56228.de.
26. Hammond FM, Sherer M, Malec JF, et al. Amantadine effect on perceptions of irritability after traumatic brain injury: results of the amantadine irritability multisite study. *J Neurotrauma.* 2015;(Journal Article). https://doi.org/10.1089/neu.2014.3803.
27. Hammond FM, Sauve W, Ledon F, Davis C, Formella AE. Safety, tolerability, and effectiveness of dextromethorphan/quinidine for pseudobulbar affect among study participants with traumatic brain injury: results from the PRISM-II open label study. *Pharm Manag.* 2018; 10(10):993–1003. https://doi.org/10.1016/j.pmrj.2018.02.010.
28. Johansson B, Wentzel AP, Andrell P, Mannheimer C, Ronnback L. Methylphenidate reduces mental fatigue and improves processing speed in persons suffered a traumatic brain injury. *Brain Inj.* 2015;(Journal Article):1–8. https://doi.org/10.3109/02699052.2015.1004747.
29. Jha A, Weintraub A, Allshouse A, et al. A randomized trial of modafinil for the treatment of fatigue and excessive daytime sleepiness in individuals with chronic traumatic brain injury. *J Head Trauma Rehabil.* 2008;23(1): 52–63. https://doi.org/10.1097/01.HTR.0000308721.77911.ea.
30. Yang T-T, Wang L, Deng X-Y, Yu G. Pharmacological treatments for fatigue in patients with multiple sclerosis: a systematic review and meta-analysis. *J Neurol Sci.* 2017; 380:256–261. https://doi.org/10.1016/j.jns.2017.07.042.
31. Zee DS. Perspectives on the pharmacotherapy of vertigo. *Arch Otolaryngol.* 1985;111(9):609–612.
32. Leddy JJ, Haider MN, Ellis M, Willer BS. Exercise is medicine for concussion. *Curr Sports Med Rep.* 2018;17(8):262–270. https://doi.org/10.1249/JSR.0000000000000505.
33. Albalawi T, Hamner JW, Lapointe M, Meehan WP, Tan CO. The relationship between cerebral vasoreactivity and post-concussive symptom severity. *J Neurotrauma.* 2017;34(19): 2700–2705. https://doi.org/10.1089/neu.2017.5060.
34. Sullivan KA, Hills AP, Iverson GL. Graded combined aerobic resistance exercise (CARE) to prevent or treat the persistent post-concussion syndrome. *Curr Neurol Neurosci Rep.* 2018; 18(11):75. https://doi.org/10.1007/s11910-018-0884-9.
35. Ritter KG, Hussey MJ, Valovich McLeod TC. Subsymptomatic aerobic exercise for patients with postconcussion syndrome: a critically appraised topic. *J Sport Rehabil.* July 2018:1–6. https://doi.org/10.1123/jsr.2017-0159.
36. Silverberg ND, Iverson GL. Etiology of the post-concussion syndrome: physiogenesis and Psychogenesis revisited. *Neuro Rehabil.* 2011;29(4):317–329. https://doi.org/10.3233/NRE-2011-0708.
37. Cicerone KD, Langenbahn DM, Braden C, et al. Evidence-based cognitive rehabilitation: updated review of the literature from 2003 through 2008. *Arch Phys Med Rehabil.* 2011;92(4):519–530. https://doi.org/10.1016/j.apmr.2010.11.015.
38. Broshek DK, De Marco AP, Freeman JR. A review of post-concussion syndrome and psychological factors associated with concussion. *Brain Inj.* 2015;29(2):228–237. https://doi.org/10.3109/02699052.2014.974674.
39. Janak JC, Cooper DB, Bowles AO, et al. Completion of multidisciplinary treatment for persistent postconcussive symptoms is associated with reduced symptom burden. *J Head Trauma Rehabil.* 2017;32(1):1–15. https://doi.org/10.1097/HTR.0000000000000202.
40. McCarty CA, Zatzick D, Stein E, et al. Collaborative care for adolescents with persistent postconcussive symptoms: a randomized trial. *Pediatrics.* 2016;138(4). https://doi.org/10.1542/peds.2016-0459.
41. Dong Y, Hu XH, Wu T, Wang T. Effect of hyperbaric oxygenation therapy on post-concussion syndrome. *Exp Ther Med.* 2018;16(3):2193–2202. https://doi.org/10.3892/etm.2018.6463.
42. Brenner LA, Stearns-Yoder KA, Hoffberg AS, et al. Growing literature but limited evidence: a systematic review regarding prebiotic and probiotic interventions for those with traumatic brain injury and/or posttraumatic stress disorder. *Brain Behav Immun.* 2017;65:57–67. https://doi.org/10.1016/j.bbi.2017.06.003.
43. Gouvier WD, Cubic B, Jones G, Brantley P, Cutlip Q. Post-concussion symptoms and daily stress in normal and head-injured college populations. *Arch Clin Neuropsychol.* 1992;7(3):193–211.
44. Miller LJ, Mittenberg W. Brief cognitive behavioral interventions in mild traumatic brain injury. *Appl Neuropsychol.* 1998;5(4):172–183. https://doi.org/10.1207/s15324826an0504_2.

CHAPTER 5

Assessment and Management of Psychiatric Symptoms Among Adults With Mild Traumatic Brain Injury

LISA A. BRENNER, PHD • JUSTIN OTIS, MD • RILEY P. GRASSMEYER, MS • RACHEL SAYKO ADAMS, PHD, MPH • SCOTT R. LAKER, MD • CHRISTOPHER M. FILLEY, MD

About 1.5 million people in the United States sustain a traumatic brain injury (TBI) each year, and 80% of these injuries are classified as being mild in severity.[1] Concussion, here considered synonymous with mild traumatic brain injury (mTBI), is a common neurologic disorder from which the great majority of affected individuals can expect to experience a prompt and complete recovery.[1] However, a certain percentage of people with a history of concussion, perhaps 10%−15%, do not improve as expected, and can suffer with a variety of persistent symptoms.[1] The term postconcussion syndrome (PCS) is commonly used to denote the constellation of symptoms that can occur in concussed individuals who do not fully recover in days to weeks, and has been thoroughly discussed in Chapter 4.

Large systematic studies have found that history of mTBI is associated with an increased risk of psychiatric disorders/outcomes, including depression, anxiety, bipolar disorder, post-traumatic stress disorder (PTSD), and suicide.[2−4] Children may also suffer from these problems after mTBI,[5] but older people are more susceptible to psychiatric sequelae, particularly depression, than younger adults,[6] emphasizing the importance of falls that are endemic in this population. Concussed athletes tend to have better psychiatric outcomes, typically recovering from all symptoms in 5−10 days, compared to 1−2 months for nonathletes.[1] Some Veterans fare considerably worse, likely in part due to frequently co-occurring emotional stress related to combat.[3] One factor consistently found to predict psychiatric status after concussion is the existence of preinjury psychiatric illness.[1] One prospective, controlled study of mTBI patients found that preexisting depression or anxiety predicted prolonged PCS whereas mTBI alone did not.[7]

Both athletes and military personnel are at greater risk for sustaining multiple mTBIs. Despite much concern about the later development of the putative neurodegenerative disease chronic traumatic encephalopathy,[3] one large meta-analysis of individuals with mTBI found no evidence that multiple concussions increased the risk of any subsequent psychiatric or neurologic disease.[4] This topic will be further discussed in Chapter 16.

This chapter will focus on behavioral/mood-related postconcussive symptoms and psychiatric conditions that frequently co-occur among those with a history of mTBI. As noted above, this topic is complicated by the reality that for many, psychiatric conditions predate their injury event. However, data also suggest that sustaining an mTBI increases one's risk for developing a new-onset psychiatric condition. For example, Bryant and colleagues[8] assessed those with mTBI who were admitted to major trauma hospitals and found that 12 months post injury, 31% reported a psychiatric disorder, and 22% developed a psychiatric disorder that they had never previously experienced. Information provided within this chapter includes epidemiologic data regarding common psychiatric symptom clusters/conditions post mTBI, including persistent PCS related to mood, mood disorders, anxiety disorders, PTSD, and substance use disorders. This is followed by sections on assessing and managing psychiatric symptoms. Finally, we discuss the relationship between history of concussion and suicide, including strategies for assessment and management (Fig. 5.1).

Concussion. https://doi.org/10.1016/B978-0-323-65384-8.00005-5
Copyright © 2020 Elsevier Inc. All rights reserved.

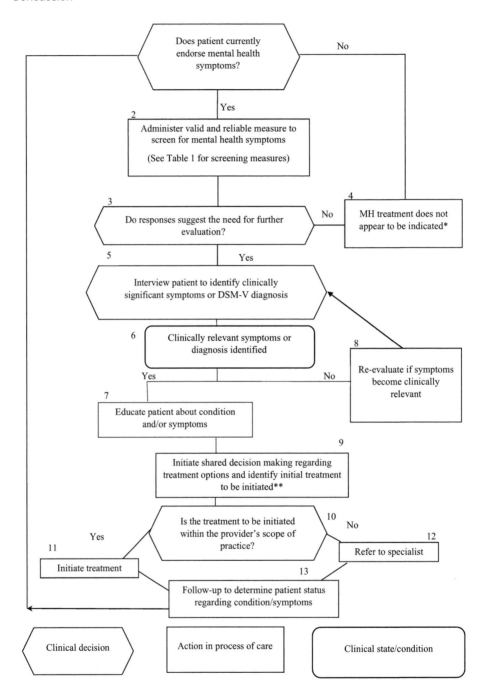

FIG. 5.1 Clinical algorithm: screening, evaluation, and treatment of psychiatric symptoms.

*If at any point other information emerges during the clinical interaction that suggests that treatment may be indicated go to Box 7

**For more information regarding shared decision making see TreatmentWorksforVets.org

EPIDEMIOLOGY

Persistent Postconcussive Symptoms Related to Mood

Mood symptoms (e.g., irritability, anxiety, depression) are prominent components of PCS, typically associated with problems, including headaches, sleep disorders, dizziness, visual disturbances, and cognitive complaints.[1] A study of people with a history of mTBI found that those who also had postinjury significant depression reported more severe PCS symptoms, compared to individuals with depression only, or mTBI only with no significant symptoms of depression.[9]

Mood Disorders

Depression is the most common psychiatric complication post TBI regardless of injury severity.[1] In patients who had a concussion, depression is also the most common psychiatric sequel, occurring at higher rates than among individuals with moderate or severe TBI.[10,11] Depression is most common in the first year post injury,[11] but may also occur long post injury, as studies have demonstrated the persistence of depression in some individuals up to 30 years after the injury.[10] A large meta-analysis also found that individuals with a history of mTBI are at increased risk for bipolar disorder compared to uninjured individuals.[4]

Anxiety Disorders

Among members of the general population, anxiety is the most common psychiatric disorder, with a reported lifetime prevalence of 29%.[12] After concussion, the development of anxiety is also common and has been estimated to develop in roughly 25% of injured persons.[13] All types of anxiety disorders can be encountered post mTBI, including generalized anxiety disorder, panic disorder, phobic disorders, and obsessive-compulsive disorder.[13] Consistent with other data underscoring the prominence of depression after mTBI, studies have indicated that individuals with anxiety after mTBI often meet criteria for major depression.[13]

Post-traumatic Stress Disorder

PTSD was formerly classified as an anxiety disorder, but the fifth edition of the Diagnostic and Statistical Manual of Mental Disorders reclassified this condition as one of the "Trauma and Stressor-related Disorders".[14] As might be expected, military populations experience a higher prevalence of PTSD after concussion secondary to shared combat-related mechanisms.[3] A systematic review of PSTD after military mTBI found that 33% −39% of those injured were affected.[15] The presence of PTSD among military personnel following an mTBI may prolong or exacerbate PCS symptoms.[16] In contrast, the largest studies of civilian mTBI have found PTSD to develop in 12%−27%,[3] with a prospective study finding that 14% of those hospitalized for mTBI met criteria for PTSD 6 months after injury.[17]

Substance Use Disorders

Persons who have experienced a TBI have higher rates of preinjury substance misuse and abuse than their peers and are often intoxicated during the injury event.[18−21] While many individuals consume less alcohol in the immediate days and months following a TBI, for some, escalation of drinking resumes over time, potentially to preinjury levels or greater.[21−24] Yet, much of what is known about postinjury drinking is drawn from studies with persons who have incurred a moderate or severe TBI, and less is known about drinking after concussion. Several large studies of military and Veteran populations that have examined postinjury substance misuse, particularly of alcohol, have found that experiencing a TBI while deployed, in which most injuries were mild, has been associated with an increased risk for postdeployment alcohol misuse,[25] binge drinking, heavy drinking (i.e., binge drinking at least weekly),[26,27] and receiving a substance use diagnosis in the Veterans Health Administration.[28] Studies with both civilian and military populations have found that the relationship between experiencing a TBI and postinjury substance misuse or abuse was independent of comorbid mental health conditions.[8,29] Because of concerns about the opioid epidemic, and increased risk for pain among individuals with a TBI,[30,31] new information is emerging about the relationship between TBI and risk for opioid use disorder.[32] While information is limited, preliminary studies have found that military members with a TBI diagnosis who received an opioid prescription were at increased risk for long-term opioid use,[33] and that persons with a TBI were at tenfold greater risk for death due to opioid overdose compared to the general population.[34] Again, it is unclear how these relationships may differ among individuals who have experienced a concussion. Lastly, there has been increasing evidence that experiencing a TBI during childhood or adolescence can increase the risk for adult substance misuse, with the majority of these studies including mild injuries.[35−39]

ASSESSMENT

Assessment of psychiatric symptoms post mTBI should be conducted via multiple modalities. Components of this process should include both a clinical interview to evaluate diagnostic criteria (i.e., the Diagnostic and Statistical Manual-5 [DSM-5]),[14] and psychometrically sound measures to evaluate symptom severity. When selecting assessment measures, it is important to consider whether study is required to determine whether they are reliable and valid for use among those with mTBI. For example, when symptoms of the psychiatric condition overlap with mTBI sequelae, such work may be of greater import. In such cases, clinically meaningful cutoffs may also be different.[10] Examples of recommended assessment measures can be found in Table 5.1.

Persistent Postconcussive Symptoms Related to Mood

The Neurobehavioral Symptom Inventory (NSI) can be used to assess postconcussive symptoms. Bahraini and colleagues evaluated the dimensionality and measurement properties of this 22-item questionnaire using a national sample of Operation Enduring Freedom/Operation Iraqi Freedom (OEF/OIF) Veterans with mTBI.[51] Findings suggested that responses can be differentiated into three unidimensional domains that include Cognitive, Mood-Behavioral, and Vestibular-Sensory symptoms. Specific items that can be used to evaluate Mood-Behavioral symptoms are 17–22.

Mood Disorder

The Beck Depression Inventory-II (BDI-II) is a frequently used measure of depressive symptoms. Research conducted among those with a history of mTBI suggests that depression can be diagnosed with a cutoff score of at least 19, which is associated with optimized sensitivity (87%) and specificity (79%).[10,52] Similar to the BDI-II, the Patient Health Questionnaire-9 (PHQ-9)[53] includes somatic items. There has been some discussion in the literature as to whether measures of depression post-TBI should include somatic symptoms, which may be related to the injury itself. Toward this end, the Traumatic Brain Injury Quality of Life (TBI-QOL) measurement, which was developed based on item response theory, includes a depression item bank. Among a sample of individuals with mixed TBI severity (18.4% mild) Cohen and colleagues compared how individuals with TBI were classified by the different measures. This group found that PHQ-9 and TBI-QOL depression bank performed similarly.[43,54]

TABLE 5.1
Frequently Used Scales to Measure Psychiatric Symptoms.

Symptom	Measure	Number of Items	Time to Administer
Anxiety	Neurobehavioral Symptom Checklist (NSC)[40]	5	30 minutes
	Beck Anxiety Inventory (BAI)[41]	21	5–10 minutes
	General Anxiety Disorder-7 item (GAD-7)[42]	7	5–10 minutes
	Traumatic Brain Injury Quality of Life (TBI-QOL)[43]	20	5–10 minutes
Depression	Beck Depression Inventory (BDI-II)[44]	21	5–10 minutes
	Patient Health Questionnaire-9 (PHQ-9)[45]	9	5–10 minutes
	TBI-QOL[43]	20	5–10 minutes
Post-traumatic stress	PTSD Checklist for DSM-5 (PCL-5)[46]	20	5–10 minutes
Substance use disorders	The AUDIT Alcohol Consumption Questions (AUDIT-C)[47]	3	5 minutes
	The Drug Abuse Screening Test (DAST-10)[48]	10	5–10 minutes
	CRAFFT Screening Interview[49]	10	5–10 minutes
	Daily Sessions, Frequency, Age of Onset, and Quantity of Cannabis Use Inventory (DFAQ-CU)[50]	37	15–20 minutes

Anxiety Disorders

The TBI-QOL[43] also includes an item bank associated with anxiety. Additional frequently used measures of anxiety include the General Anxiety Disorder-7 (GAD-7) item,[55] as well as the Beck Anxiety Inventory (BAI).[56] Whereas the TBI-QOL[43] was developed specifically for use among those with mTBI, little to no psychometric work pertaining to the use of other measures has been conducted among those with such injuries.

PTSD

As noted above, PTSD and mTBI are commonly co-occurring, particularly among those who served in Iraq and Afghanistan. The Post-traumatic Stress Disorder Checklist-5 (PCL-5) which was developed based on criteria for the DSM-5 has three versions (military, civilian, specific).[46] Although continued validation regarding cut-point scores is underway, initial work supports the use of the score of 33.

Substance Use Disorders

Alcohol misuse can be assessed with the 3-item Alcohol Use Disorders Identification Test consumption (AUDIT-C) questions, which are included in a validated 12-point scale commonly used in primary care settings and the Veterans Health Administration.[47,57] Optimal screening thresholds to identify potential alcohol misuse with maximum sensitivity and specificity are ≥ 4 for males and ≥ 3 for females. Drug use disorders can be assessed with the Drug Abuse Screening Test (DAST-10).[48] If time is limited, there is research indicating that a single screening item for drug use can be effective in primary care settings.[58] The 1-item screen is the question "How many times in the past year have you used an illegal drug or used a prescription medication for non-medical reasons?", and a response of at least one time is considered positive for drug use.

MANAGEMENT
Expectation for Recovery

Research suggests that after mTBI most individuals return to baseline functioning within 1 year.[59] As such, particularly among those with acute injuries, it is important for healthcare providers to support the expectation for a full recovery.

Psychosocial Interventions
Persistent postconcussive symptoms related to mood

To date, specific evidence-based treatments for mood-related postconcussive symptoms are limited. That

being said, expert consensus opinion supports treating persistent symptoms (e.g., depressed mood) with known evidence-based interventions.[60]

Mood and anxiety disorders

Evidence-based psychotherapies for depression and anxiety include Cognitive Behavioral Therapy (CBT) and Acceptance and Commitment Therapy (ACT). Whereas both of these interventions are in part aimed at addressing problematic thoughts, CBT targets thought content and ACT is focused on the process of thoughts. Resources for patients and clinicians regarding both of these interventions specifically focused on depression are available at http://www.TreatmentWorksforVets.org.[61]

PTSD

The two most frequently implemented evidence-based psychotherapies for PTSD include Cognitive Processing Therapy (CPT)[62] and Prolonged Exposure Therapy (PE). Whereas PE is a therapy designed to facilitate emotional processing of traumatic memories via imaginal and in vivo exposure, as well as psychoeducation and relaxation training,[63] CPT is primarily a cognitive intervention.[62] Treatment is focused on helping individuals modify trauma-related beliefs. There is evidence supporting the efficacy of both CPT and PE among those with mTBI.[64] Interestingly, both treatments seem to address post-traumatic and postconcussive symptoms.[43,65]

Substance use disorders

Evidence-based psychosocial interventions for individuals with a substance use disorder include CBTs (e.g., relapse prevention, social skills training), motivational enhancement therapy, behavioral therapies (e.g., community reinforcement, contingency approach), 12-step facilitation, brief interventions, and psychodynamic therapy/interpersonal therapy.[60,66] There have not been systematic studies to determine if the effectiveness of these interventions is impacted for those with a history of concussion. Yet, it is plausible that due to weakened executive functioning skills among some individuals with a history of mTBI, that substance use interventions should incorporate accommodations to reduce potential treatment barriers (e.g., impulsivity, planning and organization, mental flexibility).[67] It has been noted that effectiveness studies of screening and brief intervention (SBI) have largely neglected to include patients with mTBI.[68] One multisite trauma center study examined the effectiveness of an alcohol SBI using motivational interviewing among patients with and without an mTBI and found that the effectiveness was diminished among those with a history of mTBI,[69] yet it is unclear what proportion of this sample had sustained mild injuries.

Pharmacotherapy—Neurobehavioral Sequelae of Traumatic Brain Injury

A large body of research as well as clinical experience is available to guide pharmacological treatment of the sequelae of mTBI. During the past 2 decades, over 200 Phase II or higher trials for mTBI have targeted mechanisms, including damage-related tauopathy, acute intervention for physiological stabilization, cell replacement strategies for neuroplasticity, attenuating inflammation, restoring cell and tissue metabolism, and modulating neurotransmission.[70] Despite a modest number of successful studies, the most successful interventions have addressed neurotransmitter dysfunction, electrical activity, or post-traumatic depression.[70] We will review current strategies for pharmacological management of postconcussive emotional dysregulation, mood, anxiety, post-traumatic stress, and substance use disorders. It has been well established that persons with mTBI are particularly sensitive to changes in neurochemistry and in addition to specific pharmacological interventions described below, it is important to consider some general strategies when treating persons with mTBI. One should consider a treatment approach that incorporates low initial dosing and slow titration, ensuring adequate therapeutic trials, continuous reassessment, monitoring for drug-drug interactions, and augmentation when one agent is partially effective.[71]

Persistent postconcussive symptoms related to mood

Affective instability is common after concussion, particularly when injury involves frontal-subcortical circuits important for emotional regulation. Affective instability may manifest as irritability, emotional lability, or pseudobulbar affect, and pharmacological treatment routinely begins with selective serotonin reuptake inhibitors (SSRIs) for both efficacy and tolerability. Other agents to consider as second-line medications include tricyclic antidepressants, selective norepinephrine reuptake inhibitors (SNRIs), methylphenidate or amphetamines, amantadine, or antiepileptic drugs such as valproate, lamotrigine, and carbamazepine. Atypical antipsychotics such as quetiapine or aripiprazole may also be considered for severe or treatment-refractory cases.[72] A combination of dextromethorphan/quinidine has more recently demonstrated efficacy and tolerability in concussed individuals who have pseudobulbar affect.[73]

Aggression is a problematic sequel of mTBI and necessitates urgent evaluation and management. Pharmacological treatment should be tailored to the presenting etiology with careful consideration of the underlying processes involved. Aggression related to encephalopathy, flashbacks associated with PTSD, predatory aggression, and aggression associated with affective lability or poor impulse control may all be managed differently. In general, acutely aggressive behavior may be managed with typical antipsychotics such as haloperidol or atypical antipsychotics such as olanzapine, both of which are available in oral and intramuscular formulations. Short-acting benzodiazepines may also be helpful as a monotherapy or to enhance the effects of an antipsychotic, though caution should be used if encephalopathy is the underlying process. Aggression that persists over time generally requires preventative or maintenance treatment, typically with SSRIs as a first line combined with or alternatively a β-blocker. Additional considerations include amantadine, anticonvulsants such as divalproate or carbamazepine, or an atypical antipsychotic such as quetiapine, olanzapine, or risperidone.[74] Presence of persisting aggression as well as psychosis should warrant consultation with an experienced professional.

Apathy is a common neuropsychiatric sequel across a range of neurological disorders including mTBI, and, as it is notoriously difficult to treat, may be associated with significant impairment in functioning. This syndrome must first be differentiated from depression, and helpful features suggesting apathy are its lack of emotionality and paucity of goal-directed behavior. Concussion-related apathy may respond to psychostimulants such as methylphenidate and amphetamine, or even modafinil or armodafinil, although less potent agents such as fluoxetine, SNRIs, or bupropion are often attempted first. Caution must be exercised with bupropion given its propensity to lower the seizure threshold.[75]

Often accompanying apathy is fatigue, which manifests with exertion and can lead to hypersomnia. Sleep requirement can increase after concussion. Wakefulness promoting agents such as modafinil, armodafinil, methylphenidate, or amphetamines may be helpful in combating TBI-related fatigue. Modafinil or armodafinil may be particularly useful given a lower propensity for abuse or tolerance, additional cognitive enhancing effects, and a more favorable side effect profile compared to methylphenidate or amphetamine.[76]

Insomnia is a common problem after concussion, and a number of pharmacological agents may be helpful as an adjunctive to behavioral interventions. Trazodone is a sedating antidepressant medication that is well tolerated and free of dependence potential and minimally anticholinergic effects, and is an effective first-line therapy at dosages ranging from 25 to 150 mg at the hour of sleep (QHS).[71] Melatonin may be effective in doses up to 10 mg QHS and may help with headaches of many types as well as insomnia.[77] Over-the-counter sleep medications should be avoided, as these most often achieve sedation using anticholinergic medications combined with alcohol. Short-acting sedative-hypnotics such as zolpidem, eszopiclone, ramelteon, lorazepam, temazepam may be helpful for short-term use, but the risk of dependence, cognitive impairment, and behavioral issues rises with chronic use.[71] Quetiapine may be particularly helpful in the case of associated PTSD as well as with paranoia or aggression.[74] The novel orexin receptor antagonist suvorexant has shown promise in treating insomnia as well as in delirium prevention, although no studies have been performed directly with TBI.[78]

Mood disorders

Pharmacotherapy for depression includes agents such as SSRIs, SNRIs, tricyclic and tetracyclic antidepressants, atypical or novel antidepressants (mirtazapine, vortioxetine, bupropion), monoamine oxidase inhibitors, and stimulants. SSRIs and SNRIs are common first-line choices, and selection should minimize anticholinergic activity to reduce cognitive impairment. Electroconvulsive therapy has been used successfully for treatment-refractory depression in TBI.[79] Repetitive transcranial magnetic stimulation has shown efficacy in treatment-refractory Major Depressive Disorder, and a recent randomized, controlled double-blind pilot study demonstrated efficacy for treatment-refractory depression associated with TBI.[80] Pharmacological management of post-traumatic onset of bipolar disorder and mania should warrant consultation with a mental health professional given the scarcity of direct evidence and risks of pharmacotherapy in this population.

Anxiety disorders

The mainstay of treatment for anxiety disorders should be nonpharmacological approaches founded on evidence-based treatment of the particular disorder. Pharmacotherapy may be necessary with increased severity or persistence of symptoms,[81] in which case SSRIs or buspirone represent first-line treatments.

PTSD

Management of PTSD should follow an approach similar to that used for anxiety disorders, using non-pharmacological methods either alone or in combination with an SSRI or buspirone. The α-1 receptor antagonist prazosin may be used for nightmares or night terrors associated with PTSD, and some efficacy has been demonstrated.[82]

Substance use disorders

Nonpharmacological approaches such as CBT may be most effective. This modality may be used alone, or combined with agents such as naltrexone, acamprosate, gabapentin, disulfiram, topiramate, buprenorphine or methadone maintenance therapy.[83,84]

SUICIDE

There is significant interest in the role of mTBI as a risk factor for death by suicides. Inherent challenges associated with this work are related to time between history of injury and suicidal behavior, as well as measuring the impact of additional factors including pre- and postinjury psychiatric history and exposure to multiple mTBIs.[85,86] Additional methodological issues are related to the heterogeneity of populations sustaining such injuries (e.g., adolescent athletes, military personnel). Although it is likely that there are specific factors (pre/post injury) that increase risk among select cohorts, studies to date have yet to allow us to answer such questions. Nonetheless, Fralick and colleagues[86] recently conducted a systematic review which suggests that history of mTBI is associated with a twofold increased risk for suicide.[86]

The findings of Fralick and colleagues[86] support screening for both suicide risk and risk factors among those with concussion, particularly those expressing emotional distress. Although limited work has been conducted to validate measures specifically for those with a history of concussion, tools such as the Columbia-Suicide Severity Rating Scale − Screener Recent[87] have been implemented in a wide range of settings, with diverse populations.[88] Depending on the individual's responses, between three and eight items are administered. For those individuals with positive screens, a more comprehensive evaluation is indicated. In addition, hopelessness has long been identified as a powerful risk factor for suicide.[89] As such, the Beck Hopelessness Scale (BHS)[90] may have utility in identifying those at risk. The BHS is a 22-item measure that generally can be completed in less than 5 minutes.

In terms of management, clinicians are encouraged to both address drivers of suicide, such as mood and anxiety symptoms (see above), as well as to engage patients in evidence-based activities known to increase safety. Several examples include Safety Planning[91] and lethal means safety counseling. Safety planning is a six-step process in which the patients and providers (1) identify personalized warning signs (thoughts, feelings, and behaviors associated with suicidal thoughts), (2) determine internal coping strategies, (3) and (4) identify family members and friends who can act as distractors, as well as provide support during a suicidal crisis, (5) list mental health professional resources to contact during a crisis, and (6) engage in activities to make the environment safer.[92] Step six of safety planning can be further expanded to include lethal means counseling, a practice in which healthcare providers engage patients in collaborative decision-making regarding safe gun storage practices, as well as other strategies to reduce exposure to lethal means (e.g., firearms, medications) during high risk periods.[93]

CONCLUSION

As highlighted above, a wide range of factors contribute to psychiatric symptoms following mTBI. Clinicians are encouraged to screen for such conditions among their patients with a history of mTBI, as well as evaluate and manage accordingly. Existing research provides sufficient support for addressing symptoms in an evidence-informed manner.

REFERENCES

1. Katz DI, Cohen SI, Alexander MP. Mild traumatic brain injury. *Handb Clin Neurol.* 2015;127:131–156.
2. Carroll LJ, Cassidy JD, Cancelliere C, et al. Systematic review of the prognosis after mild traumatic brain injury in adults: cognitive, psychiatric, and mortality outcomes: results of the International Collaboration on Mild Traumatic Brain Injury Prognosis. *Arch Phys Med Rehabil.* 2014;95(3 suppl):S152–S173.
3. Chapman JC, Diaz-Arrastia R. Military traumatic brain injury: a review. *Alzheimers Dementia.* 2014;10(3 suppl):S97–S104.
4. Perry DC, Sturm VE, Peterson MJ, et al. Association of traumatic brain injury with subsequent neurological and psychiatric disease: a meta-analysis. *J Neurosurg.* 2016;124(2):511–526.
5. Brent DA, Max J. Psychiatric sequelae of concussions. *Curr Psychiatr Rep.* 2017;19(12):108.
6. Papa L, Mendes ME, Braga CF. Mild traumatic brain injury among the geriatric population. *Curr Transl Geriatr Exp Gerontol Rep.* 2012;1(3):135–142.
7. Meares S, Shores EA, Taylor AJ, et al. The prospective course of postconcussion syndrome: the role of mild traumatic brain injury. *Neuropsychology.* 2011;25(4):454–465.
8. Bryant RA, O'Donnell ML, Creamer M, McFarlane AC, Clark CR, Silove D. The psychiatric sequelae of traumatic injury. *Am J Psychiatry.* 2010;167(3):312–320.
9. Lange RT, Iverson GL, Rose A. Depression strongly influences postconcussion symptom reporting following mild traumatic brain injury. *J Head Trauma Rehabil.* 2011;26(2):127–137.
10. Homaifar BY, Brenner LA, Gutierrez PM, et al. Sensitivity and specificity of the Beck Depression Inventory-II in persons with traumatic brain injury. *Arch Phys Med Rehabil.* 2009;90(4):652–656.
11. Ouellet MC, Beaulieu-Bonneau S, Sirois MJ, et al. Depression in the first year after traumatic brain injury. *J Neurotrauma.* 2018;35(14):1620–1629.
12. Kessler RC, Angermeyer M, Anthony JC, et al. Lifetime prevalence and age-of-onset distributions of mental disorders in the World Health Organization's World Mental Health Survey Initiative. *World Psychiatr.* 2007;6(3):168–176.
13. Moore EL, Terryberry-Spohr L, Hope DA. Mild traumatic brain injury and anxiety sequelae: a review of the literature. *Brain Inj.* 2006;20(2):117–132.
14. American Psychiatric Association. *Diagnostic and Statistical Manual of Mental Disorders.* 5th ed. Washington, DC: American Psychiatric Association; 2013.
15. Carlson KF, Kehle SM, Meis LA, et al. Prevalence, assessment, and treatment of mild traumatic brain injury and posttraumatic stress disorder: a systematic review of the evidence. *J Head Trauma Rehabil.* 2011;26(2):103–115.
16. Brenner LA, Ivins BJ, Schwab K, et al. Traumatic brain injury, posttraumatic stress disorder, and postconcussive symptom reporting among troops returning from Iraq. *J Head Trauma Rehabil.* 2010;25(5):307–312.
17. Gil S, Caspi Y, Ben-Ari IZ, Koren D, Klein E. Does memory of a traumatic event increase the risk for posttraumatic stress disorder in patients with traumatic brain injury? A prospective study. *Am J Psychiatry.* 2005;162(5):963–969.
18. Corrigan JD. Substance abuse as a mediating factor in outcome from traumatic brain injury. *Arch Phys Med Rehabil.* 1995;76(4):302–309.
19. Cuthbert JP, Harrison-Felix C, Corrigan JD, et al. Epidemiology of adults receiving acute inpatient rehabilitation for a primary diagnosis of traumatic brain injury in the United States. *J Head Trauma Rehabil.* 2015;30(2):122–135.
20. Graham DP, Cardon AL. An update on substance use and treatment following traumatic brain injury. *Ann N Y Acad Sci.* 2008;1141:148–162.
21. Pagulayan KF, Temkin NR, Machamer JE, Dikmen SS. Patterns of alcohol use after traumatic brain injury. *J Neurotrauma.* 2016;33(14):1390–1396.
22. Bombardier CH, Temkin NR, Machamer J, Dikmen SS. The natural history of drinking and alcohol-related problems after traumatic brain injury. *Arch Phys Med Rehabil.* 2003;84(2):185–191.

23. Ponsford J, Whelan-Goodinson R, Bahar-Fuchs A. Alcohol and drug use following traumatic brain injury: a prospective study. *Brain Inj.* 2007;21(13−14):1385−1392.

24. Whelan-Goodinson R, Ponsford J, Johnston L, Grant F. Psychiatric disorders following traumatic brain injury: their nature and frequency. *J Head Trauma Rehabil.* 2009; 24(5):324−332.

25. Rona RJ, Jones M, Fear NT, et al. Mild traumatic brain injury in UK military personnel returning from Afghanistan and Iraq: cohort and cross-sectional analyses. *J Head Trauma Rehabil.* 2012;27(1):33−44.

26. Adams RS, Larson MJ, Corrigan JD, Horgan CM, Williams TV. Frequent binge drinking after combat-acquired traumatic brain injury among active duty military personnel with a past year combat deployment. *J Head Trauma Rehabil.* 2012;27(5):349−360.

27. Sayko Adams R, Corrigan JD, Mohr BA, Williams TV, Larson MJ. Traumatic brain injury and post-deployment binge drinking among male and female army active duty service members returning from operation enduring freedom/operation Iraqi freedom. *J Neurotrauma.* 2017; 34(7):1457−1465.

28. Carlson KF, Nelson D, Orazem RJ, Nugent S, Cifu DX, Sayer NA. Psychiatric diagnoses among Iraq and Afghanistan war veterans screened for deployment-related traumatic brain injury. *J Trauma Stress.* 2010; 23(1):17−24.

29. Adams RS, Larson MJ, Corrigan JD, et al. Combat-Acquired traumatic brain injury, posttraumatic stress disorder, and their relative associations with postdeployment binge drinking. *J Head Trauma Rehabil.* 2016;31(1):13−22.

30. Bertenthal D, Yaffe K, Barnes DE, et al. Do postconcussive symptoms from traumatic brain injury in combat veterans predict risk for receiving opioid therapy for chronic pain? *Brain Inj.* 2018;32(10):1188−1196.

31. Grandhi R, Tavakoli S, Ortega C, Simmonds MJ. A review of chronic pain and cognitive, mood, and motor dysfunction following mild traumatic brain injury: complex, co-morbid, and/or overlapping conditions? *Brain Sci.* 2017; 7(12).

32. Corrigan JD, Adams RS. The intersection of lifetime history of traumatic brain injury and the opioid epidemic. *Addict Behav.* 2019;90:143−145.

33. Adams RS, Thomas CP, Ritter GA, et al. Predictors of post-deployment prescription opioid receipt and long-term prescription opioid utilization among Army active duty soldiers. *Mil Med.* 2019;184(1-2):e101−e109.

34. Hammond CJ, Shah AH, Snoddon A, Patel JV, Scott DJ. Mortality and rates of secondary intervention after EVAR in an unselected population: influence of simple clinical categories and implications for surveillance. *Cardiovasc Interv Radiol.* 2016;39(6):815−823.

35. Corrigan JD, Bogner J, Holloman C. Lifetime history of traumatic brain injury among persons with substance use disorders. *Brain Inj.* 2012;26(2):139−150.

36. Corrigan JD, Bogner J, Mellick D, et al. Prior history of traumatic brain injury among persons in the traumatic brain injury model systems national database. *Arch Phys Med Rehabil.* 2013;94(10):1940−1950.

37. Corrigan JD, Hammond FM. Traumatic brain injury as a chronic health condition. *Arch Phys Med Rehabil.* 2013; 94(6):1199−1201.

38. Dams-O'Connor K, Spielman L, Singh A, et al. The impact of previous traumatic brain injury on health and functioning: a TRACK-TBI study. *J Neurotrauma.* 2013;30(24): 2014−2020.

39. McKinlay A, Corrigan J, Horwood LJ, Fergusson DM. Substance abuse and criminal activities following traumatic brain injury in childhood, adolescence, and early adulthood. *J Head Trauma Rehabil.* 2014;29(6):498−506.

40. Meterko M, Baker E, Stolzmann KL, Hendricks AM, Cicerone KD, Lew HL. Psychometric assessment of the Neurobehavioral Symptom Inventory-22: the structure of persistent postconcussive symptoms following deployment-related mild traumatic brain injury among veterans. *J Head Trauma Rehabil.* 2012;27(1):55−62.

41. Fydrich T, Dowdall D, Chambless DL. Reliability and validity of the beck anxiety inventory. *J Anxiety Disord.* 1992; 6(1):55−61.

42. Lowe B, Decker O, Muller S, et al. Validation and standardization of the generalized anxiety disorder screener (GAD-7) in the general population. *Med Care.* 2008;46(3): 266−274.

43. Tulsky DS, Kisala PA, Victorson D, et al. TBI-QOL: development and calibration of item banks to measure patient reported outcomes following traumatic brain injury. *J Head Trauma Rehabil.* 2016;31(1):40−51.

44. Further evidence for the construct validity of the Beck depression Inventory-II with psychiatric outpatients [press release]. *Psychol Rep.* 1997. US.

45. Fann JR, Bombardier CH, Dikmen S, et al. Validity of the Patient Health Questionnaire-9 in assessing depression following traumatic brain injury. *J Head Trauma Rehabil.* 2005;20(6):501−511.

46. Blevins CA, Weathers FW, Davis MT, Witte TK, Domino JL. The posttraumatic stress disorder checklist for DSM-5 (PCL-5): development and initial psychometric evaluation. *J Trauma Stress.* 2015;28(6):489−498.

47. Bush K, Kivlahan DR, McDonell MB, Fihn SD, Bradley KA. The AUDIT alcohol consumption questions (AUDIT-C): an effective brief screening test for problem drinking. Ambulatory Care Quality Improvement Project (ACQUIP). Alcohol Use Disorders Identification Test. *Arch Intern Med.* 1998;158(16):1789−1795.

48. Yudko E, Lozhkina O, Fouts A. A comprehensive review of the psychometric properties of the Drug Abuse Screening Test. *J Subst Abus Treat.* 2007;32(2):189−198.

49. Dhalla S, Zumbo BD, Poole G. A review of the psychometric properties of the CRAFFT instrument: 1999-2010. *Curr Drug Abuse Rev.* 2011;4(1):57−64.

50. Cuttler C, Spradlin A. Measuring cannabis consumption: psychometric properties of the Daily Sessions, Frequency, Age of Onset, and Quantity of Cannabis Use Inventory (DFAQ-CU). *PLoS One.* 2017;12(5):e0178194.

51. Bahraini NH, Hostetter TA, Forster JE, Schneider AL, Brenner LA. A Rasch analysis of the Neurobehavioral Symptom Inventory in a national cohort of Operation Enduring and Iraqi Freedom veterans with mild traumatic brain injury. *Psychol Assess*. 2018;30(8):1013−1027.

52. Strunk KK, Lane FC. The beck depression inventory, second edition (BDI-II): a cross-sample structural analysis. *Meas Eval Couns Dev*. 2017;50(1−2), 0748175616664010.

53. Kroenke K, Spitzer RL, Williams JB. The PHQ-9: validity of a brief depression severity measure. *J Gen Intern Med*. 2001; 16(9):606−613.

54. Cohen ML, Holdnack JA, Kisala PA, Tulsky DS. A comparison of PHQ-9 and TBI-QOL depression measures among individuals with traumatic brain injury. *Rehabil Psychol*. 2018;63(3):365−371.

55. Spitzer RL, Kroenke K, Williams JB, Lowe B. A brief measure for assessing generalized anxiety disorder. *Arch Intern Med*. 2006;166:1092−1097.

56. Steer RA, Beck AT. Beck anxiety inventory. In: Zalaquett CP, Wood RJ, eds. *Evaluating Stress: A Book of Resources*. Lanham, MD, USA: Scarecrow Education; 1997.

57. Bradley KA, DeBenedetti AF, Volk RJ, Williams EC, Frank D, Kivlahan DR. AUDIT-C as a brief screen for alcohol misuse in primary care. *Alcohol Clin Exp Res*. 2007;31(7):1208−1217.

58. Smith PC, Schmidt SM, Allensworth-Davies D, Saitz R. A single-question screening test for drug use in primary care. *Arch Intern Med*. 2010;170(13):1155−1160.

59. Iverson GL, Gardner AJ, Terry DP, et al. Predictors of clinical recovery from concussion: a systematic review. *Br J Sports Med*. 2017;51(12):941−948.

60. Department of Veterans Affairs DoD. *VA/DoD Clinical Practice Guideline for the Management of Substance Use Disorders*. 2015.

61. Center ED. Treatment Works for Vets. TreatmentWorksforVets.org.

62. Monson CM, Schnurr PP, Resick PA, Friedman MJ, Young-Xu Y, Stevens SP. Cognitive processing therapy for veterans with military-related posttraumatic stress disorder. *J Consult Clin Psychol*. 2006;74(5):898−907.

63. McLean CP, Foa EB. Dissemination and implementation of prolonged exposure therapy for posttraumatic stress disorder. *J Anxiety Disord*. 2013;27(8):788−792.

64. Chard KM, Schumm JA, McIlvain SM, Bailey GW, Parkinson RB. Exploring the efficacy of a residential treatment program incorporating cognitive processing therapy-cognitive for veterans with PTSD and traumatic brain injury. *J Trauma Stress*. 2011;24(3):347−351.

65. Wolf GK, Mauntel GJ, Kretzmer T, et al. Comorbid posttraumatic stress disorder and traumatic brain injury: generalization of prolonged-exposure PTSD treatment outcomes to postconcussive symptoms, cognition, and self-efficacy in veterans and active duty service members. *J Head Trauma Rehabil*. 2018;33(2):E53−E63.

66. Kleber HD, Mcintyre JS. *Practice Guideline for Treatment of Patients with Substance Use Disorders*. Arlington, VA: American Psychiatric Association; 2006:122.

67. Ohio Valley Center For Brain Injury Prevention and Rehabilitation. *Accommodating the Symptoms*; 2013. http://ohiovalley.org/informationeducation/accommodatingtbi/accommodationspresentation/, 2018.

68. Corrigan JD, Bogner J, Hungerford DW, Schomer K. Screening and brief intervention for substance misuse among patients with traumatic brain injury. *J Trauma*. 2010;69(3):722−726.

69. Zatzick D, Donovan DM, Jurkovich G, et al. Disseminating alcohol screening and brief intervention at trauma centers: a policy-relevant cluster randomized effectiveness trial. *Addiction*. 2014;109(5):754−765.

70. McGuire JL, Ngwenya LB, McCullumsmith RE. Neurotransmitter changes after traumatic brain injury: an update for new treatment strategies. *Mol Psychiatry*. 2018. https://doi.org/10.1038/s41380-018-0239-6.

71. Arciniegas DB. Psychopharmacology. In: Silver JM, McAllister T, Yudofsky SC, eds. *Textbook of Traumatic Brain Injury*. 2nd ed. Washington DC: American Psychiatric Publishing; 2011:553−570.

72. Arciniegas DB, Wortzel HS. Emotional and behavioral dyscontrol after traumatic brain injury. *Psychiatr Clin*. 2014; 37(1):31−53.

73. Hammond FM, Sauve W, Ledon F, Davis C, Formella AE. Safety, tolerability, and effectiveness of dextromethorphan/quinidine for pseudobulbar affect among study participants with traumatic brain injury: results from the PRISM-II open label study. *PM R*. 2018;10(10):993−1003.

74. Wortzel HS, Brenner LA, Silver JM. Traumatic brain injury. In: Arciniegas DB, Yudofsky SC, Hales RE, eds. *Textbook of Neuropsychiatry and Clinical Neurosciences*. 6th ed. Washington DC: American Psychiatric Publishing; 2018:265−286.

75. Starkstein SE, Pahissa J. Apathy following traumatic brain injury. *Psychiatr Clin*. 2014;37(1):103−112.

76. Minzenberg MJ, Carter CS. Modafinil: a review of neurochemical actions and effects on cognition. *Neuropsychopharmacology*. 2008;33(7):1477−1502.

77. Gelfand AA, Goadsby PJ. The role of melatonin in the treatment of primary headache disorders. *Headache*. 2016;56(8):1257−1266.

78. Hatta K, Kishi Y, Wada K, et al. Preventive effects of suvorexant on delirium: a randomized placebo-controlled trial. *J Clin Psychiatry*. 2017;78(8):e970−e979.

79. Jorge RE, Arciniegas DB. Mood disorders after TBI. *Psychiatr Clin*. 2014;37(1):13−29.

80. Siddiqi SH, Trapp NT, Hacker CD, et al. Repetitive transcranial magnetic stimulation with resting state network targeting for treatment-resistant depression in traumatic brain injury: a randomized, controlled, double blinded pilot study. *J Neurotrauma*. 2018;36(8):1361−1374.

81. Ponsford J, Alway Y, Gould KR. Epidemiology and natural history of psychiatric disorders after TBI. *J Neuropsychiatry Clin Neurosci*. 2018. appineuropsych18040093.

82. Singh B, Hughes AJ, Mehta G, Erwin PJ, Parsaik AK. Efficacy of prazosin in posttraumatic stress disorder: a systematic review and meta-analysis. *Prim Care Companion CNS Disord*. 2016;18(4).

83. Ray LA, Bujarski S, Grodin E, et al. State-of-the-art behavioral and pharmacological treatments for alcohol use disorder. *Am J Drug Alcohol Abuse.* 2018:1–17.

84. Dowell D, Haegerich TM, Chou R. CDC guideline for prescribing opioids for chronic pain–United States, 2016. *JAMA.* 2016;315(15):1624–1645.

85. Redelmeier DA, Bhatti JA. On the link between concussions and suicide. *JAMA Neurol.* 2018;76(2):140–141.

86. Fralick M, Sy E, Hassan A, Burke MJ, Mostofsky E, Karsies T. Association of concussion with the risk of suicide: a systematic review and meta-analysis. *JAMA Neurol.* 2019; 76(2):144–151.

87. Project TCL. Columbia-Suicide Severity Rating Scale - Recent.

88. Roaten K, Johnson C, Genzel R, Khan F, North CS. Development and implementation of a universal suicide risk screening program in a safety-net hospital system. *Jt Comm J Qual Patient Saf.* 2018;44(1):4–11.

89. Beck AT, Steer RA, Kovacs M, Garrison B. Hopelessness and eventual suicide: a 10-year prospective study of patients hospitalized with suicidal ideation. *Am J Psychiatry.* 1985; 142(5):559–563.

90. Beck AT, Steer RA, Kovacs M, Garrison B. *Manual for the Beck Hopelessness Scale.* San Antonio, TX: Psychological Corporation; 1988.

91. Stanley B, Brown GK, Brenner LA, et al. Comparison of the safety planning intervention with follow-up vs usual care of suicidal patients treated in the emergency department. *JAMA Psychiatry.* 2018;75(9):894–900.

92. Stanley BB. *G.K. Safety Planning Intervention;* 2018. http://www.suicidesafetyplan.com/.

93. Runyan CW, Brooks-Russell A, Betz ME. Points of influence for lethal means counseling and safe gun storage practices. *J Public Health Manag Pract.* 2018;25(1):86–89.

CHAPTER 6

Postconcussive Headache

NATHAN D. ZASLER, MD, FAAPM&R, FAADEP, DAAPM, CBIST •
SARA ETHEREDGE, PT, DPT, CKTP, CCI, CMTPT

INTRODUCTION

Polytrauma, including traumatic brain injury, has been associated with significant pain sequelae.[1] Postconcussive headache (PCH) has historically been viewed as a singular headache disorder with some quoting an incidence of headache occurring in nearly 90% of concussive brain injuries (CBIs) with a fairly alarming rate of chronicity. Whether PCH chronicity is a reflection of our lack of understanding of the condition and/or a consequence of suboptimal diagnoses remains to be elucidated. The idea that PCH is a singular headache disorder is now known to be an oversimplification of a much more complex and variable pathoetiology that is often mixed with diverse biopsychosocial factors that may influence symptom presentation, pain adaptation versus promulgation, and prognosis. Other factors such as base rate misattribution (e.g., migraine incidence in the military), sociocultural issues, nocebo effects, and/or compensation/litigation must also be considered.[2-4] Increased understanding regarding the array of post-traumatic headache (PTHA) pain generators following CBI has further emphasized the complexity of PCH and the interrelationships of vascular, autonomic, peripheral nerve, muscular, osseous/joint, and other contributors to such headaches.[3-5]

Risk factors for development of specific headache phenotypes may differ in different types of CBI mechanisms, including assaults, vehicular, sports, whiplash, and blast injury, but no methodologically sound data are available yet to answer this question. Theoretically, each of the aforementioned mechanisms of injury may put a patient at greater risk for certain types of post-traumatic head pain generators than others. Additionally, the acute, subacute, and chronic variants of PCH have not been studied in a manner to determine differences in incidence, prevalence, etiology, diagnostic accuracy, treatment efficacy and prognosis. Similarly, risk factors for PCH and vulnerabilities for developing so-called "chronic" PCH remain debated in part due to variable study methodology. Some literature suggests that preinjury migraine is associated with protracted recovery from sports-related CBI, greater levels of postconcussive symptom complaints, as well as more impairment on subacute neuropsychological testing (particularly in females), although controversy remains.[6,7] The bulk of the literature does note a positive association between acute headache symptom burden and protracted recovery from CBI.[6,7]

The effect genetic loading risk factors, preexisting neck pain, and/or headache associated with whiplash injury, impact preparedness, dizziness, sex, anatomic variables between males and females, cultural norms/perspectives, affective disorders, and characterological traits have on influencing PCH incidence/reporting, severity, and duration are still debated. There is some literature, however, that suggests that such factors may impact outcome. PCH can adversely impact neuropsychological testing performance, alter sleep quality and behavior (e.g., irritability and decreased frustration tolerance), as well as lead to secondary symptoms of depression and anxiety and has also been associated with poorer outcomes from CBI.[3,4]

Terminology remains in limbo and there is no international consensus on how best to "label" PCHs; however, consideration should be given to avoiding nonhelpful generic labels such as PCH or PTHA and not providing further diagnostic information. Instead, practitioners need to stipulate the presumed pain generators (e.g., cervicogenic, migraine, tension, neuralgic, etc.), which may at times be mixed in order to adequately direct treatment decisions.[8] Use of such general terms may also cause practitioners and others to misattribute the headache disorder to traumatic brain injury when, in fact, its cause may be extracerebral as in the case of impact injury, post-traumatic neuralgic or neuritic pain, referred myofascial and cervicogenic headache, among other possibilities. The phrase

Concussion. https://doi.org/10.1016/B978-0-323-65384-8.00006-7
Copyright © 2020 Elsevier Inc. All rights reserved.

"chronic PCH" should also be avoided since a chronicity label may only have been given due to an incorrect diagnosis and/or treatment, which results in persistence of the underlying pain disorder. Such labels can only serve to negatively bias evaluating clinician perspectives. It is therefore preferential to document the headache onset date and duration of symptoms as well as the specific presumed pain generators.

CLASSIFICATION CHALLENGES

Use of the current IHS (International Headache Society) International Classification of Headache Disorders (ICHD-3 and 3B) systems has its limitations with regard to how PCHs and PTHAs in general are classified. There is a lack of differentiation of the various causes of PCH/PTHA and all PTHAs are categorized under section 5 of ICHD-3 and are divided into three broad categories relative to headache being due to trauma to the head, neck, or secondary to craniotomy. The specific categories include acute as well as persistent headache attributed to traumatic injury to the head, acute as well as persistent headache attributed to whiplash, and acute as well as persistent headache attributed to craniotomy. Acute PTHA is defined as headache that resolves within 3 months from the date of injury, whereas persistent PTHA refers to headache lasting greater than 3 months (although this is somewhat distinct from typical "chronic pain" definitions that use a timeframe of greater than 6 months before chronicity is established). There is additional division of the classification system based on the severity of TBI, which is dualistic and divides TBI into two broad categories of mild TBI and moderate/severe TBI. Onset of headache must be within 7 days of injury (although to our knowledge this is empirical and not evidence-based), regaining consciousness or discontinuation of medications that might impair the ability to sense or report headache following the injury in question.[9] The 7-day onset criterion has been shown to underestimate incidence of this disorder; specifically, PCH may have its onset after 1 week post injury.[10] The terminology used in ICHD is confusing as brain injury and head injury appear to be used interchangeably and should not be since the two phenomena can occur separately or conjointly. There is no mention of the myriad other causes of PTHA such as migraine, tension-type headache (TTHA), neuralgic/neuritic headache, among numerous other conditions that are categorized elsewhere but may present following trauma.[11] Another problem with use of ICHD is the fact that it is only symptom based and does not consider physical examination findings or

any type of diagnostic testing.[8] Based on symptom profiling, ICHD-3 has the potential to incorrectly categorize secondary headache disorders due to trauma, including overdiagnosis of migraine.[3,4] As noted by Dwyer and others, no specific headache features or treatment approaches accompany the definition, which likely limits its usefulness in both research and clinical practice.[11] Whether classification systems, such as IHS ICHD-3[9] or ICD-10,[12] are truly relevant to PCH and PTHA, more generally, remains to be seen. In the context of secondary headache disorders, such classification systems may have limited value and the potential to incorrectly or inadequately classify these headache subtypes, which in turn may lead to inappropriate treatment being rendered and as a consequence a suboptimal outcome. As a consequence of these concerns, some have advocated for a more multifaceted classification system taking into consideration the nature of the brain injury and symptom-based profiles.[13]

LIMITATIONS OF EXISTING LITERATURE

Historical studies assessing incidence of headache subtypes post-TBI have relied on neurological headache classification systems such as ICHD and ICD with little or no regard to the overlap of symptoms of PCH with PCD (i.e. autonomic symptoms like photosensitivity and sonosensitivity), physical exam correlates of underlying pain generators, and/or headache pain symptom validity measures. Additionally, the role, if any, of secondary gain incentives including litigation, worker's compensation, and social security disability in headache reporting and prognosis remains to be edified. What contribution comorbid affective issues including depression, anxiety, and PTSD have on headache presentation and persistence are also unknown. Lastly, the diagnosis of concussion may be associated with nocebo effects and negative expectancy biases as related to headache reporting and prognosis that we currently have no good methods of assessing.

The literature is highly variable in study methodologies, criteria for "concussion" diagnosis, and delineation of involvement of potential secondary gain incentives that may serve to perpetuate headache complaints. For example, the study by Lane et al. found a headache persistence rate at 24 months of 70% with 90% of patients meeting criteria for migraine or probable migraine.[14] Stacey, Lucas, and Dikmen et al. assessed PTHA (very few with mTBI) natural history over 5 years and used ICHD-2 criteria and found a high rate of frequent headache at 60 months (36%)

with migraine accounting for just under 60% of headache subtypes and with close to 30% of headaches being "unclassifiable".[15] Yet, other studies show significantly lower rates of headache complaint persistence and much lower rates for migraine-type headaches.[16–18] These disparities reinforce the calls for further research on PCH using randomized controlled study protocols and broadening the scope of the assessments.

It should also be noted that cervical whiplash injury has been found to be associated with various autonomic comorbidities that may mimic postconcussive symptomatology, which can further complicate headache classification. Given the complexities of these injuries, it would be naïve to assume that headache classification is as simple as finding one thing that is causing the headache. In most cases, there are multiple pain generators and/or perpetuators that require holistic assessment and treatment. The neck should be considered a primary target for examination in the context of PCH assessment and yet, has historically received little recognition or attention.

Another significant area of concern is the nomenclature inconsistencies across studies as related to use of brain, head, and neck injury labels and criteria for the same. There is often inadequate information regarding whether subjects truly met criteria to be diagnosed with concussion, as well as a lack of documentation on comorbid injuries to the cranium, cranial adnexal structures, and/or neck. Another common oversight is the focus on CBI as the most likely explanation for the PCH. Headache onset after concussion does not mean that the concussion itself was necessarily the cause of the headache. Clinicians should understand that aside from concussion, cranial impact injuries, cranial adnexal trauma, e.g., TMJ, and cervical acceleration deceleration (whiplash) injuries, among other conditions often cause PCH and/or contribute to it. There is also likely a reporting bias relative to preexisting headache disorders as well as genetic loading risk factors, both of which likely get underreported either due to recall bias or lack of knowledge.[19] Lastly, there has been inadequate study of the potential role that prescription drug–induced headaches, and more importantly, medication overuse headaches (MOHs) play in the PCH population.

PCH PATHOETIOLOGY

Anatomic sources of head pain that may be relevant in the assessment of a patient presenting with PCH include the dura, venous sinuses, and cranial cavities, including sinuses, eye sockets, etc. The skin, nerves, muscles, and periosteum of the cranium are all pain sensitive. Cervical/cranial joint capsules (including the temporomandibular joint), cervical facets/zygapophyseal joints, peripheral nerves (supraorbital, trochlear, greater occipital, lesser occipital, as well as third occipital nerves), and the cervical sympathetic plexus may all be pain generators that produce local or referred head pain.[20,21]

Given CBI injury mechanisms, it is possible to incur various types of trauma to the aforementioned structures including but not limited to impact injuries (both long and short impulse), stretch injuries of various tissues (both rotational and linear), penetrating injuries, shearing/tearing injuries, and compression, as well as herniation-related forces. One of the most common, yet often overlooked, sources of head pain following CBI is referred cervical pain, which is typically associated with acceleration-deceleration insults or whiplash-associated disorders. Postwhiplash sequelae may include referred myofascial pain emanating from any of the four layers of the posterior cervical, as well as anterolateral cervical musculature; traumatic neuralgias (as noted above), vertebral osseous somatic dysfunction, disc herniation and/or rupture, ligamentous injury and/or facet joint trauma (with potential for osteoarthropathy and/or traumatic injury to the medial branches of the dorsal ramus). Risk factors for persistent postwhiplash symptoms including headache should be identified and addressed as apropos.[22] These injuries can be seen in the absence of CBI or as a comorbid feature and should always be considered in the context of identifying the specific pain generators contributing to the PCH even in the absence of subjective complaints of cervicalgia.

The neurobiology of PCH following a single traumatic insult may involve cerebral/intracranial, cranial as well as cranial adnexal, and cervical structures involved with encoding and processing of craniocervical noxious stimuli. Pain receptors may be activated by tissue injury and neuroinflammation and mediated by bradykinin, serotonin, substance P, histamine, leukotrienes, cytokines, and prostaglandins.[23,24] Additionally, it seems clear that there are likely both peripheral and central mediators of PCH. Acutely, it is more likely that peripheral mechanisms account for pain mediation rather than central or supraspinal causes. Cranial mechanical hyperalgesia likely related to peripheral structure injury to blood vessels, nerve fibers, and osseous structures, as well as the inflammatory cascade, likely serve as sources of peripheral pain sensitization and PCH. The aforementioned would suggest that earlier more aggressive treatments during the acute phase could prevent secondary chronification through central sensitization mechanisms. Some have speculated that central mechanisms are involved in persistent allodynia related to somatosensory cortex injury. Mechanisms of central sensitization are still being explored; however, it appears that abnormal neuronal excitability may lead to altered processing of sensory stimuli causing cortical spreading depression and trigeminal activation. There are numerous pathways in the neuromatrix that when damaged may lead to centrally mediated pain. Central sensitization contributes to both acute allodynia and headache persistence. Sensitization, whether peripheral and/or central, is not just relevant to post-traumatic migraine but may be seen in cervical whiplash injury, traumatic temporomandibular disorder, among other conditions. Repetitive concussions may promote trigeminal sensitivity and microglial proliferation, astrocytosis and neuropeptide release in the trigeminovascular system further exacerbating the underlying headache disorder.[25]

Nitric oxide synthase and calcitonin gene–related peptide have been implicated as at least potentially contributory to mediating allodynia in migraineurs following concussion, which has been linked with trigeminal neuroplastic changes.[26] Others have speculated that the pathophysiology of PTHA is shared with the pathophysiology of brain injury itself relative to inflammatory responses. These inflammatory responses could persist beyond timeframes for actual beneficial physiological effect leading to secondary injuries due to alterations in neuronal excitability, axonal integrity, central processing, as well as other changes.[27]

A key anatomic entity that must be appreciated in the pathobiology of PCH is the convergence of upper cervical and trigeminal nociceptors through the trigeminal nucleus caudalis (TNC). Nociceptive input from a variety of sources in the neck can activate the TNC via occipital and cervical afferents (whether from muscles or joints). This phenomenon may account for improvements seen in postconcussive migraine and tension headache when cervical nociceptive afferent inputs, if present, are appropriately identified and treated, leading to decreased or negated nociceptive afferent input into the TNC. Such treatment can also help modulate peripherally sensitized trigeminal branches such as the supraorbital nerves.[4]

Lastly, the disparate findings on the correlation between injury severity parameters and type, frequency, severity, and duration of PTHA seemingly begs the question of whether other non-CBI-related pain generators and/or mechanisms are involved in both the origin of PCH and its promulgation.

PCH CLINICAL PRESENTATIONS—AN OVERVIEW

Headache and neck pain are the most common physical complaints following CBI and are experienced early after injury in a very large percentage of patients and, in a smaller percentage, longer term (however, the latter literature is not as strong methodologically). The major types of headaches seen following trauma include musculoskeletal headache (including direct cranial trauma, cervicogenic headache, and TMJ disorders), neuromatous and neuralgic (nerve) headache, TTHA, migraine, as well as less common causes such as dysautonomic headaches, seizures, facial and/or skull fractures, cluster headaches, paroxysmal hemicrania, post-traumatic sinus infections, drug induced headaches, MOHs, and the surgical conditions previously mentioned. There remain controversies regarding the occurrence and causal relationship of trigeminal autonomic cephalgias such as cluster and paroxysmal hemicranias with concussion. The overlap in headache subtypes as related to cervicogenic, referred myofascial, migraine, and tension headache cannot be overemphasized in the context of both assessment and treatment implications.[28]

The majority of headaches following CBI are most likely benign and do not typically require surgical treatment; although, there are, on occasion, complications that occur after both CBI and more severe injury that may cause headache and require surgical intervention. Subdural and epidural hematomas, carotid cavernous fistulas, traumatic carotid or vertebral artery dissection, cavernous sinus thrombosis, as well as post-traumatic intracranial pressure (ICP) abnormalities (high vs. low ICP), among other conditions can all be responsible for headaches and bring with them a potential need for surgical intervention. Readers are referred to more comprehensive sources for details on the aforementioned less common etiologies of PTHA.[3]

PCH is best evaluated with time taken to acquire an adequate preinjury, injury, and postinjury history and in that context, a detailed history of the presenting headache symptoms. Equally important, but often ignored, a headache physical examination (including relevant neurological and musculoskeletal elements) should be performed. As clinically indicated, other diagnostic testing, including imaging, psychoemotional, and/or pain assessments, among other examinations, may be necessary/helpful. One of the most frequent areas of concern is whether the patient with suspected CBI requires brain/head imaging. In general, such imaging is not necessary except in cases where there are worsening headaches, medically unresponsive headaches, and/or protracted headaches after injury. The main physical findings that justify considering neuroimaging in head trauma as well as CBI include eye swelling or pupil abnormalities, diplopia or vision loss, and/or focal neurological findings.[29]

Late-onset headaches (i.e., greater than 2 months post trauma) should cue the treating clinician to think of less common injury-related conditions such as a slowly expanding extra-axial collection as a cause for the headache disorder or just as likely, a noninjury-related cause such as a space-occupying lesion (e.g., brain tumor, colloid cyst, subsequent injury), among other conditions[3]; although, late-onset headaches apportionable to the initial injury can happen even years post insult.

THE PCH HISTORY

The examination should start with taking a thorough history from the patient as related to their PCH complaint. One of the most important pieces of information to acquire in this context is to determine if the patient had any type of headache complaints preemptory to the injury in question and if so, whether the headache presentation has changed. In that context, it is also important to determine if there are genetic loading risk variables for headache such a migraine in the patient's family.[30] Important information to garner in the context of the history taking is the timing of headache onset relative to the traumatic event. Clarifying the frequency and severity of pain is also of paramount importance and ideally should include use of standardized pain rating scales and/or headache questionnaires. A nice mnemonic to assist in taking a headache history is "COLDER"…character of pain, onset, location, duration, exacerbation, and relief. Understanding how the headache has evolved post injury is also important as is acquisition of a treatment history relative to what specific treatments were prescribed and what the patient's response was to the same. As it relates to prior drug treatment, it is important to note that the clinician should edify both the dose of the medicine as well as the duration that the medicine was given to assure that an adequate trial was provided. As far as nonpharmacological treatments are concerned, the clinician should establish that there were adequate interventions utilized to address the underlying pain generators as might be the case with osteopathic, chiropractic,

physical therapy, and/or psychological management. The clinician should get as much information as possible about injury mechanisms to understand risk factors for particular PCH pain generators such as might be associated with brain injury itself, cranial impact injuries, and/or cervical whiplash. Lastly, clarification of the functional consequences of PCH is important and may include limitations in physical activity, including exercise and sexual activity, work or school pursuits, sleep quality, and mood alterations, among other factors to explore. Use of headache questionnaires to assess disability from same such as MIDAS or HIT-7, headache diaries, and tracking tools/applications for smartphones (e.g., Curelator, Headache Diary Lite Pro, iHeadache, Migraine Buddy, MigrainePal and My Migraine Triggers), although none have been validated for PCH, may further complement the information garnered during history taking.[4] Given the existing literature on the accuracy, or limits thereof, of histories provided by people with brain injury, it is important to interview corroboratory sources as well due to potential limitations in patient insight and memory.

THE PCH PHYSICAL EXAMINATION

The hands-on physical examination, which is often ignored in PTHA assessment, should take into consideration central and peripheral neurological clinical findings, as well as musculoskeletal clinical findings. The neurological evaluation should entail an elemental neurological examination of all 12 cranial nerves, funduscopic examination (to rule out papilledema), deep tendon reflexes including pathological reflex testing, sensory examination including visual field confrontational testing, motor examination and cerebellar assessment (which should also encompass measures of postural stability), assessment for meningismus, and mental status evaluation. Appropriate cognitive screening should be performed as clinically indicated. The peripheral neurological examination should include assessment for neuralgic and/or neuritic headache pain generators such as supraorbital neuralgia, temporoauricular neuralgia, and occipital neuralgia. The musculoskeletal examination should include palpatory assessment of the face, temporomandibular joints, head and craniocervical junction, cervicothoracic spine, and upper thorax at a minimum to assess for pathologic findings.

The musculoskeletal evaluation of the patient with PCH should be holistic in nature as the entire body should be screened, not just the cervical spine. Sitting and standing postures should be noted, preferably without the patient's awareness, so that the clinician can obtain a realistic view of postural habits. Details such as forward head, increased kyphosis in the thoracic spine, and increased or flattening of the lordotic curvature in the lumbar and cervical spines are important to note as well as scapular positioning. A closer inspection for body asymmetries (e.g., head tilt, shoulder droop, rotated or tilted pelvis, and leg length discrepancy) are also important to note as these asymmetries may be contributing to ongoing cervical dysfunction and pain complaints. Jaw range of motion and tracking is an often overlooked but important assessment as TMJ issues commonly refer pain into the head and have been associated with both facial trauma and cervical whiplash injuries.[3,4] The temporomandibular joints should also be auscultated, as clinically indicated, for abnormal articular sounds.

Cervical spine range of motion can provide valuable insights into dysfunction (e.g., limited right rotation and side-bending can indicate a right cervical facet dysfunction and rotation less than 45° can indicate dysfunction at C2).[31] Auscultation for bruits should be done as appropriate over the carotids, closed eyes, temporal arteries, and mastoids for assessment of arteriovenous fistulas. Palpatory examination should include the face, head (including TMJ and masticatory muscles), shoulder girdles, and neck musculature. This must be done in a controlled, layer-by-layer fashion to truly localize pathology with an eye to identifying activated trigger points and referred pain patterns. Common special tests that should be included in the musculoskeletal examination are the cervical flexion rotation test, to assess for C2 dysfunction; Spurling's test, to assess for cervical facet dysfunction; alar ligament stress test, anterior shear test, Sharp Purser test, and the tectorial membrane test to assess for upper cervical instability. When assessing facets, the examination focus should be on the first three cervical levels as these levels can directly refer pain into the head through nociceptive inputs into the trigeminocervical nucleus; although there remains some debate about whether referral of pain can occur below the C3 level. A systematic review of physical examination tests for screening for cervicogenic headache found that the cervical flexion-rotation test exhibited the highest reliability and strongest diagnostic accuracy.[32] Referred cervical myofascial pain as a consequence of cervical whiplash is a particularly common cause of PCH. This fact should emphasize the importance of a good musculoskeletal examination in any patient presenting with PCH including, of course, the neck. One can often find activated trigger points in the suboccipital musculature,

sternocleidomastoid, and/or upper trapezius muscles as common sources of referred pain into the head in such patients.

Neuralgic and neuritic pain generators associated with surgical trauma, direct scalp contusional injury, and craniocervical acceleration/deceleration forces are often overlooked. Clinicians should understand the anatomy of the peripheral nerves innervating the face and scalp including but not limited to the occipital nerves as well as their ability to be treated through interventional pain management techniques. The interconnectivity of upper cervical roots and brainstem trigeminal centers through the trigeminocervical complex is critical to keep in mind as previously noted and to understand in the context of PCH assessment when there is comorbid cervical whiplash injury.[33]

Migraine and tension headache have also been shown to not uncommonly be associated with abnormal musculoskeletal examinations of the head and neck. Given this fact, clinicians should always assess these structures even if the diagnosis of PCH falls in the migraine tension spectrum.[34] It is also important to note that patients may have had neck injuries and be unaware of that fact and even deny pain complaints referable to the same but still have pathological findings on neck examination. In patients with new-onset headache, examiners must also ascertain that they are not tender over the temporal arteries or demonstrating signs of nuchal rigidity, the latter which may be associated with a pathologic meningeal process such as meningitis.

PCH TREATMENT PRINCIPLES—AN OVERVIEW

Treatment should be instituted in a holistic fashion as early as possible with the goals of maximizing the benefit/risk ratio of any particular intervention, prescribing treatment that can be optimally complied with and educating the patient and family regarding the condition, its treatment, and prognosis in a coordinated attempt to minimize risk for longer term PCH complaints and disability as well as improve quality of life and pain adaptation.[35] Ideally, treatment should be interdisciplinary and multipronged as clinically warranted with the most essential team members being the physician, physical therapist, and psychologist.

The pharmacological management of PCH is replete with challenges due to the lack of an adequate body of evidence-based medicine examining the efficacy of pharmacotherapeutic agents in this population.[36] The general practice trend is to approach these headache disorders as they would be treated in primary headache disorders.[37] There are no FDA-approved drug treatments specific to pediatric or adult PCH or for that matter PTHA more generally. General rules of pharmacological prescription in persons after concussion are to start low, go slow, minimize polypharmacy, choose agents that will likely be effective given the specific condition being treated (as such may be available), reassess need for medication over time, monitor use/abuse as clinically indicated, and attempt to choose medications that can be taken once to twice a day at most to optimize compliance.[38]

Treatment approaches should emphasize conservative measures first as possible as interventional treatments lack methodologically sound evidence.[39] Such interventions may include physical modalities, lifestyle changes, postural education, and behavioral therapy among other treatments.[40] Knowledge regarding psychological assessment and behavioral therapies in these types of pain patients is essential to holistic management as is clinical acumen on methods to ascertain pain reporting response biases and pain catastrophizing.[41–43] Interventional procedures such as facet, peripheral nerve, as well as sphenopalatine ganglion blocks should be considered as clinically appropriate.[44] With the advent of a number of different types of neuromodulation treatments, clinicians have more treatment choices particularly for post-traumatic migraine and certain neuralgias although these interventions have yet to be studied in this patient group.

Pain medications that are not specific for the particular headache subtype should usually be avoided, particularly such agents as opiates and barbiturates, which may cause a variety of long-term adverse effects including, but not limited to, MOH, adverse endocrine effects, drug tolerance over time, impairment issues that may affect safety for driving and/or equipment use, and addiction, among other risks.[4,37] There is seldom an indication for prescribing opiates in this group of patients, particularly for longer term use. Additionally, not all pain is opiate responsive, and clinicians should therefore use caution when prescribing such agents. Patients should only be placed on chronic opioid treatment if they demonstrate true failure to respond to a variety of other pharmacotherapeutic agents with less potential short- and long-term risks, have opiate responsive pain, and are not candidates for neuromodulation, interventional pain management procedures, and/or surgery. Pediatric patients, those with significant Axis II issues, or those with a history of chronic substance abuse should generally not be considered candidates for opioid therapy.

Once central sensitization is suspected to have taken place, the prognosis becomes more guarded for complete pain resolution; however, clinicians must be familiar with methodologies for modulating this type of complication in the context of PCH. A multipronged approach has been shown to have the best results by focusing on specific targets for desensitization including both bottom-up and top-down strategies such as oral medications, topical analgesic therapies, as well as metabolic and neurotrophic factors all with the goal of decreasing hyperexcitability in the central nervous system.[45]

PCH: COMMON PRESENTATIONS AND RECOMMENDED TREATMENT APPROACHES

The following will summarize the clinical presentation and treatment of the most common PCH variants. Please see Table 6.1 for an overview of headache subtypes, typical symptom presentation, examination findings, and treatment options.

Migraine
Clinical presentation
As per ICHD-3, migraine is defined based on clinical history. The patient must have at least five headache attacks that lasted for a duration of 4–72 h, with the headache having at least two of the following characteristics: unilateral (nonside alternating), location, pulsatile quality, pain intensity that is moderate or severe, and pain aggravated by activity or pain that limits activity.[9] It should be noted, however, that more than 50% of people who suffer from migraines report nonthrobbing pain at some time during the attack. During the headache there must be at least one of the following reported: nausea or emesis, and/or photophobia/phonophobia (also referred to his photosensitivity and sonosensitivity). There must not be any other explanation for the headache to classify it as migraine. Of note, migraine attacks commonly occur during waking hours but less commonly may awaken a person from sleep.

Treatment
There are three basic approaches to pharmacotherapeutic management of post-traumatic migraine. These include prophylaxis, abortive therapy, and symptomatic therapy. Successful treatment of migraines may be paradoxically achieved by reducing medication use. In medication overuse, headache worsening typically occurs because of the overuse of abortive pain medications.

TABLE 6.1
Postconcussive Headache Subtypes, Symptoms, Examination, and Treatment.

Headache Pain Generator	Presenting Symptoms	Physical Examination Caveats	Treatment Recommendations
Migraine	Unilateral location, pulsatile/throbbing pain character, pain intensity that is moderate to severe and aggravated by activity. Classically associated with nausea or emesis and or photo– and/or phonosensitivity. Typically occurs during waking hours.	Potential for associated musculoskeletal examination abnormalities of the head and neck which may compound and/or perpetuate trigeminovascular instability.	Consideration of prescription pharmacotherapeutic interventions involving symptomatic, abortive, and/or prophylactic medications including medications such as botulinum toxin. Can also consider use of naturopathic agents and over-the-counter medications including agents with caffeine. Interventional procedures including sphenopalatine ganglion blocks, occipital nerve blocks, and neuromodulation should all be considered as clinically appropriate/lifestyle changes and behavioral interventions including cognitive behavioral therapy (CBT) with stress management training, biofeedback, and relaxation training among other interventions should also be utilized as apropos. Physical therapy referral may be appropriate to treat concurrent abnormal musculoskeletal findings.
Tension-type headache (TTHA)	Pain is usually bilateral and occipitofrontal in location with a "tight band" feeling that may have a throbbing quality and is usually gradual in onset with duration being highly variable with a more constant quality but generally with mild to moderate pain intensity. Typically not aggravated by physical activity. May be associated with photo– and/or phonosensitivity. Typically made worse by lack of sleep and stress.	Potential for associated musculoskeletal examination abnormalities of the head and neck.	Consideration of prescription pharmacotherapeutic interventions for abortive as well as prophylactic therapy. Avoid use of muscle relaxants. Consider nonpharmacologic treatments including CBT, biofeedback, relaxation therapy, massage, stress inoculation treatment, and exercise among other interventions. Physical therapy referral as appropriate to treat concurrent abnormal musculoskeletal findings.
Cervicogenic	Headaches tend to be unilateral and nonalternating as far as laterality although they can on occasion be bilateral. Pain described typically is nonthrobbing, nonlancinating with moderate to severe pain intensity with episodes of varying duration. May see a variety of comorbid autonomic symptoms associated with these types of headaches (i.e., blurry vision, dizziness).	Assess for upper cervical vertebral somatic dysfunction, cervical instability (i.e., ligamentous), facet-mediated pain, neuralgic pain generators such as occipital neuralgia and/or activated myofascial trigger points in the neck and or upper shoulder girdles that may refer into the head.	Physical modalities including manual therapies and physical therapy interventions with consideration of focused exercise therapies and in some cases interventional pain management procedures. Rarely surgery.

| Neuralgia/Neuritic | Variable presentations based upon nature of nerve dysfunction from dysesthetic more diffuse pain symptoms to very focal point tenderness to shooting or lancinating-type pain with referral. Location will be variable depending upon the nerve affected. Duration can be episodic or constant. | Assess for dysesthetic areas on the scalp, positive Tinel's signs over major nerves (i.e., supraorbital, greater occipital) or their branches, nerve tenderness, as well as referred pain. | Treatment consideration should include enteral, topical, and injected medication therapies. Additionally, cryoneurolysis, radiofrequency ablation, and neuroablation can be considered, although newer techniques involving neuromodulation may provide more conservative yet effective management. |
| Medication overuse headache | Typically presents as a holocephalic, throbbing headache which can be persistent. They tend to occur daily to nearly every day and may awaken a person in the early morning. Tend to improve with pain relief medication and will return as medication wears off. May be associated with nausea, restlessness, behavioral changes, and cognitive difficulties. | Likely to find parallel physical examination abnormalities as seen with migraineurs or patients with TTHA. | Discontinuation of offending medication with replacement with alternate treatment for the suspected background headache disorder which should be initiated either during or immediately following withdrawal. Nonpharmacologic therapies such as biofeedback and targeted physical therapy may also be indicated. Support groups and behavioral techniques have also been found to enhance success of treatment in some patients. |

Migraine prophylactic therapy should be aimed at improving quality of life, decreasing abortive drug therapy usage, as well as complications, and reducing attack frequency, severity, and/or duration. There are generally considered to be three broad classes of medications currently endorsed for migraine prophylaxis. These include antiepileptic drugs (AEDs), antihypertensives, and antidepressants.[46] Botulinum toxin A has also been FDA approved for use in chronic migraine management and is typically reserved for patients who have failed three preventive medications and are experiencing chronic migraine per aforementioned criteria.

The most recent guidelines for the prevention of episodic migraines by the American Headache Society/American Academy of Neurology, the Canadian Headache Society, and the European Federation of Neurological Societies were published in 2012. The medications with the highest level of evidence for migraine prevention were sodium valproate, butterbur, topiramate, propranolol, timolol, and metoprolol.[47] Although the aforementioned guidelines included only studies published up to 2009, more recent studies have confirmed most of the findings of previous systematic reviews.

Several "migraine-specific" prophylactic drugs have recently been developed, including CGRP receptor antagonists (abortive use) and monoclonal antibodies targeting CGRP (prophylactic use). These medications target known migraine pathophysiological mechanisms. Several oral CGRP receptor antagonists are now on the market and have shown promising efficacy in treating migraine with superiority to placebo and comparability to triptans. Some trials have been discontinued because of the concerns of hepatotoxicity after taking the drug for multiple consecutive days. Four monoclonal antibodies targeting CGRP or the CGRP receptor have been tested in humans for the prevention of migraine: galcanezumab, eptinezumab, erenumab, and fremanezumab. Another major breakthrough in the treatment of migraine has been the development of 5-hydroxytryptamine 1F (5-HT1F) receptor agonists, such as lasmiditan, which are similar to triptans but without their vascular side effects. This drug class binds more specifically to the serotonin 1F receptor than do triptans, which are less specific and bind to other vasoconstricting subtypes of serotonin receptors. Still in phase III trials, this drug class may be valuable for an aging population that is no longer eligible for triptan therapy because of cardiovascular and cerebrovascular risk factors.[46]

Naturopathic agents such as feverfew and butterbar can be considered as prophylactic antimigraine alternatives with the latter agent being available commercially as Petadolex, which is a patented, standardized CO_2 rhizome root extraction. Although butterbar has been used for many years, it has recently been shown to have potential for serious hepatotoxicity. Other agents including magnesium, riboflavin, and coenzyme Q10 have been touted as also being beneficial with empirical data being best for magnesium supplementation. Further studies are required to address persistent questions about efficacy, optimal dosing ranges, and parameters for choosing one drug over another in a particular patient.

Over-the-counter medications such as Advil Migraine, Excedrin Migraine, and Motrin Migraine, which are all FDA approved, should be considered first-line migraine abortives and are oftentimes quite effective if not overused. Prescription abortive medications include ergot derivatives, dihydroergotamine derivatives, and triptans, as well as combination medications such as Treximet. Dihydroergotamine-containing compounds such as DHE-45 can be given intravenously, typically with concurrent administration of metoclopramide (Reglan), for expedient abortive management of migraine. Dihydroergotamine is also available as a nasal spray, marketed as Migranal. Ergotamine formulations include oral medications such as Cafergot, as well as Ergotamine tartrate with caffeine, in addition to Ergomar sublingual tablets and Migergot suppositories. Parenteral atypical antipsychotics may also be used for abortive purposes.

Nonsteroidal anti-inflammatory drugs (NSAIDs) can be used for both prophylaxis and abortive therapy, the latter including menstrual migraine. Midrin, which is an acetaminophen-containing compound (acetaminophen-isometheptene-dichloralphenazone) has also been used for migraine headache management but typically works better for TTHAs.

Symptomatic medications are typically used for decreasing symptoms associated with nausea and emesis that may accompany migraine headaches. Traditionally, the drugs that are used for symptomatic management include prochlorperazine (Compazine) and promethazine (Phenergan), which may be given orally or via other routes such as rectal suppository. Metoclopramide (Reglan) and domperidone (Motilium) are also used as adjutants either orally or intravenously for symptomatic control and will also facilitate intestinal drug absorption.

Newer treatment interventions can also be considered in the context of migraine management, including sphenopalatine ganglion and/or greater occipital nerve blocks as well as neuromodulation modalities such as transcutaneous magnetic stimulation (TMS) with the eNeura SpringTMS, transcutaneous direct current stimulation (tDCS) of the supraorbital nerves with Cefaly or vagal nerve stimulation with gammaCore, among other developing methodologies.[48] These modalities may be helpful in both prophylaxis and abortive treatment of migraine.

Biobehavioral interventions have also been found to be effective for migraine management and may include cognitive behavioral therapy (CBT) with stress management training, biofeedback, and root relaxation training among the most common. Ideally biobehavioral interventions should be used in conjunction with pharmacotherapeutic approaches.

Tension Headaches
Clinical presentation
By ICHD criteria, tension headaches are divided into either episodic (frequent or infrequent) or chronic and further categorized by whether or not they are associated with pericranial muscle abnormalities. These types of headaches comprise the most common primary headache disorder.[49] Episodic tension headache is usually associated with heightened motions and/or stress and tends to be of moderate intensity with a self-limiting course. Episodic tension headache tends to be responsive to over-the-counter medications although prescription medications are sometimes necessary. Chronic tension–type headache (CTTH) on the other hand recurs daily and has been shown to be correlated with abnormalities in the pericranial and cervical muscle examinations. Genetic factors seem to be more important in the pathogenesis of CTTH.[50] This type of headache is usually bilateral and occipitofrontal in location. Pain onset can have a throbbing quality and is usually more gradual than the onset seen in migraine. Duration tends to be more highly variable than other headache disorders such as migraine with a more constant quality but lower degree of severity. The headache tends to be felt as a tightening around the head ("tight hat syndrome") (although location can vary) and is typically described as nonpulsatile. TTHA is not classically aggravated by physical activity.[50] They are typically made worse by lack of sleep and stress. These types of headaches are typically not associated with nausea or vomiting although photosensitivity and sonosensitivity can be seen but must be differentiated from postconcussive impairments of the same nature as well as migrainous phenomena.[51] There is very little understood about TTHA pathoetiology in primary headache or secondary headaches such as PCH but it is likely multifactorial.

Treatment
Acute pharmacotherapy of TTHA should include NSAIDs (including acetylsalicylic acid) sometimes in conjunction with caffeine, sedatives, and/or tranquilizers. There is no scientific evidence to support the use of muscle relaxants. Prophylactic pharmacotherapy for TTHA is more diversified and without any FDA-approved drugs currently endorsed. Tricyclic antidepressants, tizanidine, botulinum toxin, and venlafaxine (the latter an SNRI) have all shown at least some benefit, with TCAs having the best evidence basis.[52] Nonpharmacological treatments for tension headache include CBT, stress inoculation treatment, biofeedback, relaxation therapy, massage, trigger point therapy, exercise, and acupuncture.[52–54] Modalities may also play a role in modulating TTHA including hot or cold packs, ultrasound, electrical stimulation, postural education, trigger point injections, occipital nerve blocks, manual medicine treatment, and stretching among other interventions.[55] Proper diet, regular exercise, and restorative sleep are crucial in any headache patient including those with tension headache.

Neuritic and Neuralgic Headache
Clinical presentation
These types of headaches may present in variable patterns depending upon the nature of the peripheral nerve injury. Small nerve fibers in the scalp may be injured in the context of penetrating injuries, surgical intervention such as craniotomies, as well as by direct impact injury resulting in scalp dysesthesia, significant tender points, and/or positive Tinel's sign over the affected region. When upper cervical distal nerve roots are involved such as greater, lesser, or third occipital nerve, the pain may be localized and noted on compression over the nerve or when more severe may radiate into the sensory distribution of the nerve. In more severe cases, there will be ipsilateral radiation into the frontotemporal scalp and occasionally retro-orbitally...both of which will be described as painful by the patient. Peripheral nerve injuries to larger nerves, whether in the face or scalp, such as the supratrochlear, supraorbital, infraorbital (face), and/or auriculotemporal nerve may present with localized as well as referred pain and may be due to peripheral nerve injury as well as central sensitization. Clinicians must be familiar with the general anatomic location of all the aforementioned nerves as well as their associated sensory distributions.

Treatment
Drug management of post-traumatic neuritic and neuralgic pain tends to emphasize focal injection

therapies and topical agents. Secondary interventions may include enteral medications such as NSAIDs, tricyclic antidepressants, SNRIs such as duloxetine or anticonvulsants such as carbamazepine, gabapentin, and pregabalin. For post-traumatic neuralgias involving larger nerves of the face, scalp, and/or craniocervical junction, local injection therapy with corticosteroids and local anesthetic remains the mainstay of treatment. Serial injections may be necessary to abate or modulate the pain generator. Greater and lesser occipital neuralgia treatment approaches may include segmental blocks at C2 and C3, cryoneurolysis, radiofrequency (RF) ablation, and neuroablation; although, newer noninvasive strategies such as neuromodulation are now showing some promise.[56] Additionally, RF lesioning as well as surgical interventions do not necessarily guarantee resolution as there is a relatively high recurrence rate. Interestingly, blocks of afferent cervical nociceptive inputs have been shown to modulate trigeminal nerve pain as well as neurogenic inflammation[28]

Diffuse neuritic pain associated with scalp injuries such as postcraniotomy pain or local blunt trauma should be addressed with compounded topical formulations. Such topical agents, typically applied as an ointment or gel, generally need to be applied 3 to 4 times per day to be optimally effective. Topical agents for neuropathic pain may include TCAs, local anesthetics, NSAIDs, AEDS such as gabapentin, clonidine, and/or ketamine hydrochloride, among other agents. There are often challenges getting insurance coverage for compounded topical pain medications. For information on local and/or regional compounding pharmacies see https://www.achc.org/pcab-accredited-providers.html.

Myofascial Pain Related Headaches
Clinical presentation
Myofascial pain typically presents with pain in the neck and upper back/shoulders with potential to refer into the base of the skull in the head in general. Myofascial pain is associated with development of painful active trigger points (as opposed to latent trigger points which do not replicate the patient's pain complaint pattern). A myofascial trigger point (sometimes just called a trigger point) is a tight knot located within a taut muscular band. The knot or nodule can be distinctly felt underneath the skin and is tender when pressed. In addition, when pressure is applied to the knot, the taut muscular band which holds the knot contracts. This creates a twitching of the muscle that can be felt or visually observed, the so-called "twitch response."[57,58]

When a trigger point is located in the neck, shoulder, and/or head muscles, it can cause referred or spreading pain that can be perceived as headache. The headache may be localized or more diffuse depending on the number and location of the aforementioned trigger points. The patient may be misdiagnosed as having tension headache with bilateral referred cervical myofascial pain unless an appropriate musculoskeletal examination is performed and even then, the conditions can be comorbid and in such cases, both need to be addressed from a treatment standpoint. It should be further noted that such myofascial trigger points can be seen in association with headache due to whiplash, migraine, and tension headache.[57,58]

Treatment
Treatment should focus on an understanding of myofascial pain disorder triggers, as well as perpetuating factos. Myofascial therapies are the mainstay of such treatment and should include specific stretching exercises, deep soft tissue work, and myofascial techniques such as trigger point acupressure, and dry needling, among other techniques as clinically indicated.[57,58] Postural reeducation can be a very important component of holistic MPD treatment since incorrect posture (i.e., forward head position or upper crossed syndrome) may perpetuate referred headache pain. Manual techniques to restore proper mobility and alignment, muscle strengthening, and individualized exercise programs should all be considered in the context of such treatment.[58]

Pharmacologic interventions for myofascial pain, although traditionally not first-line treatment, include NSAIDs, tricyclic antidepressants, and possibly, muscle relaxants. Muscle relaxants have no proven efficacy, although some resemble TCAs in their structure and clinical effect and may contribute to treatment efficacy. Antispasticity drugs are seldom used for myofascial pain, although tizanidine may have some theoretical benefit over other traditional antispasticity agents due to its antinociceptive properties garnered through its effect on blocking of substance P. For chronic intractable myofascial pain, some have advocated for use of botulinum toxins although there are inconclusive data to support this use in the head and neck regions.

Cervicogenic Headache
Clinical presentation
The clinical presentation may be confounding due to the overlap of symptoms with other possible primary as well as secondary headache disorders, including tension headache, migraine, and greater occipital neuralgia headache. In part, this confusion occurs because even the aforementioned headaches tend to be associated

with complaints of neck pain and/or with pathological cervical physical examination findings in the absence of cervicalgia. Headaches tend to be unilateral and not alternating side to side although they can be bilateral.[59–61] Headaches are typically nonthrobbing, nonlancinating, and associated with moderate to severe pain with episodes of varying duration. To further complicate things, cervicogenic headaches have also been noted to be associated with sono- and photosensitivity, nausea, dizziness, unilateral blurred vision, among other symptoms.[62] It is critical to differentiate cervicogenic headaches from other headache etiologies[63] and recognize that afferent nociceptive input into the trigeminocervical complex can aggravate or perpetuate migraine as well as tension headache.

Treatment

Conservative treatment options should be tried first, including physical therapy and manual therapies (manipulation with or without mobilization), whether chiropractic, osteopathic, or craniosacral.[54,64,65] Low load endurance craniocervical and cervicoscapular exercises have also been shown to have a role in amelioration.[54] Exercise including postural and strengthening can play a key role in ameliorating/modulating such headaches.[66] In more intractable cases, interventional pain management procedures such as anesthetic blocks of the upper cervical joints can be helpful in both assessment and treatment.[67]

Medication Overuse Headache
Clinical presentation

MOH is defined as a headache occurring at least 15 days per month in patients with preexisting headache disorders and with concurrent use of either simple analgesic agents such as ibuprofen or naproxen at least 15 days per month or other analgesic agents such as triptans or ergotamines 10 days per month for at least 3 months.[68] MOH may be seen from excessive use of a variety of analgesic and/or abortive headache agents, including ergotamines, opiates, caffeine, triptans, and/or barbiturates.[69] Overuse of these medications may lead to development of increased headaches and even CDH. Patients may become dependent on these symptomatic headache medications. The headache tends to present as holocephalic and throbbing.[70] Headache medication overuse may also make headaches refractory to prophylactic headache medication and the affected person more sensitive to headache triggers. Unfortunately, most patients are unaware of MOH, so providers should be diligent in evaluating the frequency of medication use and educating patients as well as their family about the risks of MOH if medications are not taken as prescribed.[68]

Treatment

Although withdrawal and reduction of abortive medications is considered to be the treatment of choice, there is no standard practice recommended as related to withdrawal at this time. Drug withdrawal, particularly when abrupt, normally results in worsening of headache. Alternatively, if MOH is a concern, the offending medication should be slowly weaned with concurrent alternative preventative headache management options prescribed with evidence based on randomized studies best for topiramate and onabotulinumtoxin A.[50,68] What role some of the newer generation migraine medications may have is yet to be determined. Detoxification can be done as an outpatient, in a day hospital, or in an inpatient setting depending on the severity of the MOH and the comorbidities of the specific case.

PCH NATURAL HISTORY, PROGNOSIS, AND OUTCOME

There are inadequate evidence-based studies to stipulate the natural history, prognostic factors, and long-term outcomes of PCH, in part, because PCH is not one single pathophysiological disorder but rather a symptom descriptor that may involve multiple pain generators/causes including psychogenic ones. The relative lack of prospective, controlled, and blinded studies that adequately consider variables associated with headache cause, treatment, and secondary complications only further challenges our ability to understand its natural history and provide opinions regarding prognosis. There are also multiple methodological challenges in studying an impairment that is predominantly based on subjective patient report including issues of misattribution bias (on the part of the patient as well as the assessing clinician), patient recall bias, nocebo effects of the diagnosis, cultural influences on pain perception and reporting, and potential response bias relative to symptom amplification as well as minimization (depending on incentives...which may be subconscious, conscious, or some combination of both) regarding pain reporting and/or associated pain–related disability, among other issues.

Any study of chronic PCH must also address the inherent comorbidities of the psychological and medical effects of chronic pain (and the associated stress) on not only the patient's reporting of their pain but also on a myriad of other aspects of function, including cognition, behavior, and sleep. Studies to date have not integrated data from focused headache physical assessments that take into consideration neurological and musculoskeletal findings nor have they included measures of response bias, pain validity reporting, or analysis of the potential influence of secondary gain factors in headache reporting. Additionally, studies have not linked specific examination findings with current headache classification systems (the latter of which have been criticized relative to their lack of applicability and relevance to this particular population). Importantly, historical studies have not attempted to assess the accuracy of the PCH-related diagnoses nor their historical response to treatment. Without knowing what the specific PCH pain generators are in a population and/or how they were treated, we cannot make determinations of the true incidence of "chronic" PCH. Any such conclusions would furthermore be based on the assumption or confirmation that the headache condition(s) was/were appropriately diagnosed and treated. That being said, there is no literature to the authors knowledge regarding the natural history of untreated PCH.

Based on the available studies, headache tends to improve in the months following trauma, whether to the brain, head, or neck. How much improvement is seen will be dependent on injury severity, preinjury physical and psychoemotional status, presence of complicating factors such as nocebo effects, secondary gain incentives, resilience, among other factors, as well as appropriate diagnosis of the underlying pain generators and subsequent optimal treatment for same. Appropriate and timely treatment shortens the period of impairment, associated disability, lost work hours, as well as pain and suffering. There is very limited evidence regarding the impact of ongoing litigation on the persistence of headache complaints but that which exists suggests that patients still continue to report significant symptoms even after litigation has ended.[71] Further research to confirm prior findings is strongly recommended.

A small number of patients will develop intractable and sometimes severe PCH; however, this group of patients has been poorly studied and the influence of other factors including inappropriate headache categorization and treatment, MOH, secondary gain incentives, cultural factors, preinjury genetic loading risk variables, as well as psychogenic factors in such patients remains unclear. The first prospective controlled study examining PCH persistence found that approximately 15% of patients continued to complain of headache at 3 months post injury[72]; however, accuracy of diagnosis and appropriateness of treatment were not confirmed. Kjeldgaard et al. studied "chronic PTHA" in a group with "mild head injury" and found a high correlation with unemployment and interestingly TTHA was the most common headache subtype noted with over 30% of patients having a mixed headache picture.[73] Also of note in the Kjeldgaard study was the fact that over 50% of the chronic PCH group was involved in litigation. Dumke found that headache severity was strongly correlated with a poorer prognosis for return to work; yet, based on the study it is unclear whether patients were appropriately diagnosed and treated.[74]

When properly diagnosed and treated, most patients, in our experience, are able to achieve substantive headache improvement, if not cured, particularly when PCH is addressed earlier rather than later. Good outcomes depend to a great extent on patient education and avoidance of nocebo, iatrogenic, and lexigenic effects of the injury. Additionally, work disability due to PCH, in and of itself, is very uncommon in the hands of a sophisticated practitioner with a good treatment team, unless there are significant comorbidities including mental health issues and/or secondary gain incentives.

PCH prognosis must be based on an exact understanding of headache etiology (based on history and focused examination and questionably headache classification systems), overlay as relevant of psychogenic factors (including patient preinjury characterological issues) and secondary gain incentives, response to appropriate historical treatment, and consideration of whether the correct diagnosis and treatment for the pain generator was made from the initial assessment.[4,75]

PATIENT AND FAMILY EDUCATION

Patients, as well as significant others/caretakers, need to be educated so that they understand the relevant diagnoses, treatment plan, and prognosis. Education should also be provided regarding the importance of compliance with recommended treatments and in particular medication use as related to avoidance of MOH, potential drug side-effects, and drug interactions among other issues. Clinicians should remain accessible for questions or concerns.[4,5]

CONCLUSIONS

PCH is ultimately a symptom and not a diagnosis. This complex disorder has multiple potential causes and as a result, has multiple treatments to address the headache disorder that is associated with the underlying pain generator(s). Assessing and treating PCH is a process that requires adequate time commitment and knowledge by the treating clinician…some will consider this "a pain" and if that is the case, then those clinicians should defer treatment to others who make it their business to assess and treat these types of patients and conditions. Pejorative and potentially self-prophesizing labels such as "chronic PCH" are often a misnomer due to the fact that the actual pain generators were never diagnosed correctly in the first place and should be avoided. There is in fact hope for those with PCH regardless of how long they have suffered from pain. The challenge is finding clinicians and treatment teams who understand the diversity of this class of disorders and have experience in holistic assessment and treatment of patients who have had concussions, cranial trauma, and/or whiplash injuries.

RESOURCES OF INTEREST FOR PATIENTS AND PRACTITIONERS

ACHC: Pharmacy Compounding Accreditation Board (PCAB): https://www.achc.org/pcab-accredited-providers.html.

American Council for Headache Education: www.achenet.org.

American Headache Society: https://americanheadachesociety.org.

American Migraine Foundation: https://americanmigrainefoundation.org.

BIAA (PTHA webinar): https://shop.biausa.org/product/BOB092216CD/20160922-post-traumatic-headache-recorded-webinar.

Brainline. Post-traumatic headache: https://www.brainline.org/article/post-traumatic-headache-after-tbi.

Chiropractic Canada. Clinical practice guideline for the management of headache disorders in adults: http://ccpor.ca/wp-content/uploads/CPG-for-the-Management-of-Headache-Disorders-in-Adults-2012.pdf.

National Headache Foundation: www.headaches.org.

Ontario Neurotrauma Foundation. Guideline for concussion/mild traumatic brain injury & persistent symptoms. Third edition (for adults over 18 years of age). Post-traumatic headache. HTTPS://BRAININ JURYGUIDELINES.ORG/CONCUSSION/INDEX.PHP? ID=135&TX_ONFADULTS_ADULTDOCUMENTS%5B THEME%5D=6&TX_ONFADULTS_ADULTDOCUM ENTS%5BACTION%5D=SHOW&TX_ONFADULTS_ ADULTDOCUMENTS%5BCONTROLLER%5D= THEME&CHASH=036827A60A01AE94FC9382FE19 B89508.

Practical Pain Management, Migraine tracking apps for smartphones: https://www.practicalpainmanagement.com/patient/resources/pain-self-management/9-apps-tracking-your-migraine-days.

The American Council for Headache Education (provides a listing of on-line and local support groups): www.achenet.org.

ACKNOWLEDGMENTS

We thank John Leddy, MD, FACSM, FACP, for his input on this work.

REFERENCES

1. Dobscha SK, Clark ME, Morasco BJ, Freeman M, Campbell R, Helfand M. Systematic review of the literature on pain in patients with polytrauma including traumatic brain injury. *Pain Med.* 2009;10(7):1200−1217.
2. Evans RW. Persistent post-traumatic headache, post-concussion syndrome, and whiplash injuries: the evidence for a non-traumatic basis with a historical review. *Headache.* 2010;50(4):716−724.
3. Horn LJ, Siebert B, Patel N, Zasler ND. Post-traumatic headache. In: Zasler N, Katz D, Zafonte R, eds. *Brain Injury Medicine.* 2nd ed. New York: Demos; 2013:932−953.
4. Zasler ND, Leddy JJ, Etheredge S, Martelli MF. Post-traumatic headache. In: Silver JM, McAllister TW, Arciniegas D, eds. *Textbook of Traumatic Brain Injury.* 3r^d ed. Washington, D.C: American Psychiatric Publishing, Inc.; 2019:471−490.
5. Zasler ND, Martelli MF, Nicholson K, Horn L. Post-traumatic pain disorders: medical assessment and management. In: Zasler N, Katz D, Zafonte R, eds. *Brain Injury Medicine: Principles and Practice.* 2nd ed. New York: Demos Publishers; 2013:954−973.
6. Iverson GL, Gardner AJ, Terry DP, et al. Predictors of clinical recovery from concussion: a systematic review. *Br J Sports Med.* 2017;51:941−948.
7. Terry DP, Huebschmann NA, Maxwell BA, Cook NE, et al. Pre-injury migraine history as a risk factor for prolonged return to school and sport following concussion. *J Neurotrauma.* August 2, 2018. Epub ahead of print.
8. Zasler ND. Post-traumatic headache, caveats and controversies. *J Head Trauma Rehabil.* 1999;14(1):1−8.
9. Headache Classification Committee of the International Headache Society. The international classification of headache disorders, 3rd edition (beta version). *Cephalalgia.* 2013;33(9):629−808.
10. Hoffman JM, Lucas S, Dikmen S, et al. Natural history of headache after traumatic brain injury. *J Neurotrauma.* 2011;28(9):1719−1725.
11. Dwyer B. Post-traumatic headache. *Semin Neurol.* 2018;38:619−626.

12. ICD-10. Available at: http://apps.who.int/classifications/icd10/browse/2010/en#/G44.3. Accessed December 15, 2018.

13. Lucas S, Ahn AH. Post-traumatic headache: classification by symptom-based clinical profiles. *Headache*. 2018;58:873–882.

14. Lane R, Davies P. Post-traumatic headache in a cohort of UK compensation claimants. *Cephalalgia*. 2018. Epub ahead of print.

15. Stacey A, Lucas S, Dikmen S, et al. Natural history of headache five years after traumatic brain injury. *J Neurotrauma*. 2017;34(8):1558–1564.

16. Lew HL, Lin P-H, Fuh J-L, Wang S-J, Clark DJ, Walker WC. Characteristics and treatment of headache after traumatic brain injury: a focused review. *Am J Phys Med Rehabil*. 2006;85(7):619–627.

17. Lucas S, Hoffman JM, Bell KR, Dikmen S. A prospective study of prevalence and characterization of headache following mild traumatic brain injury. *Cephalalgia*. 2014;34(2):93–102.

18. Nordhaug LJ, Hagen K, Vik A, et al. Headache following head injury: population-based longitudinal cohort study (HUNT)). *J Headache Pain*. 2018;19(1):8.

19. Silverberg ND, Iverson G, Brubacher JR, et al. The nature and clinical significance of pre-injury recall bias following mild traumatic brain injury. *J Head Trauma Rehabil*. 2016;31(6):388–396.

20. Walker W. Pain pathoetiology after TBI: neural and non-neural mechanisms. *J Head Trauma Rehabil*. 2004;19(1):72–81.

21. Zasler ND, Etheredge S. Post-traumatic headache: knowledge update. *The Pain Practitioner*. 2015;25(2):19–22.

22. Walton DM, Macdermid JC, Giorgianni AA, Mascarenhas JC, West SC, Zammit CA. Risk factors for persistent problems following acute whiplash injury: update of a systematic review and meta-analysis. *J Orthop Sports PhysTher*. 2013;43(2):31–43.

23. Elliott MB, Oshinsky ML, Amenta PS, et al. Nociceptive neuropeptide increases and periorbital allodynia in a model of traumatic brain injury. *Headache*. 2012;52(6):966–984.

24. Mayer CL, Huber BR, Peskind E. Traumatic brain injury, neuroinflammation, and post-traumatic headaches. *Headache*. 2013;53(9):1523–1530.

25. Tyburski AL, Cheng L, Assari S, et al. Frequent mild head injury promotes trigeminal sensitivity concomitant with microglial proliferation, astrocytosis and increased neuropeptide levels in the trigeminal pain system. *J Heache Pain Dec*. 2017;18(1):16.

26. Mustafra G, Hou J, Tsuda S, et al. Trigeminal neuroplasticity underlies allodynia in a preclinical model of mild closed head traumatic brain injury (cTBI). *Neuropharmacology*. 2016;107:27–39.

27. Moye LS, Pradhan AA. From blast to bench: a translational mini-review of post- traumatic headache. *J Neurosci Res*. 2017;95(6):1347–1354.

28. Giblin K, Newmark JL, Brenner GJ, Wainger BJ. Headache plus: trigeminal and autonomic features in a case of

29. Rau JC, Dumkrieger GM, Chong CD, Schwedt TJ. Imaging post-traumatic headache. *Curr Pain Headache*. 2018;30;22(10):64.

30. Bendtsen L, Birk S, Kasch H, et al. Reference programme: diagnosis and treatment of headache disorders and facial pain. Danish Headache Society, 2nd edition, 2012. *J Headache Pain*. 2012;S1:S1–S29.

31. Hutting N, Scholten-Peeters GGM, Vijverman V, et al. Diagnostic accuracy of upper cervical spine instability tests: a systematic review. *Phys Ther*. 2013;93(12):1686–1695.

32. Rubio-Ochoa J, Benitez-Martinez J, Lluch E, Santacruz-Zaragoza S, Gomez-Contreras P, Cook CE. Physical examination tests for screening and diagnosis of cervicogenic headache: a systematic review. *Man Ther*. 2016;21:35–40.

33. Watson DH, Drummond PD. The role of the trigeminocervical complex in chronic whiplash associated headache: a cross sectional study. *Headache J Head Face Pain*. 2016;56(6):961–975.

34. Watson DH, Drummond PD. Head pain referral during examination of the neck in migraine and tension-type headache. *Headache*. 2012;52(8):1226–1235.

35. Bell KR, Kraus EE, Zasler ND. Medical management of posttraumatic headaches: pharma-cological and physical treatment. *J Head Trauma Rehabil*. 1999;14(1):34–48.

36. Watanabe TK, Bell KR, Walker WC, Schomer K. Systematic review of interventions for post-traumatic headache. *Phys Med Rehabil*. 2012;4:129–140.

37. Zasler ND. Pharmacotherapy and post-traumatic cephalalgia. *J Head Trauma Rehabil*. 2011;26(5):397–399.

38. Zasler ND. Pain management in persons with traumatic brain injury. In: Zollman F, ed. *Manual of Traumatic Brain Injury Assessment and Management*. 2nd ed. New York: Demos Medical; 2016:299–307.

39. Conidi FX. Interventional treatment for post-traumatic headache. *Curr Pain Headache Rep*. 2016;20:40.

40. Fraser F, Matsuzawa Y, Lee YSC, Minen M. Behavioral treatment for post-traumatic headache. *Curr Pain Headache Rep*. 2017;21:22.

41. Martelli MF, Nicholson K, Zasler N. Psychological assessment and management of post-traumatic pain. In: Zasler N, Katz D, Zafonte R, eds. *Brain Injury Medicine*. 2nd ed. New York: Demos; 2013:974–989.

42. Minen M, Jinich S, Vallespir EG. Behavioral therapies and mind-body interventions for post-traumatic headache and post-concussive symptoms: a systematic review. *Headache*. December 1, 2018. Epub ahead of print.

43. Martelli MF, Nicholson K, Zasler ND. Assessing and addressing response bias. In: Zasler N, Katz D, Zafonte R, eds. *Brain Injury Medicine: Principles and Practice*. 2nd ed. New York: Demos; 2013:1415–1436.

44. Ashkenazi A, Blumenfeld A, Napchan U, et al. Peripheral nerve blocks and trigger point injections in headache management - a systematic review and suggestions for future research. *Headache*. 2010;50(6):943–952.

45. Nijs j, Malfliet A, Ickmans K, Baert I, Meeus M. Treatment of central sensitization in patients with unexplained chronic pain: an update. *Expert Opin Pharmacother*. 2014; 15(12):1671–1683.

46. Ong JJY, Wei DY, Goadsby PJ. Recent advances in pharmacotherapy for migraine prevention: from pathophysiology to new drugs. *Drugs*. 2018;78(4):411–437.

47. Loder E, Burch R, Rizzoli P. The 2012 AHS/AAN guidelines for prevention of episodic migraine: a summary and comparison with other recent clinical practice guidelines. *Headache*. 2012;52(6):930–945.

48. Puledda F, Shields K. Non-pharmacological approaches to migraine. *Neurotherapeutics*. 2018;15:336–345.

49. Jensen RH. Tension type headache- the normal and most prevalent headache. *Headache J Head Face Pain*. 2018; 58(2):339–345.

50. Jay GW, Barkin RL. Primary headache disorders – Part 2: tension-type headache and medication overuse headache. *Disease-a-Month*. 2017;63:342–367.

51. Kahriman A, Zhu S. Migraine and tension-type headache. *Semin Neurol*. 2018;38:608–618.

52. Ghadiri-Sani M, Silver N. Headache (chronic tension type). *BMJ Clin Evid*. 2016:1205.

53. Alonso-Blanco C, de-la-Llave-Rincón AI, Fernández-de-las-Peñas C. Muscle trigger point therapy in tension-type headache. *Expert Rev Neurother*. 2012;12(3):315–322.

54. Varatharajan S, Ferguson B, Chrobak K, et al. Are non-invasive interventions effective for the management of headaches associated with neck pain? An update of the bone and joint decade, task force on neck pain and its associated disorders by the Ontario protocol for traffic injury management collaboration. *Eur Spine J*. 2016; 25(7):1971–1999.

55. Posadzki P, Ernst E. Spinal manipulations for tension-type headaches: a systematic review of randomized controlled trials. *Complement Ther Med*. 2012;20(4):232–239.

56. Choi I, Jeon SR. Neuralgias of the head: occipital neuralgia. *J Korean Med Sci*. 2016;31(4):479–488.

57. Do TP, Heldarskard GF, Kolding LT, Hvedstrup J, Schytz H. Myofascial trigger points in migraine and tension-type headache. *J Headache Pain*. 2018;19(1):84.

58. Donnelly JM, Fernandez-de-las-Penas C, Finnegan M, Freeman JL. Myofascial pain and dysfunction. In: Travell, Simons, Simons, eds. *The Trigger Point Manual*. 3rd ed. Philadelphia, PA: Wolter Kluwer; 2019.

59. Packard RC. The relationship of neck injury and post-traumatic headache. *Curr Pain Headache Rep*. 2002;6: 301–307, 2002.

60. Becker WJ. Cervicogenic headache: evidence that the neck is a pain generator. *Headache*. 2010;50(4):699–705.

61. Bogduk N. The neck and headaches. *Neurol Clin*. 2014; 32(2):471–487.

62. Blumenthal A, Siavoshi S. The challenges of cervicogenic headache. *Curr Pain Headache Rep*. 2018;22:47.

63. Vincent MD. Cervicogenic headache: a review comparison with migraine, tension type headache and whiplash. *Curr Pain Headache Rep*. 2010;14:238–243.

64. Garcia JD, Arnold S, Tetley K, et al. Mobilization and manipulation of the cervical spine in patients with cervicogenic headache: any scientific evidence? *Front Neurol*. 2016;7:40.

65. Racicki S, Gerwin S, Diclaudio S, Reinmann S, Donaldson M. Conservative physical therapy management for treatment of cervicogenic headache: a systematic review. *J Man Manip Ther*. 2013;21(2):113–124.

66. Dunning JR, Butts R, Mourad F, et al. Upper cervical and upper thoracic manipulation versus mobilization and exercise in patients with cervicogenic headache: a multi-center randomized clinical trial. *BMC Muscoskelet Disord*. 2016;17:64.

67. Fernandez-de-las-Penas C, Cuadrado ML. Therapeutic options for cervicogenic headache. *Expert Rev Neurother*. 2014;14(1):39–49.

68. Diener HC, Holle D, Solbach K, Gaul C. Medication-overuse headache: risk factors, pathophysiology and management. *Nat Rev Neurol*. 2016;2(10):575–583.

69. Katsarava Z, Obermann M. Medication overuse headache. *Curr Opin Nueorl*. 2013;26(3):276–281.

70. Kristoffersen ES, Lundquist C. Medication-overuse headache; epidemiology, diagnosis and treatment. *Ther Adv Drug Saf*. 2014;5(2):87–99.

71. Packard RC. Post-traumatic headache: permanency and relationship to legal settlement. *Headache*. 1992;32(10): 496–500.

72. Faux S, Sheedy J. A prospective controlled study on the prevalence of post-traumatic headache following mild traumatic brain injury. *Pain Med*. 2008;9(8):1001–1011.

73. Kjeldgaard D, Forchhammer H, Teasdale T, Jensen RH. Chronic post-traumatic headache after mild head injury: a descriptive study. *Cephalalgia*. 2014;34(3):191–200.

74. Dumke HA. Post-traumatic headache and its impact on return to work after mild traumatic brain injury. *J Head Trauma Rehabil*. 2017;32(2):E55–E65.

75. Packard RC, Ham LP. Post-traumatic headache: determining chronicity. *Headache*. 1993;33(3):133–134.

CHAPTER 7

Assessment and Treatment of Sleep in Mild Traumatic Brain Injury

P.K. GOOTAM, MD • TRACY KRETCHMER, PHD •
TAMARA L. MCKENZIE-HARTMAN, PSYD • RISA NIKASE-RICHARDSON, PHD •
MARC SILVA, PHD • LAURA BAJOR, DO

INTRODUCTION

Current knowledge regarding mild traumatic brain injuries (mTBIs) and best practices for treatment is far from optimal or complete. Thus, for those endeavoring to provide the best care for those who have sustained such injuries, the path forward consists of maximizing factors known to provide an advantage toward recovery while minimizing those that are likely to hinder it. Sleep is arguably among the most important factors in recovery from TBI.[1-4]

While there is an emerging body of evidence specific to sleep disturbance in mTBI,[4-12] the vast majority of published studies do not distinguish between mTBI and moderate/severe injuries. In this chapter, we rely as much as possible on mTBI-specific data while making use of conclusions from more general TBI studies where there was no obvious reason why findings should not be extrapolated to the mTBI population.

Clinical recommendations offered (Fig. 7.1) were derived both from evidence and accepted standards of care as agreed on by members of the authorial team, who practice in the specialties of neuropsychology, psychiatry, sleep medicine, and treatment of TBIs. Such recommendations are intended for consideration and not as strict guidelines and so must be weighed against the unique factors present in a given individual's case.

RELEVANT RESEARCH REGARDING SLEEP AND TRAUMATIC BRAIN INJURIES

General

Sleep has been shown to play an essential role in the function of healthy, uninjured brains with respect to mood, cognition, and general performance.[2,13-18] There are also processes essential to brain maintenance, e.g., clearance of potentially harmful metabolites through the glymphatic system, that occur during sleep and are either degraded or do not take place at all in a state of sleep deprivation.[17,19]

Given their importance to health of uninjured brains, these processes may be even more crucial in recovery from a brain injury.[20,21] Thus, the disruption to sleep that so frequently occurs subsequent to mTBI carries risk for a "self-reinforcing spiral" since a factor necessary for recovery can be degraded by that same injury process. Left unaddressed, poor sleep may impede recovery from mTBI in the short term and while setting the stage for a protracted course of recovery and a risk for further damage in the long term, e.g., inability to clear substances such as hyperphosphorylated tau proteins and beta-amyloid has been linked to the development of dementia in older individuals.[22-24]

Anatomy of the Sleep Cycle

The normal human sleep/wake cycle occurs over a period that is slightly longer than 24 hours and is contingent on a circadian system regulated mainly by the suprachiasmatic nuclei, located in the hypothalamus.[25] Other structures involved in this system include the retinohypothalamic tract, retina, and pineal gland, which are heavily reliant on exposure to natural spectrum light and normal transcription of the proteins that act as signals within this system.[26,27] Neurotrauma can disrupt this cycle not only through direct injuries to the above mentioned structures but also through other mechanisms, such as systemic inflammation and derangement to the autonomic nervous system.[28-32]

There is preliminary evidence that circadian rhythm disorders, including delayed sleep phase or irregular sleep-wake type, occur with increased frequency in patients with TBI. These symptoms of a circadian rhythm disorder are easy to overlook and are often misattributed

Concussion. https://doi.org/10.1016/B978-0-323-65384-8.00007-9
2020 Published by Elsevier Inc.

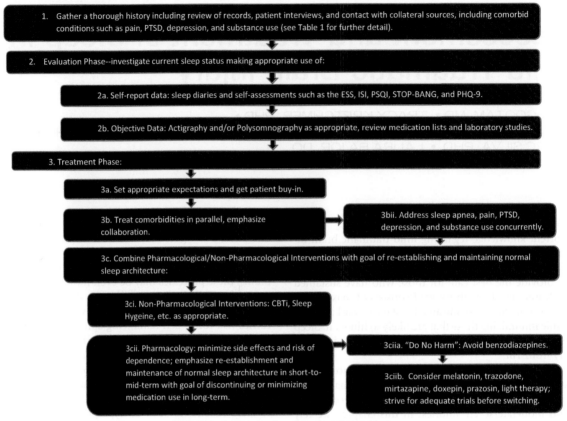

1. Gather a thorough history including review of records, patient interviews, and contact with collateral sources, including comorbid conditions such as pain, PTSD, depression, and substance use (see Table 1 for further detail).

2. Evaluation Phase--investigate current sleep status making appropriate use of:

2a. Self-report data: sleep diaries and self-assessments such as the ESS, ISI, PSQI, STOP-BANG, and PHQ-9.

2b. Objective Data: Actigraphy and/or Polysomnography as appropriate, review medication lists and laboratory studies.

3. Treatment Phase:

3a. Set appropriate expectations and get patient buy-in.

3b. Treat comorbidities in parallel, emphasize collaboration.

3bii. Address sleep apnea, pain, PTSD, depression, and substance use concurrently.

3c. Combine Pharmacological/Non-Pharmacological Interventions with goal of re-establishing and maintaining normal sleep architecture:

3ci. Non-Pharmacological Interventions: CBTi, Sleep Hygeine, etc. as appropriate.

3cii. Pharmacology: minimize side effects and risk of dependence; emphasize re-establishment and maintenance of normal sleep architecture in short-to-mid-term with goal of discontinuing or minimizing medication use in long-term.

3ciia. "Do No Harm": Avoid benzodiazepines.

3ciib. Consider melatonin, trazodone, mirtazapine, doxepin, prazosin, light therapy; strive for adequate trials before switching.

FIG. 7.1 Assessment and treatment algorithm.

to insomnia. In one study, 36% of individuals who complained of insomnia after mTBI instead met criteria for a circadian rhythm disorder.[33] The distinction is important, since treatment approaches differ.

Among military personnel, the incidence of insomnia appears to increase in a dose-dependent fashion with the number of head injuries incurred, ranging from 6% in those with no history of TBI, 20% after a single TBI, and 50% in those with multiple episodes.[34] No specific causal link should be assumed from these data given the high number of confounders present in this population, e.g., orthopedic pain, post-traumatic stress disorder, shift work, etc.

Clinical Presentations of Sleep Difficulties in TBI

Changes in consciousness and memory observable at the time of a TBI are believed to be caused by neuro-physiological disruption, e.g., increases in glucose metabolism, decreases in cerebral blood flow, and impaired

synaptic transmission and axonal functioning.[35] Problems with sleep initiation and/or maintenance are quite common during the acute phase of TBIs of all severities, as are excessive fatigue and an increased need for sleep. This is problematic, given that restorative sleep and an attentive level of wakefulness are crucial toward achieving neurocognitive rehabilitation goals in brain injured patients.[36]

Sleep-wake disturbances are among the most prevalent and residual sequelae of TBI.[37] Insomnia, excessive daytime sleepiness, increased sleep need (pleosomnia), and sleep fragmentation are commonly reported by or found in patients suffering from TBI of any severity, in both the acute and chronic phases.[8,28,38–40] In a meta-analysis of 1706 TBI patients across 21 studies, the most common sleep disturbance was insomnia (50%) followed closely by reduced sleep efficiency (49%).[38] Sleep-related breathing and movement disorders are also prevalent in the chronic phases of TBI, as the reported prevalence of obstructive sleep apnea (OSA) ranges from 25% to 35%.[38,39,41]

Distinguishing Among Insomnia, Daytime Sleepiness, and Narcolepsy

By definition, insomnia consists of difficulty initiating sleep, sleep fragmentation, and early morning awakenings. Presence of insomnia has been shown to correlate with decreased satisfaction in life, anxiety, and depression.[40a] Excessive daytime sleepiness, distinct from fatigue, is another clinically significant symptom after TBI with a frequency range reported between 50% and 80%[39,42] Excessive daytime sleepiness is often, but not always, accompanied by a short time to fall asleep on the multiple sleep latency test (MSLT). A mean sleep latency of 8 min or less is generally considered to be abnormal.[43] In addition to a reduced mean sleep latency, some patients have two or more sleep-onset rapid eye movement (REM) periods during the MSLT, fulfilling electrophysiological criteria for narcolepsy type 2 (narcolepsy without cataplexy).[44]

Prior to diagnosing narcolepsy after TBI, insufficient sleep must be ruled out as a root cause, as chronic sleep deprivation can produce increased REM sleep pressure. One prospective study found that 6% of patients met MSLT criteria for narcolepsy type 2 at a mean of 64 months after TBI, which represents a marked increase compared with the prevalence in the general population, where the rate is estimated to be less than 0.1%).[38] Other studies have also found that sleepiness persists as a chronic state for many patients.[42,45,46]

One possible neurophysiological mechanism behind excessive daytime sleepiness and sleep fragmentation in patients with TBI involves the neuropeptide orexin (also known as hypocretin). Orexin neurons in the posterior hypothalamus activate several downstream monoaminergic and cholinergic systems, driving a wake-promoting effect.[47,48] In one study involving 44 subjects who were less than 96 hours past a moderate to severe TBI, significant deficiencies in orexin were found in the cerebrospinal fluid (CSF) levels[49] Although this study did not include mTBI patients and deficits in orexin are unlikely to fully account for sleep-wake disturbances once time has passed and CSF orexin levels have returned to baseline, this mechanism is worth considering as a possible factor in sleep disturbance in mTBI.

Pleiosomnia is common after TBI. In a prospective polysomnography (PSG) study involving 65 subjects who were 6 months status post TBI, 22% reported that they needed at least two more hours of sleep in a 24-hour period than before the injury[42] This general pattern has been found in other prospective case-control studies. One longitudinal study evaluated 42 TBI patients 6 months status post injury and found

pleiosomnia of 1.2 h more on average more than matched controls. This pattern was noted to persist 18 months post injury.[45,45a]

Sleep Apnea and TBI

Sleep-related breathing disorders, including OSA and central sleep apnea, appear to occur with increased frequency after TBI. OSA, like TBI, is associated with excessive daytime sleepiness, morning headaches, increased depression or irritability, poor concentration, and memory impairment. Small studies have found an OSA prevalence ranging from 25% to 35% in TBI patients, which is higher than rates in most general population-based studies.[38,50,51] This is complicated by the significant symptom overlap between TBI, OSA, and other sleep-wake disorders.

Role of Comorbidities

Conditions that frequently occur in combination with mTBI such as post-traumatic stress disorder (PTSD), pain, and mood alteration may also contribute significantly to sleep disturbance. In the military population, the event that caused the TBI, e.g., IED blast, blunt force trauma occurring in combat, is in many cases sufficient to also trigger PTSD, and rates of comorbidity have been measured to be as high as 56%.[52,53] Features of this disorder, e.g., nightmares and hypervigilance, have a distinctly negative impact on sleep but are treatable, as discussed later in this chapter. Chronic pain is also highly prevalent in the TBI population and is known to interfere with both onset and maintenance of sleep.[54,55] There is emerging evidence regarding the neuroanatomical and neurobiological basis for comorbid pain and PTSD and potential negative impact of the comorbidity on time required for and quality of recovery.[56]

Sleep Issues Specific to mTBI

There is a stronger correlation between mTBI and sleep disturbances than with more severe TBIs[57] and those with mTBI and comorbid disorders are more likely to report higher levels of postconcussive symptoms. Insomnia complaints are more prevalent in mTBI compared with moderate or severe TBI[60]. This may contribute to hindered recovery, increased disability beliefs/rates, and more complicated treatment needs (i.e., increased medical visits).[58,59]

The most common sleep-related symptoms reported following mTBI include insomnia, fragmented sleep, feeling unrested, and excessively tired during the day, OSA, and an increased need for sleep.[4,28,38,40] While the vast majority of individuals with mTBIs will recover and experience resolution of postconcussive symptoms, including sleep difficulties, within the acute phase, many service members and veterans seen within the Veterans Health Administration (VA) system present with chronic symptomatology, defined as post concussive symptoms that extend beyond the expected 3-month recovery timeframe. A retrospective study of 202 patients (63% with mTBI) found that two-thirds complained of insomnia at a mean of 2 years post injury; furthermore, approximately one-quarter of patients with mTBI continued to complain of insomnia 5 years post injury.[60]

Major depressive disorder occurs frequently in the mTBI population.[57,61,62] Depressed mood can lead individuals to sleep either too little or too much. Given the high prevalence and potential impact of all these comorbidities on sleep in mTBI patients, it is imperative to screen thoroughly for such disorders. This begins with the taking of a targeted and thorough history that not only takes into account the circumstances and sequalae of the mTBI itself but also considers conditions that may have existed premorbidly.

COLLECTING A TARGETED HISTORY AND REVIEW OF SYSTEMS

Given the many possible contributing factors to lingering sleep disturbances, it is worth the time necessary to conduct a thorough clinical interview evaluating injury history and other details pertinent to symptom presentation. This interview should also consider factors such as overall physical health, developmental and family history, pain, mood, stress, family/social support, medications, substance use, and beliefs about current functioning. Details regarding onset (time necessary to fall asleep), maintenance (ability to remain asleep), problems related to environment (room temperature, ambient light, noise, etc.), and causes of awakenings (nightmares, hypervigilance, nocturia, etc.) can be helpful in understanding and addressing sleep difficulties. If a release of information can be obtained, speaking to a bed partner regarding witnessed sleep difficulties such as snoring, gasping, and limb jerking can be invaluable.

Information regarding sleep patterns that existed before the occurrence of an mTBI can be important in gauging the degree of sleep change since injury. Although disturbed sleep is one of the most common chronic complaints following mTBI, such symptoms rarely occur in isolation and often present in combination with cognitive concerns, PTSD, mood symptoms, headaches, chronic pain, musculoskeletal ailments,

and autonomic and endocrine problems, which tend to interact and further exacerbate sleep issues.[63] It often is not possible to know whether lingering sleep problems resulted from TBI-related brain changes or from exacerbations of comorbid conditions, whether preexisting or with onset following TBI. In such cases, it is advisable to take a multidisciplinary, "in parallel" treatment approach that addresses each of the known causes of sleep disturbance to the extent possible.[34,40,63]

When treating individuals who are military veterans or still serving on active duty, some additional factors should be considered, e.g., mechanism of concussion (blast vs. blunt injury), total number and chronological spacing of TBIs, and associated combat-related anxiety/PTSD. A study of military personnel by Bryan[34] found a history of repeated concussions to be a significant predictor of overall insomnia severity, even after controlling for depression, PTSD, and concussion symptom severity. Individuals with multiple concussions were 10 times more likely to exceed the threshold for clinical insomnia on self-report measures, suggesting that number of TBIs may be an important risk factor for reported sleep disturbance among military personnel.[34] These findings held across specific types of insomnia (onset, maintenance, and early morning awakening).

While sleep disorders following TBI are common, recent literature has indicated that specific mechanisms of injury may impact the development of distinct subtypes of sleep disorders.[41] In that study, military personnel with TBI incurred via blunt force had higher scores on the Epworth Sleepiness Scale (ESS), higher rates of poor sleep quality, and OSA, while military personnel with blast-related TBI had higher rates of insomnia and anxiety.

Clinicians gathering history via clinical interview should take care to include the specific components outlined in Table 7.1, below:

Self-Reported Data

Information from self-report questionnaires and sleep diaries may also be helpful in understanding sleep complaints. These are inexpensive and easy to acquire, though subjective in nature and reliant on accurate patient recall and motivation. While there are many self-report questionnaires that assess sleep symptoms, only the ESS, Insomnia Severity Index (ISI), and the Pittsburgh Sleep Quality Index (PSQI) have been validated among TBI patients.[63] When assessing for OSA, the STOP-BANG Sleep Apnea Questionnaire has been shown to be the most sensitive, though it has not been validated among those with TBI.[64]

TABLE 7.1
Elements of a Thorough Traumatic Brain Injury (TBI)-specific Sleep History.

Critical Elements of a Thorough Sleep/TBI History:

Description of the TBI/sleep problems and course (e.g., TBI: mechanism of injuries, spacing of injuries, sleep: frequency of problems, difficulties with onset, difficulties with maintenance, triggers, factors that improve sleep)

Analysis of the typical 24-hour period (routines, exercise, food/caffeine intake, alcohol use, tobacco use, etc.)

Consequences (i.e., fatigue, work-related errors, physical, emotional, etc.)

Previous treatments/strategies utilized and their effectiveness (i.e., medications, behavioral health, environmental, etc.)

Pre-TBI sleep history (i.e., prior sleep patterns, problems, etc.)

Medical history and current medications

Current mental status examination and history of psychological diagnoses

Sleep environment (i.e., mattress, bed partner, light, sound, temperature, routines including TV, reading, eating, etc.)

Collateral information gathered from bed partner about sleep-related movements, breathing, snoring, etc.

The PSQI is a clinical questionnaire encompassing multiple sleep domains that can be useful to guide a structured interview and has been partially validated in the TBI population.[65] The ESS is a widely used instrument for quantifying subjective sleepiness that has also been partially validated in patients with TBI.[66–68] Scores of 10 or higher are generally considered abnormal and indicative of excessive daytime sleepiness. As with other measures, ESS scores should be used in combination with other tools, as patients with TBI may over- or underestimate their degree of daytime impairment.[67] Given the frequent comorbidity of psychiatric disorders in patients with TBI, it can also be worthwhile to probe for symptoms of mood disorders and anxiety disorders. The Patient Health Questionnaire-9 (PHQ-9) is a simple, nine-item screening instrument which has proven to be reliable and valid in both primary care and traumatic brain injury treating settings.[69]

DIAGNOSTIC PHASE OF SLEEP/TBI WORKUP

Sleep-wake disorders are diagnosed using a combination of both subjective and objective data. Because subjective data may be unreliable, it is important to balance that data with objective findings such as information collected via actigraphy, PSG, the MSLT, and the maintenance of wakefulness test (MWT). Actigraphy and PSG are useful across the spectrum of sleep difficulties, while the latter two are used mainly to rule out or substantiate suspicion of narcolepsy.

Medication Reviews and Laboratory Data

Medication lists should also be fully reviewed to identify inadvertent pharmacological disrupters of the sleep-wake cycle. Many medications used in the management of acute complications of TBI are known to have negative impacts on sleep, including oral steroids, antiepileptics, opioid analgesics, benzodiazepines, antipsychotics, stimulants, and antidepressants.[70] Furthermore, use of caffeine, nicotine, alcohol, and other substances are relevant when addressing sleep impairment. If possible, obtain laboratory data to rule out occult causes of sleep disturbance such as hyper/hypothyroidism; electrolyte and mineral imbalances that may cause muscle pain or leg movement (iron, magnesium, calcium, etc); and vitamin levels important to brain health (D3, B12, folic acid).

Actigraphy

Wrist actigraphy makes use mainly of accelerometer-based movement data, which, depending on the specific device and algorithm selected, may be combined with measurements of light, heart rate, temperature, and skin conductance to generate proxy measures of day and night time rest-wake activity. While actigraphy data available as of this writing cannot provide data comparable to PSG in terms of measuring specific phases such as light, deep, and REM sleep, it offers a relatively inexpensive, nonintrusive means of collecting longitudinal data in an individual's home environment that quite helpful in generating a detailed clinical picture in terms of habits, patterns of onset and maintenance, and early morning awakenings.[71–73] Some actigraphy devices have undergone validation studies for specific populations,[74] differentiating them from "wearable" devices popular for use by the general public. While such wearables are appealing in terms of affordability and accessibility of data, they should not as of this writing be considered a substitute for data from formally validated devices and algorithms.[75]

The American Academy of Sleep Medicine has developed guidelines for use of actigraphy in assessment and treatment of sleep disorders.[76] Actigraphy has been demonstrated to be useful in the estimation of total sleep time (TST), sleep percentage/efficiency, and wake after sleep onset (WASO). However, the estimation of sleep-onset latency is less reliable, especially in persons with sleep disorders.[72] Recent work highlights their superiority to self-report (sleep logs) in mild to moderate TBI patients and validity for measuring TST and sleep efficiency in moderate to severe TBI patients; however, use in persons with motor limitations warrants caution (e.g., spasticity, paresis, agitation).[77,78]

Polysomnography

PSG studies are not necessary for all mTBI patients with sleep-wake complaints but should be obtained in select cases where warranted by history.[79] When coupled with a thorough sleep history, in-laboratory PSG is the gold standard for diagnosing sleep-related breathing disorders and periodic limb movement disorder. PSG provides information on sleep architecture measured by electroencephalography (EEG), sleep quality (e.g., TST, sleep efficiency), and physiologic parameters. To improve accessibility, several PSG testing levels are available[80] and are stratified based on instrumentation involved and whether or not the presence of a certified respiratory polysomnography technician (RPSGT) is required. The American Academy of Sleep Medicine has published practice parameters for routine use of PSG that distinguishes these levels of evaluation in the diagnostic workup and indication for follow-up testing.[79]

TREATMENT OF SLEEP PROBLEMS IN MTBI
Setting Appropriate Expectations

Once an accurate assessment of causes and patterns underlying sleep disruption has been completed, treatment planning can commence. As with any intervention, it is worthwhile to invest time in setting realistic expectations for an intervention, e.g., the goal is to improve overall sleep quantity and quality, as well as daytime function, but not necessarily for the patient to experience a "perfect" night's sleep, especially if that was not the case prior to sustaining a TBI. Given the multifactorial nature of sleep disruption in mTBI (e.g., sleep apnea, pain, mood and anxiety issues, etc.) the approach to treatment should be tailored to an individual's unique clinical picture, preferences, and ability to adhere to recommendations.

Guiding Principles

We suggest incorporation of a few guiding principles derived from research and clinical experience, beginning with the idea that, to the extent possible, underlying factors be addressed in parallel rather than sequential fashion. For example, investing time and money in diagnosis and treatment of sleep apnea may fail to provide relief if a patient's orthopedic pain or PTSD remain unaddressed and that patient cannot or will not keep a CPAP mask on through the course of a night. Such parallel treatment requires focused collaboration on the part of involved providers, e.g., coordination between primary care physicians and specialists in sleep, pain, and psychiatry, but can compress the timeline necessary for a patient to experience relief.[81,82]

A second guiding principle is that providers should not shy away from appropriate use of medication but should prescribe with the intent that medications assist patients toward a "reset" and then maintenance of normal sleep architecture and, if possible, be a temporary and not permanent measure. To this end, medications with potential for dependence such as benzodiazepines should be a last resort. Efforts to rebuild healthy habits and thought patterns, e.g., Cognitive Behavioral Therapy for Insomnia, or CBT-I and Sleep Hygiene as addressed below, should be implemented in parallel with medication use. Although not TBI specific, providers treating individuals with mTBI without the benefit of formal sleep training may find the Clinical Practice Guidelines offered by the American Academy of Sleep Medicine to be of great help (see: https://aasm.org/clinical-resources/practice-standards/practice-guidelines).

CBT-I

CBT-I is a primary intervention and standard treatment for chronic insomnia[82a–c] and has been adapted with some success in persons with TBI.[82d] CBT-I integrates both cognitive and behavioral interventions specifically targeted at improvement of insomnia. Cognitive interventions address and modify maladaptive attitudes and beliefs that prolong insomnia while behavioral interventions include stimulus control, sleep restriction, and relaxation training. Stimulus control is based on classical conditioning and aims to establish and strengthen the association of the bed and bedroom with sleep. Sleep restriction aims to limit time spent in bed while awake in order to break the association between the bed and wakefulness. (It may prove helpful to clarify to patients that sleep restriction does not actually aim to reduce sleep time and might thus have been more aptly named "bed" restriction.) Relaxation training is aimed at reducing physiological arousal with the goal of promoting sleepiness.

Sleep Hygiene

Sleep hygiene is a psychoeducational intervention that identifies habits that influence sleep quality. Sleep hygiene also includes recommendations that address behavioral and environmental factors to promote sleep[82e−f]. Examples include reducing caffeine, tobacco, and alcohol; incorporating moderate exercise into the daily routine; minimizing light and noise; avoiding naps and managing stress. Although poor sleep habits contribute to sleep disorders such as insomnia (Jansson-Fröjmark et al., 2018) and sleep apnea[82g], there is insufficient evidence to support sleep hygiene as an efficacious standalone intervention[83,83a]. Rather, sleep hygiene may best be used as an adjunct to other psychotherapeutic interventions[83].

Pharmacologic Agents

While pharmacologic intervention is often necessary and helpful in addressing sleep issues in mTBI, it should be undertaken with the thought of assisting a patient in rebuilding and solidifying sleep architecture in the short term with the goal, if possible, of minimizing use of medications in the longer term. In addition, the possible benefits of improving sleep must be weighed against risks posed by side effects and dependence. Given the sometimes paradoxical and unpredictable response of TBI patients to medications, the old dictum of "start low, go slow" definitely applies.

Avoidance of Benzodiazepines

In persons with TBI, benzodiazepines should be avoided because of cognitive side effects[83b−c] and risk of physiologic dependency and abuse. When considering any medication intended to improve sleep, no matter how benign, prescribers should make a thorough assessment of how that agent may interact with the other drugs a patient may be taking in terms of respiratory depression, daytime sedation, and other potentially harmful effects. For example, the combination of opioids prescribed to address pain and benzodiazepines intended to improve sleep poses a substantial

risk in terms of respiratory suppression and is discouraged as a matter of policy by many healthcare systems including the Veterans Administration.[84] Whatever medications are selected, after a 4−5 week trial, symptoms and effect should be reevaluated and the medication regime reconsidered[82a]. It should be noted that there is an overall paucity of research examining the efficacy and adverse effects of many pharmacological agents in persons with TBI thus marking this as an area in need of further research.

Medications to Consider—First, Do No Harm

Of the numerous medications studied, none received strong recommendations by the American Academy of Sleep Medicine[82b] and American College of Physicians[82a] due to low quality of evidence and risk of harm due to side effects. We therefore recommend as "first-line" medications with the lowest risk, e.g., melatonin, trazodone, doxepin, and mirtazapine[83c], before escalating to use of agents with a higher side effect profile. Taking a patient's comorbidities, e.g., PTSD, into consideration may help guide the selection of medications for mTBI patients with sleep issues.[85,86] Before changing from one medication to another, prescribers should ensure that an adequate trial has taken place in terms of time and titration to effective dose before moving on to another agent.

Melatonin

Melatonin was mentioned above in the list of relatively safe medications we recommend as first line and is worthy of consideration for use in TBI patients given its role in regulating circadian rhythm within the retinohypothalmic system. Melatonin production is decreased by as much as 42% and may be delayed by as much as 90 minutes past normal secretion time in TBI patients, making supplementation of this substance of possible value for mTBI patients having sleep difficulties.[30,87,88] In addition, there is recent evidence in showing that melatonin has anti-inflammatory and prorepair properties in mice with induced TBIs.[74,89,90] If a patient and provider do elect to go forward with a melatonin trial, it is more likely to be effective if the patient can achieve exposure to natural spectrum light during normal waking hours, which serves to reinforce the "circadian reset" effect of melatonin supplementation.[91] Patients should consider taking melatonin earlier in the evening than they would take other sleep-promoting medications, e.g., around the time of natural sunset. Patients should also be told that in a small minority of those who take it, melatonin may trigger headaches or nightmares.[92]

Light Exposure

Although technically not a pharmacological treatment, we include light exposure here due to low risk combined with growing evidence that light exposure without melatonin supplementation, particularly in the "blue" spectrum common during the morning hours of natural daylight, may be helpful for sleep and other problems such as daytime fatigue that are common in mTBI patients.[93–95] In addition to low inherent risk, this therapy has the advantage of having been studied specifically for the mTBI population.

Prazosin for Sleep Maintenance in Patients with Comorbid PTSD

Given the high comorbidity of PTSD with mTBI and paucity of agents that specifically address difficulties with sleep maintenance (vs. onset), it is worth mentioning that the alpha-1 antagonist prazosin has been used with good effect to assist in sleep maintenance for those suffering from nightmares and nighttime hyperarousal.[96–99] In the interest of setting appropriate expectations, it should be noted that for many individuals, prazosin does not eliminate nightmares but rather facilitates sleeping through these events, thus increasing overall sleep and REM time. The most recent evidence regarding prazosin indicates that it may be best targeted at the subpopulation with physiological symptoms that evidence a state of chronic hyperarousal,[100] e.g., patients who have hypertension despite being relatively young and fit. This finding seems to fit with the observation that prazosin can in some cases be helpful in assisting mTBI patients with PTSD in building a tolerance for wear of CPAP masks, which can be a daunting prospect for individuals with heightened nighttime arousal at baseline.

A Word Regarding Stimulants

Given the scope of this chapter (mTBI and sleep), the authors do not take a position regarding use of stimulants such as methylphenidate, dextroamphetamine, and modafinil to address daytime fatigue and inattention in the mTBI population. Given the likelihood that prescribers reading this chapter will be (or already have) asked for these medications by their mTBI patients, we do find it worth referring back to the "guiding principles" outlined at the beginning of this section: medications should be selected and prescribed with the intent of helping to reset and reinforce a normal sleep architecture, not to "mask over" symptoms caused by less-than-optimal sleep. Though individuals with mTBI and poor sleep who are struggling to maintain occupational or academic performance may understandably view stimulants as a "silver bullet," risks for further degrading sleep, for stressing the neuroendocrine system, and for abuse and diversion should be considered. If stimulants are tried, we assert that this is best done after efforts to optimize sleep are complete, or at least already underway, lest a patient comes to rely on the effects of the stimulant rather than continue to invest effort in improving their sleep.

Only one study we could locate specifically addressed use of these medications in mTBI patients,[101] while the remainder of existing literature focused on a more general TBI population.[102–105] Although there are situations where stimulant use may be appropriate in mTBI, e.g., properly diagnosed cases of narcolepsy or a preexisting attention deficit disorder, we assert that this is best and most safely undertaken after careful screening and workup that rules out factors that could be more expeditiously addressed by treating sleep deficits themselves.

CONCLUSION

To summarize the main points of this chapter, we emphasize the guiding principle that sleep problems in mTBI tend to be multifactorial, that resolution is likely to take collaboration, time, and patience on the part of both patients and providers, and that medications should be used with the intent of resetting and reinforcing a normal sleep architecture and with minimizing risk of dependence. Given this complexity, it makes sense to invest time in setting realistic expectations, taking a thorough history, and conducting a workup that takes into consideration an individual's unique comorbidities, e.g., chronic pain, PTSD, depression, sleep apnea.

REFERENCES

1. Bloomfield IL, Espie CA, Evans JJ. Do sleep difficulties exacerbate deficits in sustained attention following traumatic brain injury? *J Int Neuropsychol Soc.* 2010;16(1):17–25.
2. Macera CA, Aralis HJ, Rauh MJ, MacGregor AJ. Do sleep problems mediate the relationship between traumatic brain injury and development of mental health symptoms after deployment? *Sleep.* 2013;36(1):83–90.
3. Weymann KB, Lim MM. Sleep disturbances in TBI and PTSD and potential risk of neurodegeneration. *Curr Sleep Med Rep.* 2017;3(3):179–192.
4. Wickwire EM, Williams SG, Roth T, et al. Sleep, sleep disorders, and mild traumatic brain injury. What we know and what we need to know: findings from a national working group. *Neurotherapeutics.* 2016;13(2):403–417.

5. Chaput G, Giguère JF, Chauny JM, Denis R, Lavigne G. Relationship among subjective sleep complaints, headaches, and mood alterations following a mild traumatic brain injury. *Sleep Med.* 2009;10(7):713–716.
6. Gosselin N, Lassonde M, Petit D, et al. Sleep following sport-related concussions. *Sleep Med.* 2009;10(1):35–46.
7. Khoury S, Chouchou F, Amzica F, et al. Rapid EEG activity during sleep dominates in mild traumatic brain injury patients with acute pain. *J Neurotrauma.* 2013;30(8):633–641.
8. Rao V, Bergey A, Hill H, Efron D, McCann U. Sleep disturbance after mild traumatic brain injury: indicator of injury? *J Neuropsychiatry Clin Neurosci.* 2011;23(2):201–205.
9. Theadom A, Cropley M, Parmar P, et al. Sleep difficulties one year following mild traumatic brain injury in a population-based study. *Sleep Med.* 2015;16(8):926–932.
10. Tkachenko N, Singh K, Hasanaj L, Serrano L, Kothare SV. Sleep disorders associated with mild traumatic brain injury using sport concussion assessment tool 3. *Pediatr Neurol.* 2016;57:46–50.
11. Vagnozzi R, Signoretti S, Cristofori L, et al. Assessment of metabolic brain damage and recovery following mild traumatic brain injury: a multicentre, proton magnetic resonance spectroscopic study in concussed patients. *Brain.* 2010;133(11):3232–3242.
12. Zhou D, Zhao Y, Wan Y, et al. Neuroendocrine dysfunction and insomnia in mild traumatic brain injury patients. *Neurosci Lett.* 2016;610:154–159.
13. Belenky G, Wesensten NJ, Thorne DR, et al. Patterns of performance degradation and restoration during sleep restriction and subsequent recovery: a sleep dose-response study. *J Sleep Res.* 2003;12(1):1–12.
14. Kang JE, Lim MM, Bateman RJ, et al. Amyloid-β dynamics are regulated by orexin and the sleep-wake cycle. *Science.* 2009;326(5955):1005–1007.
15. Kuriyama K, Stickgold R, Walker MP. Sleep-dependent learning and motor-skill complexity. *Learn Mem.* 2004;11(6):705–713.
16. Stickgold R, Walker MP. Sleep-dependent memory triage: evolving generalization through selective processing. *Nat Neurosci.* 2013;16(2):139.
17. Xie L, Kang H, Xu Q, et al. Sleep drives metabolite clearance from the adult brain. *Science.* 2013;342(6156):373–377.
18. Yoo SS, Gujar N, Hu P, Jolesz FA, Walker MP. The human emotional brain without sleep—a prefrontal amygdala disconnect. *Curr Biol.* 2007;17(20):R877–R878.
19. Jessen NA, Munk ASF, Lundgaard I, Nedergaard M. The glymphatic system: a beginner's guide. *Neurochem Res.* 2015;40(12):2583–2599.
20. Iliff JJ, Chen MJ, Plog BA, et al. Impairment of glymphatic pathway function promotes tau pathology after traumatic brain injury. *J Neurosci.* 2014;34(49):16180–16193.
21. Plog BA, Nedergaard M. The glymphatic system in central nervous system health and disease: past, present, and future. *Annu Rev Pathol.* 2018;13:379–394.

22. Clark CM, Xie S, Chittams J, et al. Cerebrospinal fluid tau and β-amyloid: how well do these biomarkers reflect autopsy-confirmed dementia diagnoses? *Arch Neurol.* 2003;60(12):1696–1702.
23. Rowe CC, Ng S, Ackermann U, et al. Imaging β-amyloid burden in aging and dementia. *Neurology.* 2007;68(20):1718–1725.
24. Tarasoff-Conway JM, Carare RO, Osorio RS, et al. Clearance systems in the brain—implications for Alzheimer disease. *Nat Rev Neurol.* 2015;11(8):457.
25. Wulff K, Gatti S, Wettstein JG, Foster RG. Sleep and circadian rhythm disruption in psychiatric and neurodegenerative disease. *Nat Rev Neurosci.* 2010;11(8):589.
26. Dai J, Vliet JVD, Swaab DF, Buijs RM. Human retinohypothalamic tract as revealed by in vitro postmortem tracing. *J Comp Neurol.* 1998;397(3):357–370.
27. Hannibal J. Neurotransmitters of the retinohypothalamic tract. *Cell Tissue Res.* 2002;309(1):73–88.
28. Baumann CR. Traumatic brain injury and disturbed sleep and wakefulness. *Neuro Mol Med.* 2012;14(3):205–212.
29. Boone DR, Sell SL, Micci MA, et al. Traumatic brain injury-induced dysregulation of the circadian clock. *PLoS One.* 2012;7(10):e46204.
30. Grima NA, Ponsford JL, St Hilaire MA, Mansfield D, Rajaratnam SM. Circadian melatonin rhythm following traumatic brain injury. *Neurorehabil Neural Repair.* 2016;30(10):972–977.
31. Jaffee MS, Winter WC, Jones CC, Ling G. Sleep disturbances in athletic concussion. *Brain Injury.* 2015;29(2):221–227.
32. Williamson JB, Heilman KM, Porges E, Lamb D, Porges SW. A possible mechanism for PTSD symptoms in patients with traumatic brain injury: central autonomic network disruption. *Front Neuroeng.* 2013;6:13.
33. Williams BR, Lazic SE, Ogilvie RD. Polysomnographic and quantitative EEG analysis of subjects with long-term insomnia complaints associated with mild traumatic brain injury. *Clin Neurophysiol.* 2008;119(2):429–438.
34. Bryan CJ. Repetitive traumatic brain injury (or concussion) increases severity of sleep disturbance among deployed military personnel. *Sleep.* 2013;36(6):941–946.
35. Giza CC, Hovda DA. The new neurometabolic cascade of concussion. *Neurosurgery.* 2014;75(suppl_4):S24–S33.
36. Worthington AD, Melia Y. Rehabilitation is compromised by arousal and sleep disorders: results of a survey of rehabilitation centres. *Brain Inj.* 2006;20(3):327–332.
37. Ouellet MC, Beaulieu-Bonneau S, Morin CM. Sleep-wake disturbances after traumatic brain injury. *Lancet Neurol.* 2015;14(7):746–757.
38. Castriotta RJ, Wilde MC, Lai JM, Atanasov S, Masel BE, Kuna ST. Prevalence and consequences of sleep disorders in traumatic brain injury. *J Clin Sleep Med.* 2007;3(04):349–356.
39. Mathias JL, Alvaro PK. Prevalence of sleep disturbances, disorders, and problems following traumatic brain injury: a meta-analysis. *Sleep Medicine.* 2012;13(7):898–905.

40. Ouellet MC, Beaulieu-Bonneau S, Morin CM. Insomnia in patients with traumatic brain injury: frequency, characteristics, and risk factors. *J Head Trauma Rehabil*. 2006; 21(3):199−212.

40a. Cantor JB, Bushnik T, Cicerone K, et al. Insomnia, fatigue, and sleepiness in the first 2 years after traumatic brain injury: an NIDRR TBI model system module study. *J Head Trauma Rehabil*. 2012;27:E1.

41. Collen J, Orr N, Lettieri CJ, Carter K, Holley AB. Sleep disturbances among soldiers with combat-related traumatic brain injury. *Chest*. 2012;142(3):622−630.

42. Baumann C, Werth E, Stocker R, Ludwig S, Bassetti CL. Sleep−wake disturbances 6 months after traumatic brain injury: a prospective study. *Brain*. 2007;130(7): 1873−1883.

43. Littner MR, Kushida C, Wise M, et al. Practice parameters for clinical use of the multiple sleep latency test and the maintenance of wakefulness test. *Sleep*. 2005;28(1): 113−121.

44. Vignatelli L, Plazzi G, Bassein L, et al. ICSD diagnostic criteria for narcolepsy: interobserver reliability. *Sleep*. 2002;25(2):193−196.

45. Imbach LL, Büchele F, Valko PO, et al. Sleep−wake disorders persist 18 months after traumatic brain injury but remain underrecognized. *Neurology*. 2016;86(21): 1945−1949.

45a. Imbach LL, Valko PO, Li T, et al. Increased sleep need and daytime sleepiness 6 months after traumatic brain injury: a prospective controlled clinical trial. *Brain*. 2015;138: 726.

46. Longstreth Jr WT, Koepsell TD, Ton TG, Hendrickson AF, Van Belle G. The epidemiology of narcolepsy. *Sleep*. 2007;30(1):13−26.

47. Gooley JJ, Lu J, Chou TC, Scammell TE, Saper CB. Melanopsin in cells of origin of the retinohypothalamic tract. *Nat Neurosci*. 2001;4(12):1165.

48. Saper CB, Scammell TE, Lu J. Hypothalamic regulation of sleep and circadian rhythms. *Nature*. 2005;437(7063): 1257.

49. Baumann CR, Stocker R, Imhof HG, et al. Hypocretin-1 (orexin A) deficiency in acute traumatic brain injury. *Neurology*. 2005;65(1):147−149.

50. Guilleminault C, Yuen KM, Gulevich MG, Karadeniz D, Leger D, Philip P. Hypersomnia after head−neck trauma: a medicolegal dilemma. *Neurology*. 2000;54(3), 653-653.

51. Webster JB, Bell KR, Hussey JD, Natale TK, Lakshminarayan S. Sleep apnea in adults with traumatic brain injury: a preliminary investigation. *Arch Phys Med Rehabil*. 2001;82(3):316−321.

52. McMillan TM, Williams WH, Bryant R. Post-traumatic stress disorder and traumatic brain injury: a review of causal mechanisms, assessment, and treatment. *Neuropsychol Rehabil*. 2003;13(1−2):149−164.

53. Stein MB, McAllister TW. Exploring the convergence of posttraumatic stress disorder and mild traumatic brain injury. *Am J Psychiatry*. 2009;166(7):768−776.

54. Okura K, Lavigne GJ, Huynh N, Manzini C, Fillipini D, Montplaisir JY. Comparison of sleep variables between chronic widespread musculoskeletal pain, insomnia, periodic leg movements syndrome and control subjects in a clinical sleep medicine practice. *Sleep Medicine*. 2008; 9(4):352−361.

55. Taylor BC, Hagel EM, Carlson KF, et al. Prevalence and costs of co-occurring traumatic brain injury with and without psychiatric disturbance and pain among Afghanistan and Iraq War Veteran VA users. *Med Care*. 2012:342−346.

56. Scioli-Salter ER, Forman DE, Otis JD, Gregor K, Valovski I, Rasmusson AM. The shared neuroanatomy and neurobiology of comorbid chronic pain and PTSD: therapeutic implications. *Clin J Pain*. 2015;31(4): 363−374.

57. Kreutzer J, Seel RT, Gourley E. The prevalence and symptom rates of depression after traumatic brain injury: a comprehensive examination. *J Head Trauma Rehabil*. 2002;17(1):74−75.

58. Singh R, Mason S, Lecky F, Dawson J. Prevalence of depression after TBI in a prospective cohort: the SHEFBIT study. *Brain Injury*. 2018;32(1):84−90.

59. Vasterling JJ, Dikmen S. Mild traumatic brain injury and posttraumatic stress disorder: clinical and conceptual complexities. *J Int Neuropsychol Soc*. 2012;18(3):390−393.

60. Beetar JT, Guilmette TJ, Sparadeo FR. Sleep and pain complaints in symptomatic traumatic brain injury and neurologic populations. *Arch Phys Med Rehabil*. 1996; 77(12):1298−1302.

61. Bay E, Donders J. Risk factors for depressive symptoms after mild-to-moderate traumatic brain injury. *Brain Inj*. 2008;22(3):233−241.

62. Rapoport MJ, McCullagh S, Streiner D, Feinstein A. The clinical significance of major depression following mild traumatic brain injury. *Psychosomatics*. 2003;44(1):31−37.

63. Werner Jr JK, Baumann CR. *TBI and sleep−wake disorders: pathophysiology, clinical management, and moving towards the future*. In: *Seminars in Neurology*. Vol. 37, No. 04. Thieme Medical Publishers; August 2017:419−432.

64. Chiu HY, Chen PY, Chuang LP, et al. Diagnostic accuracy of the Berlin questionnaire, STOP-BANG, STOP, and Epworth sleepiness scale in detecting obstructive sleep apnea: a bivariate meta-analysis. *Sleep Med Rev*. 2017; 36:57−70.

65. Buysse DJ, Reynolds III CF, Monk TH, Berman SR, Kupfer DJ. The Pittsburgh Sleep Quality Index: a new instrument for psychiatric practice and research. *Psychiatr Res*. 1989;28(2):193−213.

66. Fichtenberg NL, Putnam SH, Mann NR, Zafonte RD, Millard AE. Insomnia screening in postacute traumatic brain injury: utility and validity of the Pittsburgh Sleep Quality Index. *Am J Phys Med Rehab*. 2001;80(5): 339−345.

67. Masel BE, Scheibel RS, Kimbark T, Kuna ST. Excessive daytime sleepiness in adults with brain injuries. *Arch Phys Med Rehabil*. 2001;82(11):1526−1532.

68. Mollayeva T, Colantonio A, Mollayeva S, Shapiro CM. Screening for sleep dysfunction after traumatic brain injury. *Sleep Medicine*. 2013;14(12):1235–1246.
69. Fann JR, Bombardier CH, Dikmen S, et al. Validity of the Patient Health Questionnaire-9 in assessing depression following traumatic brain injury. *J Head Trauma Rehabil*. 2005;20(6):501–511.
70. DeMartinis NA, Winokur A. Effects of psychiatric medications on sleep and sleep disorders. *CNS Neurol Disord - Drug Targets*. 2007;6(1):17–29.
71. Marino M, Li Y, Rueschman MN, et al. Measuring sleep: accuracy, sensitivity, and specificity of wrist actigraphy compared to polysomnography. *Sleep*. 2013;36(11):1747–1755.
72. Martin JL, Hakim AD. Wrist actigraphy. *Chest*. 2011;139(6):1514–1527.
73. Sadeh A. The role and validity of actigraphy in sleep medicine: an update. *Sleep Medicine Reviews*. 2011;15(4):259–267.
74. Ancoli-Israel S, Cole R, Alessi C, Chambers M, Moorcroft W, Pollak CP. The role of actigraphy in the study of sleep and circadian rhythms. *Sleep*. 2003;26(3):342–392.
75. Cook JD, Prairie ML, Plante DT. Utility of the Fitbit Flex to evaluate sleep in major depressive disorder: a comparison against polysomnography and wrist-worn actigraphy. *J Affect Disord*. 2017;217:299–305.
76. Smith MT, McCrae CS, Cheung J, et al. Use of actigraphy for the evaluation of sleep disorders and circadian rhythm sleep-wake disorders: an American Academy of Sleep Medicine systematic review, meta-analysis, and GRADE assessment. *J Clin Sleep Med*. 2018;14(07):1209–1230.
77. Nakase-Richardson R, Kamper JE, Garofano J, et al. Concordance of actigraphy with polysomnography in traumatic brain injury neurorehabilitation admissions. *J Head Trauma Rehabil*. 2016a;31(2):117–125.
78. Nakase-Richardson R, Nazem S, Forster JE, Brenner LA, Matthews EE. Actigraphic and sleep diary measures in veterans with traumatic brain injury: discrepancy in selected sleep parameters. *J Head Trauma Rehabil*. 2016b;31(2):136–146.
79. Kushida CA, Littner MR, Morgenthaler T, et al. Practice parameters for the indications for polysomnography and related procedures: an update for 2005. *Sleep*. 2005;28(4):499–523.
80. Collop NA, Anderson WM, Boehlecke B, et al. Clinical guidelines for the use of unattended portable monitors in the diagnosis of obstructive sleep apnea in adult patients. *J Clin Sleep Med*. 2007;3(7):737–747.
81. Hoge CW, Goldberg HM, Castro CA. Care of war veterans with mild traumatic brain injury-flawed perspectives. *Walter Reed Army Inst Of Research Silver Spring Md Div of Psychiatry Neurosci*. 2009;360(16):1588–1591.
82. Ryan PB, Lee-Wilk T, Kok BC, Wilk JE. Interdisciplinary rehabilitation of mild TBI and PTSD: a case report. *Brain Inj*. 2011;25(10):1019–1025.
82a. Qaseem A, Kansagara D, Forciea MA, Cooke M, Denberg TD. Clinical Guidelines Committee of the American College of Physicians. Management of Chronic Insomnia Disorder in Adults: A Clinical Practice Guideline From the American College of Physicians. *Ann Intern Med*. 2016;165(2):125–133.
82b. Sateia MJ, Buysse DJ, Krystal AD, Neubauer DN, Heald JL. Clinical Practice Guideline for the Pharmacologic Treatment of Chronic Insomnia in Adults: An American Academy of Sleep Medicine Clinical Practice Guideline. *J Clin Sleep Med*. 2017;13(2):307–349.
82c. Wilson SJ, Nutt DJ, Alford C, Argyropoulos SV, Baldwin DS, Bateson AN, Britton TC, Crowe C, Dijk DJ, Espie CA, Gringras P, Hajak G, Idzikowski C, Krystal AD, Nash JR, Selsick H, Sharpley AL, Wade AG. British Association for Psychopharmacology consensus statement on evidence-based treatment of insomnia, parasomnias and circadian rhythm disorders. *J Psychopharmacol*. 2010;24(11):1577–1601.
82d. Ouellet MC, Morin CM. Efficacy of cognitive-behavioral therapy for insomnia associated with traumatic brain injury: a single-case experimental design. *Arch Phys Med Rehabil*. 2007;88(12):1581–1592.
82e. Jansson-Fröjmark M, Evander J, Alfonsson S. Are sleep hygiene practices related to the incidence, persistence and remission of insomnia? Findings from a prospective community study. *J Behav Med*. 2019;42(1):128–138.
82f. Irish LA, Kline CE, Gunn HE, Buysse DJ, Hall MH. The role of sleep hygiene in promoting public health: A review of empirical evidence. *Sleep Med Rev*. 2015;22:23–36.
82g. Jung SY, Kim HS, Min JY, Hwang KJ, Kim SW. Sleep hygiene-related conditions in patients with mild to moderate obstructive sleep apnea. *Auris Nasus Larynx*. 2019;46(1):95–100.
83. Morgenthaler TI, Lee-Chiong T, Alessi C, et al. Practice parameters for the clinical evaluation and treatment of circadian rhythm sleep disorders. *Sleep*. 2007;30(11):1445–1459.
83a. Schutte-Rodin S, Broch L, Buysse D, Dorsey C, Sateia M. Clinical guideline for the evaluation and management of chronic insomnia in adults. *J Clin Sleep Med*. 2008;4(5):487–504.
83b. Barshikar S, Bell KR. Sleep Disturbance After TBI. *Curr Neurol Neurosci Rep*. 2017;17(11):87.
83c. Wolfe LF, Sahni AS, Attarian H. Sleep disorders in traumatic brain injury. *NeuroRehabilitation*. 2018;43(3):257–266.
84. Sun EC, Dixit A, Humphreys K, Darnall BD, Baker LC, Mackey S. Association between concurrent use of prescription opioids and benzodiazepines and overdose: retrospective analysis. *Bmj*. 2017;356:j760.
85. Bajor LA, Ticlea AN, Osser DN. The psychopharmacology algorithm project at the harvard south shore program: an update on posttraumatic stress disorder. *Harv Rev Psychiatry*. 2011;19(5):240–258.
86. Ticlea AN, Bajor LA, Osser DN. Addressing sleep impairment in treatment guidelines for PTSD. *Am J Psychiatry*. 2013;170(9), 1059-1059.

87. Grima NA, Rajaratnam SM, Mansfield D, Sletten TL, Spitz G, Ponsford JL. Efficacy of melatonin for sleep disturbance following traumatic brain injury: a randomised controlled trial. *BMC Medicine.* 2018;16(1):8.

88. Kemp S, Biswas R, Neumann V, Coughlan A. The value of melatonin for sleep disorders occurring post-head injury: a pilot RCT. *Brain Injury.* 2004;18(9):911–919.

89. Ding K, Wang H, Xu J, Lu X, Zhang L, Zhu L. Melatonin reduced microglial activation and alleviated neuroinflammation induced neuron degeneration in experimental traumatic brain injury: possible involvement of mTOR pathway. *Neurochem Int.* 2014;76:23–31.

90. Lin C, Chao H, Li Z, et al. Melatonin attenuates traumatic brain injury-induced inflammation: a possible role for mitophagy. *J Pineal Res.* 2016;61(2):177–186.

91. Lewy AJ, Ahmed S, Sack RL. Phase shifting the human circadian clock using melatonin. *Behav Brain Res.* 1995;73(1–2):131–134.

92. Wright SW, Lawrence LM, Wrenn KD, Haynes ML, Welch LW, Schlack HM. Randomized clinical trial of melatonin after night-shift work: efficacy and neuropsychologic effects. *Ann Emerg Med.* 1998;32(3):334–340.

93. Bajaj S, Vanuk JR, Smith R, Dailey NS, Killgore WD. Blue-light therapy following mild traumatic brain injury: effects on white matter water diffusion in the brain. *Front Neurol.* 2017;8:616.

94. Killgore WD, Shane BR, Vanuk JR, et al. 1143 short wavelength light therapy facilitates recovery from mild traumatic brain injury. *J Sleep Sleep Disord Res.* 2017;40(suppl_1):A426–A427.

95. Vanuk JR, Shane BR, Bajaj S, Millan M, Grandner M, Killgore WD. April). Short-wavelength light therapy as a way of improving sleep, cognition, and functional connectivity following a mild traumatic brain injury. *Sleep.* 2017;A437(40).

96. Raskind MA, Peskind ER, Hoff DJ, et al. A parallel group placebo controlled study of prazosin for trauma nightmares and sleep disturbance in combat veterans with post-traumatic stress disorder. *Biol Psychiatry.* 2007;61(8):928–934.

97. Raskind MA, Peskind ER, Kanter ED, et al. Reduction of nightmares and other PTSD symptoms in combat veterans by prazosin: a placebo-controlled study. *Am J Psychiatry.* 2003;160(2):371–373.

98. Raskind MA, Peterson K, Williams T, et al. A trial of prazosin for combat trauma PTSD with nightmares in active-duty soldiers returned from Iraq and Afghanistan. *Am J Psychiatry.* 2013;170(9):1003–1010.

99. Taylor FB, Martin P, Thompson C, et al. Prazosin effects on objective sleep measures and clinical symptoms in civilian trauma posttraumatic stress disorder: a placebo-controlled study. *Biol Psychiatry.* 2008;63(6):629–632.

100. Raskind MA, Millard SP, Petrie EC, et al. Higher pretreatment blood pressure is associated with greater posttraumatic stress disorder symptom reduction in soldiers treated with prazosin. *Biol Psychiatry.* 2016;80(10):736–742.

101. Menn SJ, Yang R, Lankford A. Armodafinil for the treatment of excessive sleepiness associated with mild or moderate closed traumatic brain injury: a 12-week, randomized, double-blind study followed by a 12-month open-label extension. *J Clin Sleep Med.* 2014;10(11):1181–1191.

102. Cantor JB, Ashman T, Bushnik T, et al. Systematic review of interventions for fatigue after traumatic brain injury: a NIDRR traumatic brain injury model systems study. *J Head Trauma Rehabil.* 2014;29(6):490–497.

103. Jha A, Weintraub A, Allshouse A, et al. A randomized trial of modafinil for the treatment of fatigue and excessive daytime sleepiness in individuals with chronic traumatic brain injury. *J Head Trauma Rehabil.* 2008;23(1):52–63.

104. Johansson B, Wentzel AP, Andréll P, Mannheimer C, Rönnbäck L. Methylphenidate reduces mental fatigue and improves processing speed in persons suffered a traumatic brain injury. *Brain Injury.* 2015;29(6):758–765.

105. McAllister TW, Zafonte R, Jain S, et al. Randomized placebo-controlled trial of methylphenidate or galantamine for persistent emotional and cognitive symptoms associated with PTSD and/or traumatic brain injury. *Neuropsychopharmacology.* 2016;41(5):1191.

CHAPTER 8

Management and Rehabilitation of Cognitive Dysfunction

LINDA M. PICON, MCD, CCC-SLP • DOROTHY A. KAPLAN, PHD • INBAL ESHEL, MA, CCC-SLP

BACKGROUND

Assessment and rehabilitation of cognitive dysfunction is a standard of practice for cognitive challenges associated with moderate to severe traumatic brain injury (TBI). Cognitive rehabilitation for moderate to severe TBI is typically offered in a standard package of inpatient, interdisciplinary rehabilitation services. Over the past decade, literature has been emerging to suggest that cognitive rehabilitation interventions may also be effective in treating patients with cognitive difficulties post concussion that extend past the acute stage. While there is no gold standard approach to the management of cognitive dysfunction associated with concussion, there is growing evidence of increased risk for chronic difficulties.

Cognitive rehabilitation, or neurorehabilitation, remains a diverse subject in both definition and practice. In general, the term refers to an array of approaches, treatment models, and domain-specific interventions aimed at optimizing function. Although there is mounting evidence supporting earlier rehabilitation, timing and duration remain largely dictated by individual patient needs, values and preferences, and clinical judgment. A report from the Institute of Medicine[1] emphasized that the limitations of the evidence to support the practice of cognitive rehabilitation at the time, particularly after mild TBI (mTBI), did not point to a lack of effectiveness. Rather, they found that the heterogeneity of interventions, functional outcomes, and patient characteristics limited the strength of available evidence. This finding resulted in a call to strengthen collaborations and advancements in the field of cognitive rehabilitation across civilian and federal agencies. Agencies such as the National Institute of Health (NIH), the National Institute on Disability, Independent Living and Rehabilitation Research (NIDILRR—NIDRR at the time) and the TBI Model

Systems, the Departments of Defense (DoD) and Veterans Affairs (VA), and the Defense and Veterans Brain Injury Center (DVBIC) remain instrumental to the advancement of the practice of cognitive rehabilitation. Over the last decade, legislation, research collaborations, and various task forces have propelled forward the science and practice of cognitive rehabilitation for mTBI.

Cooper and colleagues conducted the Study of Cognitive Rehabilitation Effectiveness,[2] a landmark study informing best cognitive practices in a military sample with history of mTBI. Clinical consensus documents and randomized controlled trials (RCTs) in mTBI (or mild to moderate) groups continue to shape the evidence for cognitive rehabilitation.

PERSISTENT COGNITIVE DIFFICULTIES AND CONCUSSION

Cognitive impairment is one of the more persistent and disabling of all postconcussive symptoms. Following mTBI, cognitive deficits are seen in reaction time, attention, mental efficiency, processing speed, delayed memory, and executive function.[3] While 80%—85% of patients who sustain a single mTBI achieve complete symptom resolution within a few days to a few months, there is a subgroup of patients who present with persistent cognitive complaints chronically that interfere with relationships, work, activities of daily living, and quality of life.[4–8] Some research suggests that for this subset of individuals with mTBI, the concussion is not simply a transient syndrome but may reflect a chronic and evolving condition.[9] The TRACK TBI (Transforming Research and Clinical Knowledge in Traumatic Brain Injury) multicenter study of a large cohort of mTBI patients admitted to trauma center emergency rooms showed that many patients experienced elevated levels

Concussion. https://doi.org/10.1016/B978-0-323-65384-8.00008-0
2020 Published by Elsevier Inc.

of cognitive symptoms at 1 year with no overall improvement from the initial evaluation. Nearly one quarter of the patients experienced persistent functional impairment at work or in daily activities.[10]

Premorbid risk factors for persistence of cognitive dysfunction following mTBI include a prior brain injury or neuropsychiatric disorder and comorbid physical or psychological health conditions. A history of three or more lifetime concussions has been shown to be associated with decreased cognitive efficiency.[11] Recovery from mTBI takes longer when coupled with other traumatic injury, sleep deprivation, prolonged physiological and psychological stressors, or emotional distress.[12-14] Acute post-traumatic stress and pain show strong associations with attentional functioning following mTBI[15] and comorbid post-traumatic stress disorder (PTSD) is associated with poorer scores on processing speed and executive functioning measures.[16] Motor vehicle crash as the type of injury event, older age, and female gender are additional factors that may affect the clinical course of cognitive recovery.[3,4,17-19]

KEY EVIDENCE AND EMERGING TRENDS

Prior evidence supported providing psychoeducation for the early management of cognitive symptoms associated with mTBI.[20] As additional evidence emerged, approaches to rehabilitation for chronic cognitive symptoms underscored a "focus on function" over traditional systematic improvement of domain-specific neuropsychological impairments. Clinical practice emphasized symptom-driven interventions that were individualized to meet functional everyday needs. In that way, preferred approaches to cognitive rehabilitation for mTBI underscore functional improvement by (1) practicing strategies to minimize the effects of cognitive difficulties, (2) training in assistive technologies to overcome cognitive challenges, and (3) coaching on self-management of cognitive slips.[21-23] Awareness of cognitive difficulties and their impact on functional activity is keen following concussion, such that psychoeducation remains a necessary component of cognitive interventions for this population. The emphasis of education is on developing an accurate understanding of cognitive effects and their management, and setting a positive expectation of functional recovery.

Key findings from published clinical trials reveal emerging trends that guide effective cognitive rehabilitation:

Cognitive Rehabilitation Improves Cognitive Functioning

A systematic review by Wilson and colleagues in 2016[24] examined seven RCTs, two in military populations and

five in civilian populations. The authors reported that varied cognitive rehabilitation interventions fared well for mild to moderate TBI. They concluded that studies in this review reported statistically significant findings on some of the primary measures examined, which included measures related to memory and executive functions. Although none of the studies found interventions to effectively improve all of the outcomes measured, most nonsignificant trends favored cognitive rehabilitation interventions over control interventions. There is no clear indication to date as to the active ingredients or dosing of effective cognitive rehabilitation interventions.

Clinician-Directed Interventions Maximize Rehabilitation Effectiveness

Clinical research evidence suggests that clinician-directed cognitive rehabilitation that is goal-driven and focused on return to function is more effective than self-administered computer-based treatments, psychoeducation, and medical management alone.[25,26]

In a systematic review, Cooper and colleagues concluded that cognitive interventions directed by a clinician achieve superior outcomes on functional cognitive measures compared to nontherapist-directed cognitive rehabilitation.[27] Moreover, in secondary analysis of SCORE! trial findings, Vanderploeg and colleagues[28] reported that self-administered computerized cognitive rehabilitation was negatively associated with cognitive and neurobehavioral outcomes.

Cognitive Rehabilitation Should Be Time-Limited and Focused on Function

Evidence to date for all severities of TBI points to cognitive rehabilitation that has an established end-point based on achievement of measurable goals that focus on reducing limitations and maximizing activity participation. Rather than describe neuropsychological impairment, impactful outcome metrics may include those that measure a reduction in functional limitations related to home and community reintegration.[29]

Interdisciplinary and Integrated Cognitive Interventions May Facilitate Functional Improvement

Studies reporting on the negative impact of comorbid pain and PTSD on rehabilitation outcomes highlight the benefits of interdisciplinary interventions to maximize outcomes.[30,31] Recent RCTs examined treatment of psychological symptoms concurrently with rehabilitation of cognitive-related symptoms after mTBI and provide some support for cognitive rehabilitation integrated with emotional regulation, self-analysis, and psychological health interventions.[2,32–34] Other RCTs provide support for integrated cognitive and psychological rehabilitation, as well as supported employment interventions.[28]

ASSESSMENT FOR COGNITIVE REHABILITATION

Neurocognitive testing focuses on the domains of attentional, learning/memory, and executive function with the exact choice of tests tailored to the individual patient. A comprehensive neuropsychological test battery provides the complexity of tasks needed to assess executive functions such as working memory and decision-making, the time to adequately assess memory, instructions in both auditory and visual modalities, and the opportunity to observe the patient's approach to test taking and problem-solving.[35]

Computerized neurocognitive assessment tests (NCATs) are routinely used in sports concussion with the Immediate Post-Concussion and Cognitive Testing Test Battery (IMPACT) the most frequently administered NCAT at all levels of athletics. The military uses the Automated Neuropsychological Assessment Metrics (ANAM) and mandated predeployment baseline testing during the OEF/OIF conflicts. Performance validity testing is critical in either computerized or traditional neuropsychological testing. Importantly, effort is a more potent predictor of neurocognitive performance post concussion than self-reported symptom severity, demographic factors, or injury characteristics.[27,36]

Objective multimodal cognitive assessments may be more sensitive to subtle executive dysfunction because these assessments simulate the multitasking demands of unstructured, complex, real-life activities.[37] The Multiple Errands Test[38] and the Assessment of Military Multitasking Performance[39] are examples of multitasking assessments. However, these tests are complex to administer and score; further research is needed to determine their clinical feasibility and validity. Virtual reality–based neuropsychological assessments may potentially offer an option for more ecologically valid assessments of executive function.

Objective neuropsychological assessment of cognitive functioning provides important information; however, some studies find a low rate of agreement between cognitive test scores and self-reported cognitive difficulties, and a large minority of patients with persistent postconcussive symptoms score within normal limits on neurocognitive tests.[40] As such, formal objective assessment is only one piece of the assessment puzzle;

multimodal and functional assessments play a unique and critical role as well.

Functional assessments are another mechanism for gathering relevant information; in this case, information regarding how the patient performs everyday tasks that require higher order cognitive skills and emotional regulation. Typically, functional assessments are completed via structured observation and documentation of an individuals' behaviors while performing functional tasks, with the intent of capturing how cognitive issues arise in real-life contexts.[41] This approach is in contrast to formal neuropsychological testing, in which the impact of cognitive challenges on function is primarily inferred. The 2016 VA/DoD CPG on mTBI suggests that "if cognitive testing is done, it should emphasize focused assessment of functional limitations to guide interventions."[22] Functional cognitive assessments can assist in planning cognitive rehabilitation treatment targets and can also help build awareness of specific cognitive challenges.

In combination with objective tests and the patient's self-reported complaints, multifactorial assessments provide a rich source of information for identifying the reasons for the cognitive failures and relevant treatment goals. A multidisciplinary team is best positioned to provide and integrate the findings from such a multifactorial assessment approach into effective treatment planning for cognitive rehabilitation.

REHABILITATION OF COGNITIVE SYMPTOMS IN THE SUBACUTE PERIOD POST CONCUSSION

Almost all the literature on cognitive rehabilitation for mTBI is with patients in the chronic stage of recovery from concussion and many months to years post injury. However, a subgroup of patients present several weeks to months after a concussion seeking treatment for seemingly lingering cognitive symptoms. Some of these patients will present with known risk factors for persistence of the cognitive symptoms. Good clinical sense does not preclude treating these patients simply because they are not yet 3 months post injury. The risk for chronicity may be abated if the patient can experience some success in managing the cognitive symptoms and achieve a state of greater self-efficacy.

For the purposes of this discussion, we consider the subacute phase to be the period beyond the initial 6 weeks of recovery and extending to 3 months post injury. Education is a critical part of management during the subacute phase of concussion recovery and includes providing the patient with information about the usual trajectory course for cognitive symptoms post injury and factors that may influence symptom mitigation. Risk management is an approach that communicates expectation of recovery, normalizes the patient's recovery experience, and orients the patient to a cognitive rehabilitation treatment approach based on the patient's functional cognitive difficulties while not attributing the etiology to any specific cause. Motivational interviewing may help in promoting active patient engagement in goal setting.[21]

During the subacute phase, it is important to address other symptoms that may be affecting the patient's cognitive function, such as headaches, vestibular disturbance, sleep difficulties, mood disturbance, fatigue, and pain. If these symptoms have not been treated, particularly if they are severe or refractory, a referral to a provider is indicated. The patient may require subsequent follow-up to reassess cognitive functioning. Cognitive rehabilitation interventions in the subacute period are brief and focus on strategies of self-management of specific functional difficulties.

Subacute postconcussive patients should be assessed for risk factors that predict symptom persistence, including a history of prior TBI and psychological health comorbidities or a history of previous neurological or psychiatric problems. A more comprehensive approach to cognitive rehabilitation may be warranted, particularly for patients with psychological health comorbidities. Integrated and holistic treatment of this patient often includes the involvement of a multidisciplinary team, management of comorbid conditions, and the addition of a psychotherapy component that addresses emotional self-regulation.

REHABILITATION OF CHRONIC POSTCONCUSSION COGNITIVE DIFFICULTIES

There has a burgeoning literature in the past decade on the treatment of executive and attentional dysfunction following mTBI. Attentional control is inherently related to and underlies executive functions, such as inhibitory control and task prioritization.[42] Executive functioning difficulties may manifest as difficulties with problem-solving, goal setting, self-monitoring, reasoning, and emotional regulation.[43] Executive functioning also affects important aspects of behavior including decision-making, motivation, cognitive flexibility, impulse control, and emotional self-regulation[44,45] and may even affect response to psychotherapy in patients with TBI.[46] There is a direct relationship between attention and cognitive, metacognitive and emotional processes.[47]

Six RCTs[2,32,33,48–50] demonstrate the effectiveness of metacognitive approaches for management of difficulties in attention and executive functions. In addition, two small crossover design studies[51,52] demonstrate the efficacy of an executive interventions. Strategic Memory Advanced Reasoning Training (SMART) teaches metacognitive strategies to improve cognitive control functions.[50] SMART emphasizes strategic attention, integrated reasoning, and cognitive flexibility ("innovation") applied to daily functioning.

Compensatory strategy development, metacognitive strategies, and emotional regulation training are key components of cognitive rehabilitation for improved executive function in the mTBI population. The curriculum for Compensatory Cognitive Training (CCT), a revised version of CogSMART,[33] includes time management, goal setting, and self-monitoring.[49] Executive function strategies taught in both the traditional and integrated interventions of the SCORE study[2] similarly include goal setting, planning, and organization (including time management).

In addition to problem-solving and individualized compensatory strategy training, some interventions also include skill development and training in emotional regulation and behavioral control. The integrated arm of Short-term Executive Plus (STEP) program focuses on planning and self-monitoring,[32] while SMART emphasizes strategic attention, integrated reasoning, and cognitive flexibility ("innovation") applied to daily functioning.[50] Likewise, SCORE is multimodal and includes psychotherapy in addition to cognitive rehabilitation. Patients in the integrated treatment approach participate in psychotherapy and homework related to cognitive behavioral therapy and mindfulness-based training.[2]

AN INTEGRATED APPROACH

Given the common clinical presentation in patients with chronic cognitive dysfunction post concussion and psychological health comorbidities, evidence-based treatments that integrate treatment for both the cognitive difficulties and the psychological heath condition offer a needed option. Almost 2/3 of OEF/OIF/OND veterans with a history of mTBI who seek VA care are also diagnosed with PTSD; these veterans experience significant difficulty in occupational and social functioning.[53,54]

Holistic treatment is delivered in an interdisciplinary rehabilitation program that addresses common cognitive difficulties along with the confounding effects of other health conditions including emotional distress, other postconcussive symptoms, and any life stressors. The treatment plan is individualized based on a comprehensive assessment with increased self-efficacy and effectiveness in managing cognitive difficulties as an overarching goal. Self-awareness of one's strengths and weaknesses is foundational for self-management.[55] Goal attainment scaling (GAS) and motivational interviewing may facilitate clinician and patient collaboration in setting individualized goals personalized to the patient's circumstances.

Integrated approaches within the setting of a therapeutic milieu offer advantages for comprehensive treatment for many patients with chronic cognitive and affective symptoms. In this comprehensive rehabilitation model, a team of therapists and rehabilitation specialists works collaboratively to ensure that each patient receives the most appropriate cognitive rehabilitation content and efficient delivery methods.[56] Treatment is individualized, guided by a consideration of the individual's goals, and addresses both the cognitive and behavioral aspects of executive functioning. Integrated cognitive rehabilitation has also employed mindfulness-based stress reduction and emotional regulation training to target postconcussive symptoms.[2,32]

These RCTs show that patients receiving high-intensity, multicomponent interventions experience decreased cognitive difficulties and improve on executive function measures compared to comparison groups. In addition to affecting cognitive functioning these interventions may also decrease emotional distress; for example, patients in the SMART intervention experienced significantly decreased depression over an educational intervention group, gains that were maintained at a 3-month follow-up. The SCORE trial demonstrated that both traditional and integrated cognitive rehabilitation treatments have superior outcomes to computer-based cognitive rehabilitation, with integrated cognitive rehabilitation the most effective in reducing psychological distress and emotional symptoms.[2]

In a recently published RCT, Jak and colleagues[57] evaluated the effectiveness of integrating components of Cognitive Symptom Management and Rehabilitation Therapy (CogSMART) into cognitive processing therapy (CPT), an evidence-based psychotherapy intervention. The 12-week hybrid treatment, SMART-CPT, was delivered as typically structured CPT, but augmented with cognitive compensatory elements from CogSMART. Both CPT and SMART-CPT resulted in clinically significant improvements in PTSD, postconcussive symptoms, and quality of life. SMART-CPT, however, also improved cognitive functioning in the domains of attention/working memory, verbal learning/memory, and novel problem solving.

IMPLEMENTING COGNITIVE REHABILITATION FOR CONCUSSION

Cognitive rehabilitation for mTBI is functionally focused on meaningful goals and activities. It requires careful assessment followed by thoughtful, shared decision-making with the patient about evidence-based treatment options. The patient's history, environment, goals and values, and available resources need to be considered. Treatment options selected should be clinician-directed and individualized to meet real-life needs. Beyond these specific treatment elements, however, there are overarching factors related to the approach and delivery of cognitive rehabilitation that can have a substantial impact on patient improvement and return to function.

For example, the invaluable patient-clinician relationship, also known as therapeutic alliance, is a potent factor in cognitive rehabilitation outcome. This cooperative agreement and collaboration sets the stage for patient buy-in, commitment, and satisfaction with treatment. Trust must be cultivated early in the process, fostering an environment of respect, understanding, and a genuine desire to effect change in areas of concern for the patient. Establishing this type of dynamic requires empathic listening and validation of the patient's real-life roadblocks and challenges, followed by an intentional crafting of meaningful goals. Transparency and collaborative decision-making promote patient motivation and engagement. Other factors, such as fostering resilience, confidence, and adaptability can positively influence the trajectory of cognitive rehabilitation.

Well-worded and time limited goals set the stage for realistic expectations and are key to a successful therapeutic experience. To achieve behavior change and functional improvement, the clinician and patient must engage in guided, systematic practice of skills, compensatory strategies and training in the use of assistive technologies to support application and minimize abandonment. Practice can occur in individual and group sessions. While individual sessions can provide the ideal setting for learning new skills and habits, group sessions can provide opportunities for practice, feedback and peer support. Throughout the therapeutic process, the patient is taught to self-monitor, self-evaluate, and help to generate solutions and next steps. Doing so cultivates an attitude of self-reliance and

TABLE 8.1
Practical Components of Cognitive Rehabilitation and Suggested Interventions or Resources.

Process	Suggested Resources

Assessment
▶ Clinical and psychosocial history including history of prior concussion/traumatic brain injury (TBI), psychological health disorder, other health-related issues, presence of life stressors, emotional distress,
▶ Cognitive complaints and examples of cognitive failures
▶ Current needs, perception of reason for everyday cognitive failures and cognitive challenges
   ◆ Tie problems and needs to impact on real-life situation, work/school, relationships, etc.
▶ Cognitive focused treatment to date
▶ Other factors affecting cognition
▶ Current use of strategies and technology
▶ Management of associated conditions (e.g., sleep, psychological health conditions, sensory deficits).
   ◆ Consult with other providers. Refer for management of any untreated, associated conditions.
▶ Formal evaluation
   ◆ Consider a combination of validated and functional measures that can inform both neuropsychological and everyday performance.
   ◆ Consult with other members of the interdisciplinary team, if available. Particularly important for patients with comorbid conditions, in the chronic stage of recovery, or whom have a history of prior treatment dissatisfaction (e.g., Neuropsychology, occupational therapy, speech-language pathology.)
	Motivational Interview
	Mild TBI (mTBI) rehabilitation toolkit[23]
	VA/DoD mTBI clinical practice guidelines[22]
	Ontario neurotrauma foundation: Guideline for concussion/mild traumatic brain injury and persistent symptoms (3rd edition, for adults over 18 years of age)[58]
	NOTE: Presence of coexisting conditions that are medically managed does not preclude cognitive rehabilitation. Severe associated problems such as psychosis and debilitating substance dependence may benefit from stabilization to ensure valid cognitive assessment.

Education
▶ Needs assessment and evaluation findings
   ◆ Discuss potential treatment plan
   ◆ Set realistic expectations of treatment plan (including effort and time commitment)
	DVBIC SCORE study manual[59]
	Clinician's guide to cognitive rehabilitation[21]
	Compensatory cognitive training (CCT) facilitator and participant manuals[49]

Goal setting ▶ Establish SMART* goals (tied to real-life, patient-identified functional challenges and activities. Include time to achieve) ◆ Discuss the application of compensatory strategies and technologies to relevant goals	Motivational interview Goal attainment scaling mTBI rehabilitation toolkit[23] DVBIC SCORE study manual[59] Clinician's guide to cognitive rehabilitation[21] *SMART—Specific, Measurable, Achievable, Relevant, Time-bound

Implementation of treatment plan

► Assistive technology

◆ Begin training on use of current technology as a cognitive tool

◆ Discuss and explore additional technology, if needed

◆ Practice (guided and systematic) to increase understanding of use during cognitive challenges and to ensure positive behavior change

◆ Encourage self-monitoring

• Teach how to self-assess and adjust.

• Promote anticipating strategy use and predicting performance in novel situations.

► Compensatory strategy training with focus on executive function training

◆ Match to functional challenge

◆ Practice (guided and systematic) to increase understanding of use during cognitive challenges and to ensure positive behavior change.

◆ Encourage self-monitoring.

• Teach how to self-assess and adjust.

• Promote anticipating strategy use and predicting performance in novel situations.

► Introduce domain-specific treatment interventions (such as attention process training), as needed.

Additional considerations for patients with chronic, refractory cognitive difficulties and comorbid conditions:

► Holistic, integrated cognitive rehabilitation approach

◆ Emotional regulation training

◆ Mindfulness-based interventions

◆ Cognitive behavioral therapy

► Case management

► Referral for pharmacological evaluation

► Discharge assessment

► Summary/review of compensatory strategies and cognitive technologies

► Determine need/consider postdischarge follow-up appointment(s)

VA/DoD mTBI clinical practice guidelines[22]
mTBI rehabilitation toolkit[23]
CogSmart[33,34]
Clinician's guide to cognitive Rehabilitation[21]
CCT[49]
DVBIC SCORE study manual[59]
Optimizing cognitive rehabilitation[60]
ACRM cognitive rehabilitation manual[61]
Ontario neurotrauma foundation: Guideline for concussion/mild traumatic brain injury and persistent symptoms[58]
NOTE: Consider benefits of manualized treatment approach matched to patient characteristics and goals

DVBIC SCORE study manual[59]
SMART-cognitive processing therapy[57]

Clinician's guide to cognitive rehabilitation[21]
Goal attainment scaling
Self-report outcome measure or questionnaire

independence and centers the treatment around the end goal of self-management from the onset.

The general process of cognitive rehabilitation includes evaluation, education, intervention and outcomes assessment. However, as in all areas of rehabilitation, cognitive rehabilitation is a dynamic and interactive process. It is patient-centric and guided by a constant needs assessment that helps direct next steps. Components of the process may be repeated over the course of treatment or overlap based on residual needs, goals and progress. The following table aims to highlight major components and practical considerations for cognitive rehabilitation, albeit not strictly in sequential order (Table 8.1).

PHARMACOLOGICAL MANAGEMENT OF PERSISTING COGNITIVE DIFFICULTIES POST CONCUSSION

There are no Food and Drug Administration (FDA)-approved medications for the treatment or prevention of concussion and none specifically developed to enhance cognitive recovery from concussion. Methylphenidate, a stimulant used to treat narcolepsy and attention deficit hyperactivity disorder, is often used by prescribing providers with patients complaining of cognitive symptoms post concussion. A recent meta-analysis of treatment outcome showed a significant benefit of methylphenidate for enhancing sustained attention, but not for memory or processing speed, in mixed samples of mild to moderate TBI patients.[61] One RCT with a sample that included mTBI patients suggested a synergistic effect of methylphenidate and a metacognitive rehabilitation approach[62]; however, more research is needed to recommend this as a clinical practice. Some providers prescribe amantadine, a catecholaminergic agent, for executive function difficulties; however, there is only limited evidence of efficacy.[63–65] While many patients use supplements and vitamins, unlike prescription medication, supplements are not reviewed for safety and quality by the FDA and there is no current evidence for a role in the treatment of cognitive difficulties post concussion.[66,67] As many patients with persisting postconcussion symptoms have comorbid psychological health conditions such as depression and PTSD, medication management with evidence-based pharmacological agents for these conditions should be considered and may improve cognitive function. In addition, the patient's complete list of medications should be assessed for the potential of negative effects on cognition and the possibility of another medication for the condition considered. Prescribing and nonprescribing providers need to work collaboratively to monitor and frequently assess the benefits and side effects of pharmacological agents and their impact on the patient's response to cognitive rehabilitation.

CONCLUSION

There is scant research about patient characteristics that predict a positive response to cognitive rehabilitation post-concussion. There is also very little known about treatment dose or the components of cognitive interventions that are most beneficial for the post-concussion population. The effect of psychological health as a possible moderator variable to cognitive rehabilitation response creates an added layer of complexity in the management of postconcussive cognitive symptoms.

Although questions about specific interventions remain unanswered empirically, the evidence to date supports time-limited, clinician-supported, functional and goal-driven interventions with a focus on executive functions, compensatory strategy, and assistive technology training and self-management. Early interventions provide the ideal setting for psychoeducation, support, and development of individualized skills and strategies that can enhance recovery and optimize function. Refractory cognitive-symptom management may require a comprehensive, holistic approach that incorporates aspects of behavioral and emotional well-being. In this respect, emerging evidence supports cognitive rehabilitation within a team milieu, as well as integrated programs that target cognitive-symptom management in a broader, whole health context. From this broader perspective, cognitive rehabilitation incorporates integrated approaches and cognitive-specific interventions to achieve a common goal.

REFERENCES

1. Institute of Medicine IOM. *Cognitive Rehabilitation Therapy for Traumatic Brain Injury: Model Study Protocols and Frameworks to Advance the State of the Science: Workshop Summary.* Washington, DC: The National Academies Press; 2013.
2. Cooper DB, Bowles AO, Kennedy JE, et al. Cognitive rehabilitation for military service members with mild traumatic brain injury: a randomized clinical trial. *J Head Trauma Rehabil.* 2017;323:E1–e15.
3. Belanger HG, Curtiss G, Demery JA, et al. Factors moderating neuropsychological outcomes following mild traumatic brain injury: a meta-analysis. *J Int Neuropsychol Soc.* 2005;11:215–227.
4. Rabinowitz AR, Levin HS. Cognitive sequelae of traumatic brain injury. *Psychiat Clin N Am.* 2014;371:1–11. https://doi.org/10.1016/j.psc.2013.11.004.

5. Carroll L, Cassidy JD, Peloso P, et al. Prognosis for mild traumatic brain injury: results of the WHO collaborating centre task force on mild traumatic brain injury. *J Rehabil Med*. 2004;360:84–105. https://doi.org/10.1080/165019 60410023859.

6. Schretlen DJ, Shapiro AM. A quantitative review of the effects of traumatic brain injury on cognitive functioning. *Int Rev Psychiatry*. 2003;15(4):342–349.

7. Ruff R. Two decades of advances in understanding of mild traumatic brain injury. *J Head Trauma Rehabil*. 2005;201:5–18. https://doi.org/10.1097/00001199-200 501000-00003.

8. Bigler ED, Farrer FJ, Pertab JL, James K, Petrie JA, Hedges DW. Reaffirmed limitations of meta-analytic methods in the study of mild traumatic brain injury: a response to Rohling et al. *Clin Neuropsychol*. 2013;27: 176–214.

9. Failla MD, Wagner AK. Models of posttraumatic brain injury neurorehabilitation. In: Kobeissy FH, ed. *Brain Neurotrauma: Molecular, Neuropsychological, and Rehabilitation Aspects*. Boca Raton FL: CRC Press/Taylor & Francis; 2015 (Chapter 35). PubMed PMID: 26269917.

10. McMahon P, Hricik A, Yue JK, et al. Symptomatology and functional outcome in mild traumatic brain injury: results from the prospective TRACK-TBI study. *J Neurotrauma*. January 1, 2014;311:26–33.

11. Spira JL, Lathan CE, Bleiberg J, Tsao JW. The impact of multiple concussions on emotional distress, post-concussive symptoms, and neurocognitive functioning in active duty United States marines independent of combat exposure or emotional distress. *J Neurotrauma*. 2014;3122: 1823–1834. https://doi.org/10.1089/neu.2014.3363. Epub 2014 Oct 9. PubMed PMID: 25003552; PubMed Central PMCID: PMC4224036.

12. Iverson GL. Outcome from mild traumatic brain injury. *Curr Opin Psychiatr*. 2005;18:301–317.

13. Meyer K, Jaffee MS. Military personnel and veterans with traumatic brain injury. In: Arciniegas DB, Zasler ND, Vanderploeg RD, Jaffee MS, Garcia TA, eds. *Management of Adults with Traumatic Brain Injury*. American Psychiatric Publishing; 2013.

14. Belanger HG, Kretzmer T, Vanderploeg RD, French LM. Symptom complaints following combat-related traumatic brain injury: relationship to traumatic brain injury severity and posttraumatic stress disorder. *J Int Neuropsychol Soc*. 2010;161:194–199.

15. Massey JS, Meares S, Batchelor J, Bryant RA. An exploratory study of the association of acute posttraumatic stress, depression, and pain to cognitive functioning in mild traumatic brain injury. *Neuropsychology*. July 2015;294:530–542.

16. Nelson LA, Yoash-Gantz RE, Pickett TC, Campbell TA. Relationship between processing speed and executive function performance among OEF/OIF veterans: implications for post-deployment rehabilitation. *J Head Trauma Rehabil*. 2009;24:32–40.

17. King NS. A systematic review of age and gender factors in prolonged post-concussion symptoms after mild head injury. *Brain Inj*. 2014;28(13–14):1639–1645.

18. Pertab JL, James KM, Bigler F. Limitations of mild brain injury meta-analyses. *Brain Inj*. 2009;23:498–508.

19. Ponsford J, Willmott C, Rothwell A, et al. Factors influencing outcome following mild traumatic brain injury in adults. *J Int Neuropsychol Soc*. 2000;65:568–579. https://doi.org/10.1017/S13556177007=655066.

20. Gravel J, D'Angelo A, Carriere B, et al. Interventions provided in the acute phase for mild traumatic brain injury: a systematic review. *Syst Rev*. 2013;2:63.

21. Working Group to Develop a Clinician's Guide to Cognitive Rehabilitation for mTBI: Application for Service members and Veterans. *Clinician's Guide to Cognitive Rehabilitation in Mild Traumatic Brain Injury: Application for Military Service Members and Veterans*. Rockville, MD: American Speech-Language-Hearing Association; 2016. Available from: http://www.asha.org/uploadedFiles/ASHA/Practice_Portal/Clinical_Topics/Traumatic_Brain_Injury_in_Adults/Clinicians-Guide-to-Cognitive-Rehabilitation-in-Mild-Traumatic-Brain-Injury.pdf.

22. Department of Veterans Affairs VA, Department of Defense DoD. *VA/DoD Clinical Practice Guideline for the Management of Concussion-Mild Traumatic Brain Injury. Version 2*; 2016. Retrieved from: https://www.healthquality.va.gov/guidelines/Rehab/mtbi/.

23. Weightman M, Radomski MV, Mashima PA, Roth CR. *Mild Traumatic Brain Injury Toolkit*. Washington, DC: Army Borden Institute; 2014. Retrieved from: http://www.cs.amedd.army.mil/FileDownloadpublic.aspx?docid=e454f2ce-00ae-4a2d-887d-26d5474c8d1a.

24. Wilson SH, Roth M, Lindblad AS, Weaver LK. Review of recent non-hyperbaric oxygen interventions for mild traumatic brain injury. *Undersea Hyper Med*. 2016;435: 615–627.

25. Fetta J, Starkweather A, Gill JM. Computer-based cognitive rehabilitation interventions for traumatic brain injury: a critical review of the literature. *J Neurosci Nurs*. 2017;494: 235–240.

26. Leopold A, Lourie A, Petras H, Elias E. The use of assistive technology for cognition to support the performance of daily activities for individuals with cognitive disabilities due to traumatic brain injury: the current state of the research. *NeuroRehabilitation*. 2015;373:359–378.

27. Cooper DB, Bunner AE, Kennedy JE, et al. Treatment of persistent post-concussive symptoms after mild traumatic brain injury: a systematic review of cognitive rehabilitation and behavioral health interventions in military service members and veterans. *Brain Imaging Behav*. 2015;9(3): 403–420.

28. Vanderploeg RD, Cooper DB, Curtiss G, Kennedy JE, Tate DF, Bowles AO. Predicting treatment response to cognitive rehabilitation in military service members with mild traumatic brain injury. *Rehabil Psychol*. 2018;632: 194–204.

29. Burleigh SA, Farber RS, Gillard M. Community integration and life satisfaction after traumatic brain injury: long-term findings. *Am J Occup Ther*. January 1998;521:45–52.

30. Cifu DX, Taylor BC, Carne WF, et al. Traumatic brain injury, posttraumatic stress disorder, and pain diagnoses

in OIF/OEF/OND Veterans. *J Rehabil Res Dev.* 2013;509: 1169–1176.

31. Lew HL, Otis JD, Tun C, Kerns RD, Clark ME, Cifu DX. Prevalence of chronic pain, posttraumatic stress disorder, and persistent postconcussive symptoms in OIF/OEF veterans: polytrauma clinical triad. *J Rehabil Res Dev.* 2009;466:697.

32. Cantor J, Ashman T, Dams-O'Connor K, et al. Evaluation of the short-term executive plus intervention for executive dysfunction after traumatic brain injury: a randomized controlled trial with minimization. *Arch Phys Med Rehabil.* 2014;951:1–9.

33. Twamley EW, Jak AJ, Delis DC, Bondi MW, Lohr JB. Cognitive symptom management and rehabilitation therapy CogSMART for veterans with traumatic brain injury: pilot randomized controlled trial. *J Rehabil Res Dev.* 2014;511: 59–70.

34. Twamley EW, Thomas KR, Gregory AM, et al. CogSMART compensatory cognitive training for traumatic brain injury: effects over 1 year. *J Head Trauma Rehabil.* 2015; 306:391–401.

35. Kontos AP, McAllister-Deitrick J, Sufrinko AM. Predicting post-concussion symptom risk in the ED. *Pediatr Neurol Briefs.* 2016;303:19. https://doi.org/10.15844/pedneurbriefs-30-3-2. PubMed PMID: 27397114; PubMed Central PMCID: PMC4936970.

36. Cooper DB, Vanderploeg RD, Armistead-Jehle P, Lewis JD, Bowles AO. Factors associated with neurocognitive performance in OIF/OEF service members with post-concussive complaints in postdeployment clinical settings. *J Rehabil Res Dev.* 2014;517:1023–1034. https://doi.org/10.1682/JRRD.2013.05.0140. PubMed PMID: 25479335.

37. Frisch S, Förstl S, Legler A, Schöpe S, Goebel H. The interleaving of actions in everyday life multitasking demands. *J Neuropsychol.* 2012;6:257–269. https://doi.org/10.1111/j.1748-6653.2012.02026.x.

38. Shallice T, Burgess PW. Deficits in strategy application following frontal lobe damage in man. *Brain.* 1991;114: 727–741. https://doi.org/10.1093/brain/114.2.727.

39. Radomski MV, Weightman MM, Davidson LF, et al. Development of a measure to inform return to-duty decision making after mild traumatic brain injury. *Mil Med.* 2013;178:246–253. https://doi.org/10.7205/MILMED-D-12-00144.

40. French LM, Lange RT, Brickell TA. Subjective cognitive complaints and neuropsychological test performance following military-related traumatic brain injury. *J Rehabil Res Dev.* 2014;51(6):933–950. https://doi.org/10.1682/JRRD.2013.10.0226.

41. Mortera MH. *The Mortera-Cognitive Screening Measure M-CSM.* New York: Programs in Occupational Therapy, Columbia University; 2004.

42. Diamond A. Executive functions. *Annu Rev Psychol.* 2013; 64:135–168. https://doi.org/10.1146/annurev- psych-113011-143750.

43. Hartikainen KM, Waljas M, Isoviita T, et al. Persistent symptoms in mild to moderate traumatic brain injury associated with executive dysfunction. *J Clin Exp Neuropsychol.* 2010;327:767–774.

44. Lezak MD, Howieson DB, Bigler ED, Tranel D. *Neuropsychological Assessment.* 5th ed. Vol. 2012. Oxford University Press; 2012.

45. Bogdanova Y, Verfaellie M. Cognitive sequelae of blast-induced traumatic brain injury: recovery and rehabilitation. *Neuropsychol Rev.* 2012;221:4–20. https://doi.org/10.1007/s11065-012-9192-3.

46. Crocker LD, Jurick SM, Thomas KR, et al. Worse baseline executive functioning is associated with dropout and poorer response to trauma-focused treatment for veterans with PTSD and comorbid traumatic brain injury. *Behav Res Ther.* September 2018;108:68–77. https://doi.org/10.1016/j.brat.2018.07.004. Epub 2018 Jul 19. PubMed PMID: 30031369.

47. Drigas A, Karyotaki M. Attentional control and other executive functions. *Int J Emerg Technol Learn iJET.* 2017;1203: 219–233.

48. Nelson LA, MacDonald M, Stall C, Pazdan R. Effects of interactive metronome therapy on cognitive functioning after blast-related brain injury: a randomized controlled pilot trial. *Neuropsychology.* 2013;276:666–679.

49. Storzbach D, Twamley EW, Roost MS, et al. Compensatory cognitive training for Operation Enduring Freedom/Operation Iraqi Freedom/Operation New Dawn veterans with mild traumatic brain injury. *J Head Trauma Rehabil.* 2017;321:16–24.

50. Vas A, Chapman S, Aslan S, et al. Reasoning training in veteran and civilian traumatic brain injury with persistent mild impairment. *Neuropsychol Rehabil.* 2016;264:502–531.

51. Novakovic-Agopian T, Chen AJ, Rome S, et al. Rehabilitation of executive functioning with training in attention regulation applied to individually defined goals: a pilot study bridging theory, assessment, and treatment. *J Head Trauma Rehabil.* 2011;265:325–338. https://doi.org/10.1097/HTR.0b013e3181f1ead2.

52. Chen AJ, Novakovic-Agopian T, Nycum TJ, et al. Training of goal-directed attention regulation enhances control over neural processing for individuals with brain injury. *Brain.* 2011;134(Pt 5):1541–1554.

53. Fulton JJ, Calhoun PS, Wagner HR, et al. The prevalence of posttraumatic stress disorder in Operation Enduring Freedom/Operation Iraqi Freedom OEF/OIF Veterans: a meta-analysis. *J Anxiety Disord.* 2015;31:98–107.

54. Wrocklage KM, Schweinsburg BC, Krystal JH, et al. Neuropsychological functioning in veterans with posttraumatic stress disorder: associations with performance validity, comorbidities, and functional outcomes. *J Int Neuropsychol Soc.* 2016;22:399–411.

55. O'Keeffe F, Dockree P, Moloney P, Carton S, Robertson IH. Awareness of deficits in traumatic brain injury: a multidimensional approach to assessing metacognitive knowledge and online-awareness. *J Int Neuropsychol Soc.* 2007; 131:38–49.

56. Institute of Medicine IOM. *Cognitive Rehabilitation Therapy for Traumatic Brain Injury: Evaluating the Evidence.* Washington, DC: The National Academies Press; 2011.

57. Jak AJ, Jurick S, Crocker L, et al. SMART-CPT for veterans with co-morbid post-traumatic stress disorder and history

of traumatic brain injury: a randomized controlled trial. *J Neurol Neurosurg Psychiatry.* 2018;0:1—9. https://doi.org/10.1136/jnnp-2018-319315.

58. Ontario Neurotrauma Foundation. *Guideline for Concussion/Mild Traumatic Brain Injury and Persistent Symptoms: Third Edition, for Adults over 18 Years of Age.* 2018.

59. Study of Cognitive Rehabilitation Effectiveness Study Manual. *Defense and Veterans Brain Injury Center;* 2015. http://dvbic.dcoe.mil/study-manuals.

60. Sohlberg MM, Turkstra LS. *Optimizing Cognitive Rehabilitation: Effective Instructional Methods.* New York, NY: Guilford Press; 2011.

61. Haskins EC, Cicerone K, Trexler L, American Congress of Rehabilitation Medicine, et al. *Cognitive Rehabilitation Manual: Translating Evidence-Based Recommendations into Practice.* Reston, VA: ACRM; 2012.

62. Huang CH, Huang CC, Sun CK, Lin GH, Hou WH. Methylphenidate on cognitive improvement in patients with traumatic brain injury: a meta-analysis. *Curr Neuropharmacol.* 2016;14:272—281.

63. McDonald BC, Flashman LA, Arciniegas DB, et al. Methylphenidate and memory and attention adaptation training for persistent cognitive symptoms after traumatic brain injury: a randomized, placebo-controlled trial. *Neuropsychopharmacology.* 2017;42(9):1766—1775.

64. Kraus MF, Smith GS, Butters M, et al. Effects of the dopaminergic agent and NMDA receptor antagonist amantadine on cognitive function, cerebral glucose metabolism and D2 receptor availability in chronic traumatic brain injury: a study using positron emission tomography (PET). *Brain Inj.* 2005;19(7):471—479.

65. Writer BW, Schillerstrom JE. Psychopharmacological treatment for cognitive impairment in survivors of traumatic brain injury: a critical review. *J Neuropsychiatry Clin Neurosci.* 2009;21(4):362—370.

66. Scher LN, Loomis E, McCarron RM. Traumatic brain injury: pharmacotherapy options for cognitive deficits. *Current Psychiatry.* 2011;10(2):21—37.

67. Ashbaugh A, McGrew C. The role of nutritional supplements in sports concussion treatment. *Curr Sports Med Rep.* 2016;15(1):16—19.

FURTHER READING

1. Defense Health Agency, Defense and Veterans Brain Injury Center. Cognitive rehabilitation for service members and veterans following mild to moderate traumatic brain injury. 2019:1—30. Retrieved from https://dvbic.dcoe.mil/system/files/resources/2688.1.1.2_CogRehab_CR_508.pdf.

CHAPTER 9

Neurosensory Deficits Associated with Concussion (Auditory, Vestibular, and Visual Dysfunction)

CHIEMI TANAKA, PHD • JAMES W. HALL III, PHD • TERRI K. POGODA, PHD • HENRY L. LEW, MD, PHD

Impairments in the auditory, vestibular, and visual domains are among the most common sensory deficits observed following concussion/mild traumatic brain injury (mTBI). This chapter will briefly discuss the assessment, management, and rehabilitation of patients with mTBI when presenting with auditory, vestibular, and visual sensory dysfunction/impairments occurring in isolation or combination with concussion.

AUDITORY DYSFUNCTION AFTER CONCUSSION/MTBI

Hearing loss (HL), auditory processing disorders (APDs), and related disorders, such as tinnitus and decreased sound tolerance disorders, are not uncommon following traumatic brain injury (TBI). The likelihood of HL, and the type of HL, varies depending on the nature and severity of head injury. For example, blunt injury or focal head injury involving temporal bone fracture is almost always associated with damage to peripheral auditory structures, including the middle ear, cochlea, and less often neural pathways.[1] Closed head injury, on the other hand, may be associated with damage to the middle ear and cochlea,[2] but it is also likely to produce dysfunction within the central auditory nervous system.[3–5] Prior to about the year 2000, the literature on head injury and hearing was mostly limited to studies of relatively small numbers of civilians, children, and adults, with trauma secondary to motor vehicle accidents, gunshot wounds, assaults, and miscellaneous accidental etiologies (see Chen et al.[6] for review). More recently, however, dozens of publications describe in considerable detail comprehensive investigations of HL, APD, and related auditory disorder of tinnitus in large populations of military personnel following blast injuries from explosive devices.[3,7–11]

Our review focuses mostly on this latter substantial clinical experience and, specifically, on papers describing HL and related auditory disorders in mTBI, covering a test battery appropriate for comprehensive and accurate assessment of auditory function in adults with mTBI, research studies of peripheral and central auditory function and related disorders, and an update on the serious problems of two related disorders: tinnitus and decreased sound tolerance. Finally, this section concludes with a discussion of rehabilitation options for persons with mTBI. Major steps and procedures important in auditory assessment and management in adult patients with mTBI are summarized in Fig. 9.1.

Test Battery for Auditory Assessment
Behavioral auditory tests
Hearing assessment is optimally conducted with a test battery consisting of procedures requiring a behavioral response from the patient and with objective auditory procedures (see Hall[12] and Lew et al.[13] for a detailed review). Auditory tests are summarized in Table 9.1. Common behavioral tests include pure tone audiometry and speech audiometry.

Pure tone audiometry is invariably included in the test battery for hearing assessment of older children and adults. However, pure tone audiometry has at least eight serious limitations as a clinical measure of auditory function: (1) Test signals are the simplest of sounds presented in an extremely quiet listening condition rarely encountered during everyday communication, (2) Only audibility of simple sounds is measured, not processing of complex sounds like speech, (3)

Concussion. https://doi.org/10.1016/B978-0-323-65384-8.00009-2
Copyright © 2020 Elsevier Inc. All rights reserved.

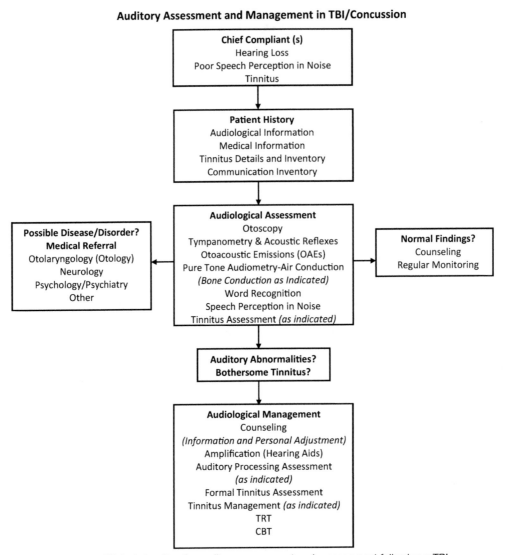

Auditory Assessment and Management in TBI/Concussion

Chief Compliant (s)
Hearing Loss
Poor Speech Perception in Noise
Tinnitus

Patient History
Audiological Information
Medical Information
Tinnitus Details and Inventory
Communication Inventory

Audiological Assessment
Otoscopy
Tympanometry & Acoustic Reflexes
Otoacoustic Emissions (OAEs)
Pure Tone Audiometry-Air Conduction
(Bone Conduction as Indicated)
Word Recognition
Speech Perception in Noise
Tinnitus Assessment *(as indicated)*

Possible Disease/Disorder?
Medical Referral
Otolaryngology (Otology)
Neurology
Psychology/Psychiatry
Other

Normal Findings?
Counseling
Regular Monitoring

Auditory Abnormalities?
Bothersome Tinnitus?

Audiological Management
Counseling
(Information and Personal Adjustment)
Amplification (Hearing Aids)
Auditory Processing Assessment
(as indicated)
Formal Tinnitus Assessment
Tinnitus Management *(as indicated)*
TRT
CBT

FIG. 9.1 Clinical algorithm for auditory assessment and management following mTBI.

Thresholds are obtained only for a very limited sample of 6–8 octave frequencies from within the range of 20 to 20,000 frequencies that can be detected by a young normal hearer, (4) pure tone audiometry has relatively poor sensitivity to cochlear auditory dysfunction, i.e., patients with modest but clinically significant cochlear damage may have normal pure tone test findings, (5) pure tone audiometry findings are typically normal in persons with APD involving the central nervous system (CNS), (6) Abnormal pure thresholds offer very little clue as to the site of dysfunction within the auditory system, (7) Test performance is poorly related to communication ability, and (8) Results are heavily influenced by listener variables that are common in persons with TBI, as detailed below.

Speech audiometry includes procedures for the detection, perception, and recognition of speech signals like words. Speech audiometry as typically performed clinically is also characterized by several limitations in patients with TBI, in addition to the listener variables affecting any behavioral auditory test. Perception of single syllable words is to a large extent dependent on hearing sensitivity in the higher frequency region (2000–4000 Hz, the frequency region involved in

TABLE 9.1
Brief Description of Auditory Procedures Applied in the Assessment of Adult Patients With Traumatic Brain Injury.

OBJECTIVE AUDITORY TESTS[a]

Tympanometry

- Clinical evidence first reported in 1970
- Highly sensitive measure of middle ear function
- Confirms perforations of the tympanic membrane
- Useful in differentiating among different types of middle ear disorders
- Devices available for automated measurements by nonaudiological personnel

Acoustic Stapedial Reflex Measurement

- Clinical evidence since the early 1970s
- Measures function of multiple sensory and neural auditory structures including cochlea, 8th (auditory) cranial nerve, and pathways in lower auditory brainstem
- Confirmation of normal versus abnormal cochlear auditory function
- Devices available for automated measurements by nonaudiological personnel

Otoacoustic Emissions

- Clinical evidence since the early 1980s
- Highly sensitive measure of cochlear (outer hair cell) function
- Useful in early detection of cochlear damage secondary to noise exposure and acoustic trauma
- Devices available for automated measurements by nonaudiological personnel

Auditory Brainstem Response

- Clinical evidence since the early 1970s
- Sensitive measurement of neural pathways from 8th (auditory) cranial nerve through midbrainstem
- Confirmation, and estimation of degree, of sensory hearing impairment
- Differentiation of type of hearing loss (i.e., conductive, sensory, mixed sensory plus conductive, neural)
- Can be recorded from patients who sedated, under anesthesia, or comatose

Cortical Auditory Evoked Responses

- Clinical evidence since the early 1960s
- Measurement of central nervous system including auditory regions of thalamus and temporal lobe
- Measurement of auditory processing with speech stimulation
- Results correlate with communication and cognitive outcome in traumatic brain injury

BEHAVIORAL AUDITORY TESTS

Pure Tone Audiometry

- Clinical evidence since the 1930s
- Most commonly performed auditory test
- Estimation of auditory thresholds for air conduction pure tone signals at octave frequencies from 250 Hz through 8000 Hz, and sometimes higher frequencies
- Estimation of auditory thresholds for bone conduction pure tone signals at octave frequencies from 500 Hz through 4000 Hz
- Generally conducted in a sound-treated room
- Determines level of sound required for audibility of speech
- Valid test performance is limited to patients who are alert, cooperative, motivated, and cognitively intact

Speech Reception Threshold

- Clinical evidence since the 1940s
- Commonly performed auditory test
- Measurement of speech threshold in dB HL using standardized two-syllabus words
- Valid test performance is limited to patients who are alert, cooperative, motivated, and cognitively intact
- Generally conducted in a sound-treated room

Continued

Word Recognition

- Clinical evidence since the 1940s
- Commonly performed auditory test
- Measurement at suprathreshold level (e.g., 40 dB HL) of ability to correctly repeat or otherwise demonstrate recognition of standardized single-syllabus words presented in quiet
- Results are reported in percent correct usually for a list of 25 words
- Valid test performance is limited to patients who are alert, cooperative, motivated, and cognitively intact
- Generally conducted in a sound-treated room

Speech Perception in Noise

- Clinical evidence since the 1960s
- Measurement at suprathreshold level of ability to correctly repeat or otherwise demonstrate recognition of words or sentences presented in background noise or speech
- Results are reported in percent correct or in terms of performance as a function of the signal-to-noise ratio
- Valid test performance is limited to patients who are alert, cooperative, motivated, and cognitively intact
- Generally conducted in a sound-treated room

Auditory Processing Tests

- Clinical evidence since the 1950s
- Measurement of ability perform tests using speech or nonspeech signals in the evaluation of various auditory processes, such as auditory discrimination, temporal auditory processing, auditory sequencing, and integration or separation of binaural auditory information

[a] Objective tests can be applied with all patients. Results are not influenced by listener variables such as motivation, cooperation, attention, language functioning, or cognitive status.

age-related and noise-induced HL). Consequently, deficits in word recognition performance may reflect preexisting HL that is not related to TBI. Also, scores of word recognition tests in quiet are not well correlated with a patient's ability to communicate effectively in typical listening conditions. That is, word recognition scores are often quite good in patients who have difficulty with speech perception in noisy environments. Finally, word recognition in quiet is an ineffective measure of auditory processing and insensitive to central auditory nervous system abnormalities.

Listener variables include patient state of alertness, cooperation, motivation, language functioning, developmental age, and cognitive factors such as attention, memory, and processing speed. In patients with a history of TBI, there is always a possibility that one or more listener variables will compromise the validity of findings for behavioral auditory assessment with procedures like pure tone and speech audiometry. The most likely erroneous outcome is an apparent HL, speech perception deficit, or APD when, in fact, the patient's poor test performance is compromised by one of the listener variables.

Objective auditory tests

Objective tests are electroacoustic or electrophysiologic measures of auditory function that do not require a behavioral response from the patient. Valid objective auditory test results can be obtained from patients who are sleeping, sedated, anesthetized, or comatose. The listener variables already cited have no effect on the outcome of objective auditory tests. As summarized in Table 9.1, objective auditory tests often recorded clinically are aural immittance measures (tympanometry and acoustic stapedial reflex measurement), otoacoustic emissions (OAEs), and auditory evoked responses (auditory brainstem response [ABR] and cortical auditory evoked responses). A detailed description of these tests is far beyond the scope of this chapter. Readers interested in learning more about objective auditory measures are referred to a recent review[13] and several recent textbooks.[12,14,15] There are also in the literature many hundreds of articles describing research evidence in support of the clinical application of each of the tests.

Patterns of Auditory Dysfunction

Over two-thirds of veterans with mTBI report hearing problems. Unfortunately, the majority of those reporting problems are not referred for audiological assessment. Furthermore, up to one-half of those who are referred for assessment do not follow through with the assessment. Therefore, accurate data are lacking on the prevalence of HL in representative unselected populations of persons with mTBI. And, to our knowledge, there are no published statistics from large civilian patient populations on reported hearing difficulties or compliance with recommendations for audiological assessment among individuals with mTBI. Our discussion here focuses on auditory status of persons with mTBI who report hearing difficulties and who then undergo formal audiological assessment. The review largely pertains to male veterans whose mTBI resulted from blast injuries and, less often, other etiologies such as falls and motor vehicle accidents.

Peripheral auditory dysfunction

Peripheral auditory abnormalities are often encountered and well recognized in persons with TBI.[3,7] Tympanic membrane (TM) perforation is documented in about one-third of persons with TBI secondary to blast injury. Indeed, perforation of the TM is the most common injury in blast survivors and the most common of all blast-related ear injuries. Perforations are invariably detected with otoscopic examination and easily confirmed with tympanometry. Fortunately, TM perforations only produce a temporary mild HL, as they usually heal spontaneously. Blasts with very high dynamic pressures may produce a disruption or discontinuity of the ossicular chain connecting the TM to the inner ear. Ossicular chain discontinuities are associated with abnormally high middle ear compliance on tympanometry plus a rather distinct audiogram pattern characterized by severe high-frequency conductive HL.

Head trauma and acoustic trauma with exposure to high pressure levels in blasts produces structural and functional inner ear (cochlear) damage. Depending on the severity of the injury, the prevalence of sensory HL ranges from 35% to over 50%. Although degree of HL varies depending on severity of injury, the majority of persons have hearing thresholds better than 60 dB HL.[10] In most cases, the amount of HL progressively increases for higher test frequencies (above 2000 Hz). Permanent sensory HL in some persons with TBI may include contributions from etiologies other than trauma. Age-related cochlear deficits can be confidently ruled out in military personnel with TBI because most are young adults, and about three-quarters are age 30 years or less. However, it is reasonable to suspect that military personnel with combat-related TBI are at considerable preinjury risk for noise-induced HL,

mostly in the frequency region of 3000−6000 Hz. In addition, intensive and longer term care of severely injured persons commonly includes treatment of infections and other medical complications with potentially ototoxic drugs including aminoglycoside antibiotic drugs, other antibiotics (e.g., vancomycin), plus loop diuretics.[7,8] We should emphasize the important role of OAEs in early detection, diagnostic confirmation, and close monitoring of cochlear HL, regardless of the etiology.

Auditory dysfunction beyond the audiogram

There is a common and rather prominent theme in the literature on auditory dysfunction in mTBI. Not all persons who report hearing problems have evidence of sensory HL on pure tone audiometry. For example, according to Lew et al.[3] roughly 1 in 10 persons complaining of HL had normal audiograms. Terms such as "subclinical HL" or "hidden HL" are sometimes for persons with hearing complaints yet normal audiogram. However, clear evidence of auditory dysfunction can usually be found when an appropriately comprehensive test battery is employed. Clinical experience in varied patient populations, and published research on hearing in TBI, provide multiple logical explanations for why pure tone audiometry underestimates auditory dysfunction.

OAEs are more sensitive to cochlear dysfunction than pure tone audiometry.[15] There is evidence that distortion product OAEs are abnormal in more than 80% of patients with TBI, whereas only about one-third of these patients have abnormal findings on pure tone audiometry. In other words, some patients with hearing complaints yet a normal audiogram have cochlear dysfunction that interferes with their everyday communication. In addition to the direct effects of trauma on physiology of the inner ear, two etiologies are most likely for cochlear auditory dysfunction in patients with clinically normal hearing sensitivity: outer hair cell dysfunction secondary to chronic or acute exposure to high intensity noise and ototoxicity.

Central auditory dysfunction

Lew et al.[3] speculate on the possibility that some patients with mTBI who complain of hearing problems even though they show no evidence of a deficit on pure tone audiometry might have central APDs. Research findings in recent years confirm this suspicion. Persons with mTBI report difficulty with hearing speech in noisy environments.[16] Formal assessment of auditory processing confirms marked abnormalities in persons with TBI secondary to blast exposure, including below normal performance for speech perception in noise, temporal processing deficits, and selected dichotic listening tasks.[4] By definition, one would suspect that trauma causing clinically documented brain injury would in many, perhaps most, cases be associated with central auditory nervous system dysfunction.

It should be stressed that cognitive factors and other listener variables (e.g., motivation, cooperation, and perhaps language impairment) play a role in the depressed central auditory processing abilities of some persons with TBI. Clinical experience and research in children with APDs consistently confirms the likelihood of comorbid conditions, often referred to as coexisting disorders.[12,17] In pediatric populations, including children with a history of head injury, language and cognitive impairments are among the two disorders most commonly coexisting with auditory processing deficits. One might reasonably ask whether poor performance on demanding listening tests in persons with mTBI reflects a true auditory deficit or, rather, whether the poor test performance is a product of injury-related cognitive and/or language impairment. With selection of an appropriate battery of auditory tests and with careful analysis of patterns of test performance, it is usually possible to verify that abnormal performance is indeed specific to the auditory system (see Table 9.1). In addition, studies of central auditory function measured electrophysiological techniques, such as the ABR and cortical auditory evoked responses, provide objective evidence of auditory specific dysfunction within the CNS.[18–20]

One point must be reemphasized at this juncture. The research literature provides ample support for the inclusion of measures of central auditory processing within the test battery for hearing assessment of persons with TBI. The test battery for auditory assessment in TBI should routinely include multiple behavioral and objective procedures for documenting peripheral and CNS dysfunction. Findings from these tests have diagnostic value, and they contribute importantly to decisions on rehabilitation of persons with TBI.

Rehabilitation Options for Auditory Dysfunction

Strategies and techniques for management and treatment of persons with HL and other auditory disorders in persons with mTBI vary depending on the type and extent of auditory dysfunction. Of course, a substantial proportion of persons with TBI sustain damage in multiple regions of the auditory system from the TM in the middle ear to the temporal lobe in the cerebral cortex.

These persons will obtain maximum benefit only if a variety of rehabilitation options are implemented by a multidisciplinary team of medical and nonmedical health professions.[7–9] Rehabilitation options for auditory disorders secondary to TBI are summarized in Table 9.2.

Surgical management is usually the most appropriate option for persons with middle ear disorders, such as TM perforation or discontinuity of the ossicular chain.[21] Bone anchor hearing aids and middle ear implants may provide considerable communication benefits for persons with permanent conductive HL (see Table 9.2). Not surprisingly, trauma sufficient to produce significant structural damage to the TM and middle ear often results in inner ear dysfunction.

First-line management for one of the most common types of auditory dysfunction, permanent sensory HL due to inner ear damage, is a combination of counseling and hearing aid use (see Table 9.2). Hearing aid technology has advanced remarkably in recent years. Small, discrete, digitally programmable hearing aids are readily available to persons with documented HL. Almost all persons with sensory HL will enjoy enhanced communication with proper amplification. The benefits of amplification are optimized when combined with family-centered audiological counseling that includes educational information about the HL and hearing aid use plus personal adjustment counseling to improve acceptance of amplification. On occasion, severe head trauma produces a profound bilateral permanent HL that cannot be adequately managed even with powerful amplification. Cochlear implantation, along with intensive rehabilitation, is generally a viable and beneficial option for this relatively small population of persons with TBI.

As noted in Table 9.2, there are now a number of effective nonmedical options for intervention in persons with central APDs following TBI. Research in recent years has confirmed the effectiveness of rehabilitation for APDs.[17] Taking advantage of the well-established principle of neural plasticity, these options for treatment and management can produce lasting improvements in central auditory nervous system function and, therefore, effective and efficient communication skills. The use of frequency modulated (FM) technology to improve speech perception in noise and computer-based auditory training programs can produce remarkable improvements in relatively short periods of time. There is growing appreciation for the importance and effectiveness of these approaches in the rehabilitation of persons following TBI.[7–9,16]

TABLE 9.2
Summary of Options for Rehabilitation of TBI Patients With Auditory Dysfunction.

PERIPHERAL AUDITORY DYSFUNCTION

Hearing Aids (Amplification)

- Digital technology amplifies intensity of speech and other sounds to improve audibility (ability to hear even faint sounds)
- An option for persons with permanent sensory hearing loss that interferes with communication
- A variety hearing aid styles and features are available
- Audiologists custom program or "fit" hearing aids for patients with different degrees and configurations of hearing loss

Cochlear Implants

- Surgical implantation of device to electrically stimulate auditory nerve
- An option for patients with permanent profound sensory hearing loss or deafness
- Audiologist programs cochlear implants for maximum benefit of each patient
- Intensive auditory rehabilitation is required following implantation

Other Implantable Devices

- bone anchored hearing aid for patients with conductive or mixed hearing loss
- middle ear implantable hearing aids for patients with conductive or sensory hearing loss

Hearing Assistance Technology

- FM technology with remote microphones to enhance communication by improving speaker-to-noise difference
- Hearing aid compatible telephones including Bluetooth technology with smartphones
- Text telephones for transcription of spoken speech
- Devices for amplification of sound from television and real-time captioning

Audiological (Aural) Rehabilitation

- Counseling about hearing loss including information (education) counseling to explain hearing loss and management options and personal adjustment counseling to help patient and family adjust to and maximally manage the hearing loss
- Instruction in compensatory strategies to enhance communication
- Speech (lip) reading instruction
- Group aural rehabilitation classes

CENTRAL AUDITORY DYSFUNCTION (AUDITORY PROCESSING DISORDERS)

FM Technology

- Remote microphone (s) for speaker (s) and earpieces for patient to enhance speaker speech in noisy listening settings
- Group amplification systems for enhanced communication during classroom instruction, meetings, etc.

Compensatory Techniques and Strategies

- Instruction in compensatory strategies to enhance communication

Auditory Training

- Computer-based auditory training programs to improve multiple auditory processing skills, e.g., speech perception in noise and temporal auditory processing
- Auditory training for specific deficits, e.g., dichotic listening programs

Post-Traumatic Tinnitus and Disorders of Sound Tolerance

Discussion of HL and related disorders in TBI would not be complete without mention of tinnitus and disorders of decreased sound tolerance. Briefly, tinnitus is the perception of sound in the absence of an external sound source.[12,22] It is sometimes referred to as a "phantom auditory perception." However, imaging and electrophysiological studies have confirmed clinical impressions that tinnitus is associated with neural activity in the auditory system, much like activity produced by the perception of external sounds. The origin of tinnitus is most often damage to the inner ear although tinnitus may also result from brain injury without inner ear dysfunction. Bothersome and even debilitating tinnitus invariably includes a physiological and psychological reaction to the tinnitus sound that is mediated in regions of the CNS not traditionally associated with auditory pathways, specifically the limbic system and the autonomic nervous system.

Tinnitus is a very common health complaint of persons with TBI. Among veterans, tinnitus and HL are the first and second most common service-connected disabilities, respectively. Furthermore, the comorbidity of bothersome tinnitus and/or reduced tolerance to loud sounds, and post-traumatic stress disorder (PTSD) following brain injury is also now well recognized.[11,23] It is important to point out that some persons with TBI who experience debilitating problems with reduced tolerance to everyday sounds have no complaints of tinnitus.[23–25]

The topic of tinnitus in persons with TBI warrants at least a book chapter, if not an entire book. Here, we will briefly make the three simple points: (1) Tinnitus and/or disorders of sound tolerance are real in persons with TBI and they warrant immediate medical and audiological attention, (2) Persons complaining of bothersome tinnitus and/or disorders of sound tolerance in persons with TBI should always be referred to audiology and otolaryngology for formally diagnostic auditory evaluation to include an index of the impact of either or both disorders on quality of life, and (3) Evidence-based effective and efficient management strategies should be implemented for patients diagnosed with bothersome tinnitus and/or disorders of sound tolerance, including, for example, audiological counseling, progressive tinnitus management,[26–30] and cognitive behavioral therapy.

VESTIBULAR DYSFUNCTION AFTER CONCUSSION/MTBI IN ADULTS

The vestibular system is known as a sensorimotor system with numerous functions such as detection of motion and position of the head and body, maintenance of balance and equilibrium of the body, orientation in space, ocular stability during movement, multisensory integration, and higher-level cognitive-perceptual functions. Surprisingly, the vestibular, vision, and somatosensory/proprioception input all contribute to balance in this multimodal system. As a result of concussion/mTBI, patients may experience a variety of vestibular symptoms, including vertigo, dizziness, lightheadedness, imbalance, unsteadiness, clumsiness, visual disorientation, and altered spatial orientation through structural/cellular damage to the vestibular system and/or due to functional/psychiatric causes.

Among a sample of Post-9/11 veterans evaluated for deployment-related TBI, 22.4% self-reported vestibular impairment. Among these veterans, 20.7% self-reported either dual sensory impairment (DSI) or multisensory impairment (MSI) that included the auditory and/or visual domains.[31] Although vestibular dysfunction has been reported as a problem following blast-related mTBI,[32] symptom complaints of feeling dizzy or loss of balance did not differ among veterans with blast- or non–blast-related TBI. This may be a function of recovery over time, since veterans were assessed months to years after any deployment-related injuries.

In a study that included objective vestibular testing, different symptom profiles were associated with blunt and blast trauma among those with mTBI. Compared to those with blunt trauma, individuals with blast exposure exhibited more constant imbalance problems, significant headache, and disequilibrium.[32] A review of vestibular disorders after TBI revealed that blast TBI appears to induce diffused damage to the vestibular and balance system from peripheral to central.[33] Regarding sports-related concussion, dizziness/balance difficulties were reported in 77% of college football players at the time of injury, and were the second common concussion-related symptoms, following headache.[34] Dizziness/balance symptoms are fairly common complaints after a sports-related concussion in high school and university student athletes.[35]

The majority of patients with vestibular dysfunction following mTBI recover spontaneously due to vestibular compensation, but some develop chronic and persistent vestibular symptoms, which are associated with preinjury factors (i.e., age, gender, concussion history, other preexisting factors), injury-related factors (i.e., amnesia/loss of consciousness, dizziness, behavioral, headaches/migraines), and postinjury comorbidities (i.e., anxiety, depression, pain, PTSD).[36] One study reported that 59% of patients with untreated mTBI had persistent vertigo 5 year post injury,[37] and 32% of patients who had minor head injury reported dizziness at 5 years post injury.[38] Unfortunately, many patients with chronic vertigo following concussion are unable to return to work. Another study reported psychological distress (significantly higher anxiety and depression), greater psychosocial dysfunction, and failure to return to work after mild to moderate TBI.[39] It was noted that vestibular dysfunction may generate anxiety since the vestibular system is capable of generating strong negative emotions due to its close alignment to the noradrenergic and limbic systems. Therefore, we need to be aware that consequences of vestibular symptoms following concussion/mTBI could be profound.

Vestibular Symptoms After Concussion/mTBI

Common complaints from patients with concussion/mTBI history are vertigo, dizziness, and imbalance. These symptoms could be intermittent, episodic, or persistent, and their onset may be immediate or delayed. Severity of the symptoms ranges from mild to very severe, and the vestibular symptoms may be spontaneous or activated by specific triggers such as body/head position and vision/sound introduction. In addition, different types of nystagmus (rapid involuntary eye movements) may be accompanied with other vestibular symptoms.

The term "dizzy" reported by a patient in a clinical setting implies and covers numerous symptoms. It is very important to understand as a clinician what "dizzy" is referring to. According to the Bárány Society, key vestibular symptoms are categorized into four types (vertigo, dizziness, vestibulovisual symptoms, and postural symptoms) and their subtypes (Table 9.3). Vertigo and dizziness are further classified into spontaneous or triggered. It is encouraged that universally understandable medical language be used to document patients' description of their symptoms.

Pathology of Vestibular Dysfunction After Concussion/mTBI

In general, peripheral vestibular pathology can be unilateral/bilateral and involve the peripheral vestibular end organs and/or central vestibular nerves. Dizziness/imbalance after concussion/mTBI may be related to damage to the peripheral vestibular system produced by head injury, but the pathophysiologic mechanism of trauma to the peripheral vestibular system is not

TABLE 9.3
Vestibular Symptom Terms and Definitions According to the Bárány Society.

Symptom	Definition	Subtypes
Vertigo	Sensation of motion of self when no motion is present or altered sensation of motion when motion occurs. The motion sensation may be rotary, translational, or tilt. A similar sensation of motion of the environment is a vestibulovisual symptom (external vertigo)	Spontaneous vertigo Triggered vertigo • Positional vertigo • Head-motion vertigo • Visually induced vertigo • Sound-induced vertigo • Valsalva-induced vertigo • Orthostatic vertigo • Other triggered vertigo
Dizziness	A disturbed or altered sensation of spatial orientation without false or altered movement	Spontaneous dizziness Triggered dizziness • Positional dizziness • Head-motion dizziness • Visually induced dizziness • Sound-induced dizziness • Valsalva-induced dizziness • Orthostatic dizziness • Other triggered dizziness
Vestibulovisual symptoms	Visual symptoms that result from vestibular pathology or visual-vestibular interactions. Symptoms arising from ocular pathology are not included	External vertigo Oscillopsia Visual lag Visual tilt Movement-induced blur
Postural symptoms	Balance-related symptoms that occur while in an upright posture. For example, unsteadiness is a sensation of swaying or rocking when sitting, standing, or walking. Symptoms that occur only when changing positions (e.g., standing up from sitting) are classified as orthostatic, not postural	Unsteadiness Directional pulsion Balance-related near-fall Balance-related fall

From Bisdorff A. Vestibular symptoms and history taking. *Handb Clin Neurol.* 2016;137:83–90; with permission.

well understood except for temporal bone fracture. Blast exposure could cause rupture of the saccule and utricle. Benign paroxysmal positional vertigo (BPPV) was reported to be the most common vestibular disorder following head injury. Other peripheral pathology associated with mTBI is labyrinthine concussion, posttraumatic Meniere's disease, perilymphatic fistula, and superior canal dehiscence syndrome.

Regarding central vestibular pathology, dizziness following mTBI is reported to result from brain injury or central dysfunction,[40] but the precise mechanism is unknown. Abnormal postural stability is a common complaint following head trauma or blast exposure and may suggest multisensory or central involvement. It is also known that mTBI can cause white matter abnormalities and diffuse axonal injury.[41] Moreover, ocular motor dysfunction indicated by saccadic dysmetria, gaze-evoked nystagmus, or saccadic pursuit after concussion/mTBI may be indicative of damage to CNS pathways (i.e., cerebral hemispheres, cerebellum, and brainstem).

Vestibular Assessment After Concussion/ mTBI

The diagnosis of vestibular function is very complex since the vestibular system involves a multimodal and multilevel process. Proper management of the vestibular symptoms requires ruling out nonvestibular causes of dizziness such as orthostatic hypotension, cervical vertigo, postconcussion syndrome, TBI, ototoxic drug exposure, and visual impairment. Generally, assessment of vestibular dysfunction consists of case history, vestibular physical examination, targeted computerized testing, radiology testing including targeted computerized tomography scanning or magnetic resonance imaging, and administration of questionnaires such as the Dizziness Handicap Inventory[42] and Activities-Specific Balance Confidence scale.[43]

Head trauma is known to cause BPPV (positional vertigo) by dislodging otoconia from the utricular otolithic membrane, collecting in the semicircular canals (SCs). Typical symptoms of BPPV is recurrent brief episodes of vertigo (a spinning sensation) when a head position is changed (i.e., rolling over in bed). Diagnosis of BPPV is usually obtained by the Dix-Hallpike test.

Following the physical examination, quantification of vestibular deficits can be performed using targeted computerized testing. Both peripheral and central pathology should be ruled out. Typically, a combination of different types of targeted testing is employed for comprehensive assessment of vestibular dysfunction (Fig. 9.2), including videonystagmography, rotational chair testing, subjective visual vertical, video head impulse testing, vestibular evoked myogenic potential, computerized dynamic visual acuity and Gaze Stability Test, and computerized dynamic posturography. Audiometric and visual assessments in combination with vestibular evaluation are considered to be important to rule out DSI/MSI. For those who need further information, refer to free webinars available for vestibular

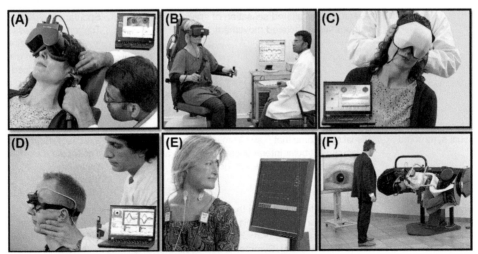

FIG. 9.2 Examples of targeted computerized testing for vestibular dysfunction. **(A)** videonystagmography caloric test; **(B)** rotational chair testing; **(C)** subjective visual vertical; **(D)** video head impulse testing; **(E)** vestibular evoked myogenic potential; **(F)** TRV chair for benign paroxysmal positional vertigo; with permission by Interacoustics A/S, Denmark.

assessments from Interacoustics Academy website[44] or a comprehensive textbook.[45]

Management and Rehabilitation of Vestibular Dysfunction After Concussion/mTBI

Based on the proper diagnosis, physicians consider the best options for individuals with vestibular dysfunction to manage and rehabilitate the symptoms. Typical treatment options include pharmacologic intervention, vestibular rehabilitation, surgical treatment for disabling dizziness and vertigo, and psychologic intervention.

Recommendations for dizziness and balance dysfunction through exercises existed as early as the 1950s and nowadays physicians and therapists have been practicing vestibular rehabilitation therapy in many countries. Ideally, an interdisciplinary team approach should be taken by including physicians (otolaryngologist, neurologist, psychiatrist) and comedicals (audiologist and either a physical or occupational therapist) due to the complex nature of these conditions.[46] Evidence strongly suggests that an individualized, specific, and targeted vestibular exercise program is better than a generic one.[47]

Prior to initiating vestibular exercises in rehabilitation, it is important to rule out BPPV. In a recent medical record review of positional vertigo following head injury versus idiopathic BPPV, TBI-related BPPV accounted for 8.5%−20% of all BPPV cases.[48] The treatment of BPPV called canalith repositioning treatment is well established and widely used. Different methods for repositioning are employed, depending on which SC is involved. For example, BPPV of the posterior SC is treated by the maneuver described by Epley.[49] Recently, mechanical canal positioning device was introduced (Fig. 9.2F), which made the maneuver easier to perform.[50]

A Cochrane review revealed moderate to strong evidence that vestibular rehabilitation is effective for unilateral peripheral vestibular dysfunction (i.e., canalith repositioning maneuvers for BPPV, vestibular rehabilitation for balance and impairment of the vestibulo-ocular reflex).[51] Moreover, two guidelines reported the effectiveness of BPPV treatment using vestibular rehabilitation. There is additional evidence that vestibular rehabilitation following concussion/mTBI is effective.[52−56] However, compared to peripheral vestibular dysfunction, rehabilitation for central vestibular dysfunction was reported to show insufficient compensation, longer treatment, and progression at slower rate.[57] In addition, some emerging evidence in sport-related concussion suggests that earlier activity rather than rest may be warranted for optimal recovery following head injury.[58] For further information regarding vestibular rehabilitation specific to concussion/mTBI population, refer to review papers[36,59] and a textbook specific to vestibular rehabilitation is also available.[60]

As discussed earlier, there is a possibility that vestibular dysfunction may generate anxiety. Anxiety management and behavioral/cognitive therapy may be used concurrently to enhance the effectiveness of vestibular rehabilitation in the mTBI population. It should also be noted that vestibular symptoms such as vertigo, dizziness, and unsteadiness may result from functional and psychiatric disorders.[61] If any signs are observed, referral to a specialist is warranted to better determine etiology.

Fig. 9.3 shows a clinical algorithm for vestibular dysfunction following mTBI provided by the Defense Centers of Excellence (DCoE) for Psychological Health and TBI (open to public at https://pueblo.gpo.gov/DVBIC/pdf/DV-9004.pdf). A review of published literature along with the proceedings of a consensus conference was the basis of this recommendation. Another clinical algorithm is available for diagnosis and management of dizziness in the emergency department at https://www.ncbi.nlm.nih.gov/pmc/articles/PMC2676794/pdf/nihms102245.pdf [62] and Water Reed Army Medical Center is also providing a clinical algorithm for blast-related TBI and vestibular dysfunction.[63]

VISUAL DYSFUNCTION AFTER CONCUSSION/MTBI
Visual Impairment and TBI

The goal of vision rehabilitation is to restore function in individuals who are blind or visually impaired so they may independently engage in activities of daily living. The National Eye Institute[64] indicates that more than two-thirds of individuals with visual impairment are older than 65 years, and the leading causes include age-related macular degeneration, glaucoma, and diabetic retinopathy. Visual impairment can be due to birth defects, aging, disease complication, or acquired through injury.[64] For more than a decade, the effects of visual impairment among Post-9/11 veterans has been a keen interest, as general military and combat conditions have placed US service members at increased risk for ocular trauma or damage to the visual pathway through blast, projectile (e.g., shrapnel, bullets), or blunt force exposures (e.g., motor vehicle accident), which may also lead to mTBI. Recent research has shown that among a cohort of Post-9/11 service

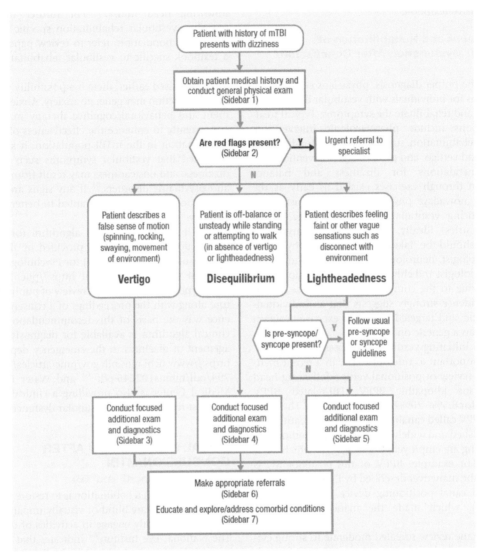

FIG. 9.3 Clinical algorithm for vestibular dysfunction following mTBI. For information about Sidebar 1 to 7, visit website below. (From Defense Centers of Excellence (DCoE) for Psychological Health and TBI. *Assessment and Management of Dizziness Associated with mTBI. DCoE Clinical Recommendation*, September 2012. Publicly available at https://pueblo.gpo.gov/DVBIC/pdf/DV-9004.pdf.)

members with deployment-related mTBI, there was a high prevalence of visual symptoms (subjective visual complaints, blurred vision at near, reading problems, eye strain, light sensitivity) and visual dysfunctions (post-trauma vision syndrome, accommodative deficit, vergence deficit, vertical deviation, version deficit, visual field defect, and diplopia).[65] There was also high prevalence of dizziness, which was more common in

blast-related mTBI compared to non–blast-related mTBI, as well as headache, which was not significantly associated with injury mechanism.[65] Although ocular diagnoses in this mTBI cohort were low, those with blast-related mTBI were more likely to have dry eye, retinopathies, and optic neuropathies relative to those with nonblast exposure. Capo-Aponte and colleagues[65] noted that one-third of the patients had significant visual sequelae and complaints more than 1 year post injury, emphasizing the need for specialized vision rehabilitation care in the military and VA.

In another sample of Post-9/11 Veterans with TBI history, with or without co-occurring PTSD, objectively measured binocular and oculomotor function deficits were prevalent and did not differ as a function of PTSD.[66] However, on subjective measures of visual problems, compared to Veterans with TBI alone, a higher rate of Veterans with TBI and comorbid PTSD reported problems with light sensitivity, blurred vision, reading performance deficits, and diplopia. Because of the high prevalence of co-occurring TBI and PTSD in Post-9/11 Veterans, clinicians treating this population should be aware of the influence of comorbid conditions when considering diagnosis and treatment. Veterans who experience injury to the brain, damage to other organ systems, and events that lead to psychological trauma will benefit from an interdisciplinary team approach to help interpret sensory and other deficits.[67] An algorithm that provides clinical recommendations for eye and vision care for service members or veterans with a history of blast exposure and/or possible TBI may be seen in Fig. 9.4.

DSI in Civilian and General Veteran Samples
One combination of DSI is impaired hearing and vision, a condition in which orientation to and interaction with one's surroundings can be compromised, thus negatively impacting quality of life. DSI is thought to cause more impairment than either auditory or visual impairment alone,[68] and can affect the patient's ability to optimally participate in rehabilitation. In adults 65 years and older, DSI is associated with numerous negative health outcomes, including communication difficulty, cognitive decline, dementia, depression, functional impairment, and reports of loneliness.[69–71] In a nationally representative sample of nearly 200,000 US adults, self-report data revealed a 3.3% DSI prevalence, ranging from 1.3% in those 18–44 years old, to 16.6% in those 80 years and older.[72] In a separate nationally representative sample of US adults in which objective assessments of hearing and vision were reviewed, it was estimated that 1.5 million Americans 20 years or older had DSI, with the highest percentage observed among those 80 years or older (11.3%).[73] DSI was observed in less than 1% of those younger than 70 years. Finally, in a retrospective review of 400 out of 1472 Veterans who were enrolled in Department of Veterans Affairs (VA) audiology and optometry outpatient clinics, overall DSI prevalence ranged from 5.0% to 7.4%, depending on the

operational definition of auditory impairment, as measured by either pure tone average (PTA) or high-frequency PTA (HFPTA).[74] DSI prevalence was 0% among Veterans less than 65 years, but on average ranged from 1% (PTA) to 4% (HFPTA) among those 65–74 years, 9% (PTA) to 13% (HFPTA) among those 75–84 years, and 22% (PTA) to 26% (HFPTA) among those 85 years and older. Altogether, these subjective and objective prevalence rates, stratified by age group, were similar across civilian and Veteran samples and suggest that DSI is relatively uncommon and primarily observed among those in their 80s and higher.

DSI in Post-9/11 Veterans
Among Post-9/11 Veteran cohorts that were younger than 40 years, self-report and clinical evaluation data revealed a different DSI pattern from those described above. In a sample of 62 Post-9/11 Veterans with blast-related TBI (mean age = 27.3, SD = 7.0 years) who were admitted to a VA Polytrauma Rehabilitation Center, each received an audiology and vision assessment. For the audiology consult, each Veteran underwent immittance and PTA evaluation. HL was classified based on the poorest audiometric threshold in the poorer ear, and categorized as mild: 26–40 dB; moderate: 41–60 dB; severe: 61–90 dB; and profound: >90 dB. For visual assessments, ICD-9 levels of moderate, severe, and profound visual impairment were combined into a "visual impairment" category, based on visual acuity ranging from <20/63 to 20/1000. Those with hemianopsia comparable with a visual impairment of <20 degrees were also categorized as being impaired, and blindness was classified as a visual acuity of <20/1000 or bilateral enucleation. Based on these classifications, 19% had hearing impairment only, 34% had vision impairment only, and 32% had DSI.[75] DSI was associated with reduced gain in total functional independence[76] between admission and discharge. Similarly, in an outpatient sample of 21,627 Post-9/11 Veterans who completed a VA Comprehensive TBI Evaluation, 12,521 were determined to have experienced deployment-related TBI, and 9106 did not have any TBI history. Categorization of auditory and hearing impairment were based on self-report of moderate to very severe problems on two Neurobehavioral Symptom Inventory (NSI)[77] items: "hearing difficulty" and "vision problems, blurring, trouble seeing," respectively. DSI was self-reported to be between 22.7% (no TBI or blast exposure) to 35.4% (TBI and blast exposure).[78] Across the sample, self-reported sensory impairment rates were 34.6% for DSI, 31.3% for auditory impairment only,

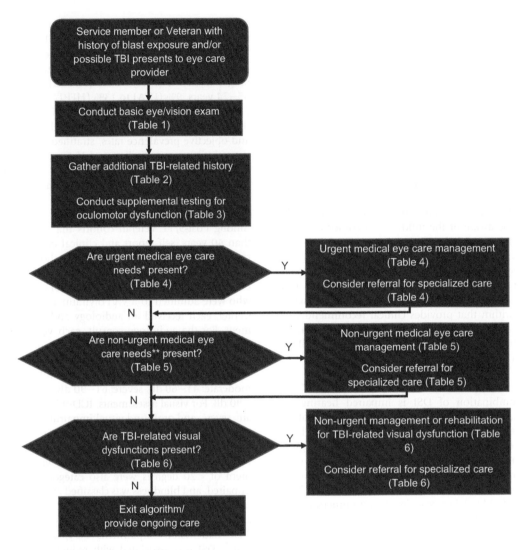

*Urgent medical eye care needs: Conditions indicating possible ocular, cranial nerve or structural brain injury, which may be sight- or life-threatening, that require immediate management by the eye care provider and/or referral to more specific specialized care

**Non-urgent medical eye care needs: Potentially chronic eye or visual conditions for which management by the eye care provider or referral to more specific specialized care may be addressed over a course of time

FIG. 9.4 Algorithm for eye and vision care following blast exposure and/or possible traumatic brain injury. The "Clinical Recommendation for Eye Care Providers: Eye and Vision Care Following Blast Exposure and/or Possible Traumatic Brain Injury" is from the Department of Defense Walter Reed National Military Medical Center Vision Center of Excellence. (For information about Tables 1–6, visit the publicly available website at: https://vce.health.mil/Clinicians-and-Researchers/Clinical-Practice-Recommendations/Eye-Care-and-TBI.)

9.9% for visual impairment only, and 24.2% for none to mild sensory impairment, again suggesting a high rate of perceived DSI in a young (mean age = 31.3, SD = 8.6 years) Veteran cohort.

Understanding and Anticipating Current and Future Rehabilitation Needs

There are clear differences in methodology (clinical evaluation vs. self-report), sampling (inpatient vs. outpatient, civilian vs. Veteran), and definitions of impairment among the abovementioned DSI studies. Notwithstanding, the VA and other medical facilities that provide audiology and vision treatment to Post-9/11 Veterans must understand their current clinical profile and rehabilitation needs. Saunders and Echt[68] describe research and practical considerations in various domains, including training providers to recognize DSI, communicating important health information clearly to patients with DSI, and maximizing their adherence to instructions. As the DSI literature reviewed above was primarily cross-sectional, it is critical for future research to study long-term outcomes of DSI among the Post-9/11 Veteran cohort: how sensory impairment progresses with age, and how it may manifest or interact with TBI, PTSD, and other co-occurring conditions that are common in this cohort, so that clinicians can meet the future rehabilitation needs of this complex population.

REFERENCES

1. Honeybrook A, Patki A, Chapurin N, Woodard C. Hearing and mortality outcomes following temporal bone fractures. *Craniomaxillofacial Trauma Reconstr.* 2017;10(4):281−285.
2. Hall III JW, Huangfu M, Gennarelli TA, Dolinskas CA, Olson K, Berry GA. Auditory evoked responses, impedance measures, and diagnostic speech audiometry in severe head injury. *Otolaryngol Head Neck Surg.* 1983;91(1):50−60.
3. Lew HL, Jerger JF, Guillory SB, Henry JA. Auditory dysfunction in traumatic brain injury. *J Rehabil Res Dev.* 2007;44(7):921−928.
4. Gallun FJ, Diedesch AC, Kubli LR, et al. Performance on tests of central auditory processing by individuals exposed to high-intensity blasts. *J Rehabil Res Dev.* 2012;49(7):1005−1025.
5. Gallun FJ, Lewis MS, Folmer RL, et al. Implications of blast exposure for central auditory function: a review. *J Rehabil Res Dev.* 2012;49(7):1059−1074.
6. Chen JX, Lindeborg M, Herman SD, et al. Systematic review of hearing loss after traumatic brain injury without associated temporal bone fracture. *Am J Otolaryngol.* 2018;39(3):338−344.
7. Meyers PJ, Wilmington DJ, Gallun FJ, Henry JA, Fausti SA. Hearing impairment and traumatic brain injury among soldiers: special considerations. *Semin Hear.* 2009;30:5−27.
8. Fausti SA, Wilmington DJ, Gallun FJ, Myers PJ, Henry JA. Auditory and vestibular dysfunction associated with blast-related traumatic brain injury. *J Rehabil Res Dev.* 2009;46(6):797−810.
9. Gallun FJ, Papesh MA, Lewis MS. Hearing complaints among veterans following traumatic brain injury. *Brain Inj.* 2017;31(9):1183−1187.
10. Oleksiak M, Smith BM, St Andre JR, Caughlan CM, Steiner M. Audiological issues and hearing loss among Veterans with mild traumatic brain injury. *J Rehabil Res Dev.* 2012;49(7):995−1004.
11. Swan AA, Nelson JT, Swiger B, et al. Prevalence of hearing loss and tinnitus in Iraq and Afghanistan veterans: a chronic effects of Neurotrauma Consortium study. *Hear Res.* June 2017;349:4−12.
12. Hall III JW. *Introduction to Audiology Today.* Boston, MA: Pearson Educational; 2014.
13. Lew HL, Tanaka C, Hirohata E, Goodrich GL. Auditory, vestibular, and visual impairments. In: Cifu DX, ed. *Braddom's Physical Medicine and Rehabilitation.* 5th ed. Philadelphia: Elsevier; 2016:1137−1161.
14. Hall III JW. *eHandbook of Auditory Evoked Responses.* Kindle Direct Publishing; 2015. e as a digital eBook from Amazon.com using this link: http://www.amazon.com/dp/B0145G2FFM.
15. Dhar S, Hall III JW. *Otoacoustic Emissions: Principles, Procedures, and Procedures.* San Diego, CA: Plural Publishing; 2018.
16. Hoover EC, Souza PE, Gallun FJ. Auditory and cognitive factors associated with speech-in-noise complaints following mild traumatic brain injury. *J Am Acad Audiol.* 2017;28(4):325−339.
17. American Academy of Audiology Clinical Practice Guidelines. *Diagnosis and Management of Children and Adults with Central Auditory Processing Disorder.* August 2010.
18. Harris DP, Hall 3rd JW. Feasibility of auditory event-related potential measurement in brain injury rehabilitation. *Ear Hear.* 1990;11(5):340−350.
19. Lew HL, Lee EH, Pan SS, Date ES. Electrophysiologic abnormalities of auditory and visual information processing in patients with traumatic brain injury. *Am J Phys Med Rehabil.* 2004;83(6):428−433.
20. Vander Werff KR, Rieger B. Brainstem evoked potential indices of subcortical auditory processing after mild traumatic brain injury. *Ear Hear.* 2017;38(4):e200−e214.
21. Diaz RC, Cervenka B, Brodie HA. Treatment of temporal bone fractures. *J Neurol Surg B Skull Base.* 2016;77(5):419−429.
22. Baguley D, McFerran D, Hall D. Tinnitus. *Lancet.* 2013;382(9904):1600−1607.
23. Moring JC, Peterson AL, Kanzler KE. Tinnitus, traumatic brain injury, and posttraumatic stress disorder in the military. *Int J Behav Med.* 2018;25(3):312−321.
24. Landon J, Shepherd D, Stuart S, Theadom A, Freundlich S. Hearing every footstep: noise sensitivity in individuals

following traumatic brain injury. *Neuropsychol Rehabil.* 2012;22(3):391−407.

25. Callahan ML, Binder LM, O'Neil ME, et al. Sensory sensitivity in operation enduring freedom/operation Iraqi freedom veterans with and without blast exposure and mild traumatic brain injury. *Appl Neuropsychol Adult.* 2018;25(2):126−136.

26. Henry JA, Zaugg TL, Schechter MA. Clinical guide for audiologic tinnitus management I: assessment. *Am J Audiol.* 2005;14(1):21−48.

27. Henry JA, Zaugg TL, Schechter MA. Clinical guide for audiologic tinnitus management II: treatment. *Am J Audiol.* 2005;14(1):49−70.

28. Henry JA, Zaugg TL, Myers PM, Kendall CJ. *How to Manage Your Tinnitus: A Step-by-step Workbook.* 3rd ed. San Diego, CA: Plural Publishing; 2010.

29. Henry JA, Zaugg TL, Myers PM, Kendall CJ. *Progressive Tinnitus Management: Clinical Handbook for Audiologists.* San Diego, CA: Plural Publishing; 2010.

30. Henry JA, Thielman EJ, Zaugg TL, et al. Telephone-based progressive tinnitus management for persons with and without traumatic brain injury: a randomized controlled trial. *Ear Hear.* 2019. https://doi.org/10.1097/AUD.0000000000000609.

31. Pogoda TK, Hendricks AM, Iverson KM, et al. Multisensory impairment reported by veterans with and without mild traumatic brain injury history. *J Rehabil Res Dev.* 2012;49(7):971−984.

32. Hoffer ME, Balaban C, Gottshall K, Balough BJ, Maddox MR, Penta JR. Blast exposure: vestibular consequences and associated characteristics. *Otol Neurotol.* 2010;31(2):232−236.

33. Franke LM, Walker WC, Cifu DX, Ochs AL, Lew HL. Sensorintegrative dysfunction underlying vestibular disorders after traumatic brain injury: a review. *J Rehabil Res Dev.* 2012;49(7):985−994.

34. Guskiewicz KM, McCrea M, Marshall SW, et al. Cumulative effects associated with recurrent concussion in collegiate football players: the NCAA Concussion Study. *JAMA.* 2003;290(19):2549−2555.

35. Lovell MR, Iverson GL, Collins MW, et al. Measurement of symptoms following sports-related concussion: reliability and normative data for the post-concussion scale. *Appl Neuropsychol.* 2006;13(3):166−174.

36. Gurley JM, Hujsak BD, Kelly JL. Vestibular rehabilitation following mild traumatic brain injury. *NeuroRehabilitation.* 2013;32(3):519−528.

37. Berman JM, Fredrickson JM. Vertigo after head injury–a five year follow-up. *J Otolaryngol.* 1978;7(3):237−245.

38. Masson F, Maurette P, Salmi LR, et al. Prevalence of impairments 5 years after a head injury, and their relationship with disabilities and outcome. *Brain Inj.* 1996;10(7):487−497.

39. Chamelian L, Feinstein A. Outcome after mild to moderate traumatic brain injury: the role of dizziness. *Arch Phys Med Rehabil.* 2004;85(10):1662−1666.

40. Schultz BA, Cifu DX, McNamee S, Nichols M, Carne W. Assessment and treatment of common persistent sequelae following blast induced mild traumatic brain injury. *NeuroRehabilitation.* 2011;28(4):309−320.

41. Hayes JP, Miller DR, Lafleche G, Salat DH, Verfaellie M. The nature of white matter abnormalities in blast-related mild traumatic brain injury. *Neuroimage Clin.* 2015;8:148−156.

42. Jacobson GP, Newman CW. The development of the dizziness Handicap inventory. *Arch Otolaryngol Head Neck Surg.* 1990;116(4):424−427.

43. Powell LE, Myers AM. The activities-specific balance confidence (ABC) scale. *J Gerontol A Biol Sci Med Sci.* 1995;50A(1):M28−M34.

44. Interacoustics A/S. Interacoustics academy webinar page. https://www.interacoustics.com/academy/webinars.

45. Jacobson GP, Shepard NT, eds. *Balance Function Assessment and Management.* 2nd ed. San Diego, CA: Plural Publishing; 2016.

46. Whitney SL, Sparto PJ. Principles of vestibular physical therapy rehabilitation. *NeuroRehabilitation.* 2011;29(2):157−166.

47. Black FO, Pesznecker SC. Vestibular adaptation and rehabilitation. *Curr Opin Otolaryngol Head Neck Surg.* 2003;11(5):355−360.

48. Ahn SK, Jeon SY, Kim JP, et al. Clinical characteristics and treatment of benign paroxysmal positional vertigo after traumatic brain injury. *J Trauma.* 2011;70(2):442−446.

49. Epley JM. The canalith repositioning procedure: for treatment of benign paroxysmal positional vertigo. *Otolaryngol Head Neck Surg.* 1992;107(3):399−404.

50. Richard-Vitton T, Petrak M, Beck DL. The TRV chair: introductory concepts. *Hear Rev.* 2013;20(12):52−54.

51. Hillier SL, McDonnell M. Vestibular rehabilitation for unilateral peripheral vestibular dysfunction. *Cochrane Database Syst Rev.* 2011;(2):CD005397.

52. Alsalaheen BA, Mucha A, Morris LO, et al. Vestibular rehabilitation for dizziness and balance disorders after concussion. *J Neurol Phys Ther.* 2010;34(2):87−93.

53. Gottshall KR, Hoffer ME. Tracking recovery of vestibular function in individuals with blast-induced head trauma using vestibular-visual-cognitive interaction tests. *J Neurol Phys Ther.* 2010;34(2):94−97.

54. Weightman MM, Bolgla R, McCulloch KL, Peterson MD. Physical therapy recommendations for service members with mild traumatic brain injury. *J Head Trauma Rehabil.* 2010;25(3):206−218.

55. Moore BM, Adams JT, Barakatt E. Outcomes following a vestibular rehabilitation and aerobic training program to address persistent post-concussion symptoms. *J Allied Health.* 2016;45(4):e59−e68.

56. Kontos AP, Collins MW, Holland CL, et al. Preliminary evidence for improvement in symptoms, cognitive, vestibular, and oculomotor outcomes following targeted intervention with chronic mTBI patients. *Mil Med.* 2018;183(suppl_1):333−338.

57. Shepard NT, Telian SA. Programmatic vestibular rehabilitation. *Otolaryngol Head Neck Surg.* 1995;112(1):173−182.

58. DiFazio M, Silverberg ND, Kirkwood MW, Bernier R, Iverson GL. Prolonged activity restriction after concussion: are we worsening outcomes? *Clin Pediatr.* 2016;55(5): 443–451.

59. Broglio SP, Collins MW, Williams RM, Mucha A, Kontos AP. Current and emerging rehabilitation for concussion: a review of the evidence. *Clin Sports Med.* 2015;34(2):213–231.

60. Herdman SJ, Clendaniel R. *Vestibular Rehabilitation.* 4th ed. Philadelphia: F.A. Davis Co.; 2014.

61. Dieterich M, Staab JP, Brandt T. Functional (psychogenic) dizziness. *Handb Clin Neurol.* 2016;139:447–468.

62. Kerber KA. Vertigo and dizziness in the emergency department. *Emerg Med Clin N Am.* 2009;27(1):39–50 (viii).

63. Scherer MR, Schubert MC. Traumatic brain injury and vestibular pathology as a comorbidity after blast exposure. *Phys Ther.* 2009;89(9):980–992.

64. National Eye Institute. *Vision Research: Needs, Gaps, and Opportunities.* Bethesda, MD: National Institutes of Health; 2012.

65. Capó-Aponte JE, Jorgensen-Wagers KL, Sosa JA, et al. Visual dysfunctions at different stages after blast and non-blast mild traumatic brain injury. *Optom Vis Sci.* 2017; 94(1):7–15.

66. Goodrich GL, Martinsen GL, Flyg HM, Kirby J, Garvert DW, Tyler CW. Visual function, traumatic brain injury, and posttraumatic stress disorder. *J Rehabil Res Dev.* 2014;51(4):547–558.

67. Lew HL, Weihing J, Myers PJ, Pogoda TK, Goodrich GL. Dual sensory impairment (DSI) in trauma brain injury (TBI) - an emerging interdisciplinary challenge. *NeuroRehabilitation.* 2010;26(3):213–222.

68. Saunders GH, Echt KV. An overview of dual sensory impairment in older adults: perspectives for rehabilitation. *Trends Amplif.* 2007;11(4):243–258.

69. Schneider JM, Gopinath B, McMahon CM, Leeder SR, Mitchell P, Wang JJ. Dual sensory impairment in older age. *J Aging Health.* 2011;23(8):1309–1324.

70. Davidson JGS, Guthrie DM. Older adults with a combination of vision and hearing impairment experience higher rates of cognitive impairment, functional dependence, and worse outcomes across a set of quality indicators. *J Aging Health.* August 1, 2017. https://doi.org/10.1177/0898264317723407.

71. Yamada Y, Denkinger MD, Onder G, et al. Dual sensory impairment and cognitive decline: the results from the Shelter study. *J Gerontol A Biol Sci Med Sci.* 2016;71(1): 117–123.

72. Caban AJ, Lee DJ, Gomez-Marin O, Lam BL, Zheng DD. Prevalence of concurrent hearing and visual impairment in US adults: the National Health Interview Survey, 1997-2002. *Am J Public Health.* 2005;95(11):1940–1942.

73. Swenor BK, Ramulu PY, Willis JR, Friedman D, Lin FR. The prevalence of concurrent hearing and vision impairment in the United States. *JAMA Intern Med.* 2013;173(4): 312–313.

74. Smith SL, Bennett LW, Wilson RH. Prevalence and characteristics of dual sensory impairment (hearing and vision) in a veteran population. *J Rehabil Res Dev.* 2008;45(4): 597–609.

75. Lew HL, Garvert DW, Pogoda TK, et al. Auditory and visual impairments in patients with blast-related traumatic brain injury: effect of dual sensory impairment on functional independence measure. *J Rehabil Res Dev.* 2009;46(6): 819–826.

76. Corrigan JD, Smith-Knapp K, Granger CV. Validity of the functional independence measure for persons with traumatic brain injury. *Arch Phys Med Rehabil.* 1997;78(8): 828–834.

77. Cicerone KD, Kalmar K. Persistent postconcussion syndrome: the structure of subjective complaints after mild traumatic brain injury. *J Head Trauma Rehabil.* 1995; 10(3):1–17.

78. Lew HL, Pogoda TK, Baker E, et al. Prevalence of dual sensory impairment and its association with traumatic brain injury and blast exposure in OEF/OIF veterans. *J Head Trauma Rehabil.* 2011;26(6):489–496.

CHAPTER 10

Rehabilitation and Management of Fatigue

THOMAS J. BAYUK, DO • JEFFREY D. LEWIS, MD, PHD

INTRODUCTION

Fatigue is one of the most common symptoms following mild traumatic brain injury (mTBI). In a prospective, case-control study of 122 consecutive mTBI patients assessed in the Emergency Department, fatigue was reported in 22% of patients 3 months following the injury, versus 11% of controls.[1] In this cohort, memory difficulty, sleep disturbance, and fatigue were the most common symptoms, and the severity of symptoms correlated with disability.

The rehabilitation and management of fatigue following mTBI can be challenging, as TBI-related fatigue can be prolonged and refractory to treatment. Measuring response to treatment is limited by the lack of validated outcome measures for fatigue, although we will discuss several self-assessment instruments in this chapter. Another challenge is the relatively few interventional studies for fatigue in mTBI, as most studies include mixed-severity populations of TBI patients or include only moderate to severe TBI. We have included studies completed in more severely injured TBI populations, but will highlight the relatively few studies completed in mTBI patients.

Fatigue is a common symptom in a number of diseases, including multiple sclerosis, chronic pain, and cancer. In fact, a number of the scales used in TBI-related fatigue were originally developed to measure fatigue in multiple sclerosis and cancer. Although several theories for fatigue of central origin have been proposed that may apply universally, it is not known if fatigue following mTBI is mechanistically different from other conditions. Given the potential applicability, however, we include literature regarding fatigue from other neurologic conditions and cancer to discuss interventions for which there are limited data in mTBI.

PATHOPHYSIOLOGY OF TBI-RELATED FATIGUE

The pathophysiology of mTBI is complex and understanding its relationship to fatigue is difficult, and not completely known. In the acute phase following mTBI, cell membrane disruption leads to changes in intra- and extracellular potassium and calcium, as well as fluctuations in the neurotransmitter glutamate.[2] This ultimately leads to disruption of normal cellular function. Changes are also observed in glucose metabolism. Initially, there is an increase in cerebral glucose metabolism, possibly as a response to increased energy needed to restore membrane disruption. This is then followed by a prolonged period of decreased cerebral glucose metabolism, of which the reason and mechanism is not entirely known, although decreases in cerebral blood flow are thought to play a role.[2]

Components of cellular dysfunction that occur after a biomechanical force to the brain have been speculated to cause specific symptoms. Headache may result from the propagation of ionic depolarization very early after an injury. This phenomenon has similar characteristics to the spreading depression, or Leao spread, seen with migraine.[3] Neural dysfunction and axonal injury leading to impaired neurotransmission may be responsible for symptoms of impaired cognition and memory. A definitive underlying mechanism for fatigue as a symptom of mTBI remains elusive, however. While an energy mismatch has been described in the very early phases of the neurometabolic cascade, it is not necessarily linked to fatigue. Neuroinflammation has been proposed as a possible mechanism for TBI-related fatigue; however, there has been an inability to reconcile persistent fatigue following resolution of neuroinflammatory features.[4]

Concussion. https://doi.org/10.1016/B978-0-323-65384-8.00010-9
Copyright © 2020 Elsevier Inc. All rights reserved.

Once normal metabolic rates are restored, etiologies of persistent fatigue become even more elusive. Irreparable microstructural injury to neurofilaments and microtubules may result from shear and stretch of axons during the biomechanical force exerted on the brain during TBI. Subsequent disruption of normal axonal function and neurotransmission may be a contributing factor responsible for various persistent symptoms, seen after an mTBI.[3]

FATIGUE ASSESSMENT INSTRUMENTS

Patients often report fatigue without provider prompting, and the symptom can then be measured with a number of self-report scales. A wide range of fatigue assessment tools are available and have been qualitatively compared in a large review.[5] The most commonly used patient-reported measures of fatigue are based upon a causal formative measurement model, in which fatigue is inferred from responses about functions likely to be affected. Fatigue has been modeled as unidimensional, bidimensional (e.g., cognitive vs. physical), and multidimensional latent construct in the various fatigue measures.

Screening for fatigue can be completed as part of a larger symptom inventory. The Rivermead Postconcussion Questionnaire (RPQ) has items for fatigue (tiring more easily) and sleep disturbance. The questionnaire asks about severity of each symptom compared to preinjury baseline (0 = not experienced at all, 1 = no more of a problem, 2 = a mild problem, 3 = a moderate problem, 4 = a severe problem). The RPQ is a commonly used measure for outcome assessment.[6]

Another commonly used multisymptom measure is the Neurobehavioral Symptom Inventory (NSI). The NSI is structurally similar to the RPQ and asks patients to rate the degree to which symptoms have been disturbing (0 = none, 1 = mild, 2 = moderate, 3 = severe, 4 = very severe). The NSI has separate questions about fatigue and sleep disturbance and asks about severity of symptoms since time of injury.

One limitation of both the RPQ and NSI is that both instruments ask patients to compare symptoms to their preinjury baseline and may be susceptible to recall or attribution bias. Another limitation is that overreporting of postconcussive symptoms has been described with these multisymptom self-report measures,[7] and so the degree of fatigue may be exaggerated.

The Fatigue Severity Scale (FSS) is a self-report, 9-item instrument based upon a causal model of fatigue and asks questions related to physical function, duty performance, and interference with social life. The FSS has been used primarily in studies of moderate to severe TBI, but has been used in mTBI studies as well.[8] A score of 4 or greater is considered to be clinically significant.

An example of a multidimensional fatigue self-report instrument is the Modified Fatigue Impact Scale (MFIS). The MFIS is a 21-item instrument that asks about the effect of fatigue on cognitive, physical, and social functioning. The psychometric properties of the MFIS were determined in a sample of 106 US veterans with a history of mild-moderate TBI (92% mTBI).[9] Using a Principal Components Analysis method, the questions were loaded on two factors, called cognitive and physical/activities. In this study, a cutoff score of 29 for MFIS Total Score provided a sensitivity of 85% and specificity of 80% for differentiating fatigued and nonfatigued patients.

The Visual Analog Scale of Fatigue (VAS-F) is an 18-item inventory asking patients to rate their sense of different experiences expressed on a scale of 0−10 (e.g., not at all tired vs. extremely tired, not at all active vs. extremely active). The construct is different from the other fatigue instruments in that it asks about the direct experience rather than the impact of fatigue on the ability to complete activities of daily living, utilizing a reflective rather than causal model. The VAS-F has been reported to be less sensitive to fatigue in TBI patients than the FSS.[10]

The various fatigue scales tend to be highly intercorrelated. The appropriate choice of scale is dependent upon the intent of the assessment. For screening, one or two questions in a larger symptom inventory may be preferred. In patients with significant fatigue in which repeat assessments are being performed, a unidimensional scale may be useful. For research purposes in which the investigator wishes to determine if an intervention affects different aspects of fatigue, a multidimensional inventory will be most useful.

SLEEP AND TBI-RELATED FATIGUE

Differentiating symptoms of sleep disruption and fatigue is difficult. The term fatigue is often used to describe the effects of various sleep disorders such as insomnia, hypersomnia, obstructive sleep apnea, periodic limb movements, and narcolepsy. Post-traumatic sleep disturbance can occur following TBI, including mTBI. The reported prevalence of post-traumatic sleep disturbance varies from 30% to 70%.[11] This inevitably leads to the co-occurrence of sleep and non–sleep-related fatigue, which can be difficult to distinguish with commonly used fatigue measures.[12] In a cross-sectional study of 334 participants assessed at 1 and 2 years after TBI, insomnia and fatigue occurred together in a significant number of participants; however, fatigue was found more frequently without insomnia.[13] In this study, fatigue was related to disability severity whereas insomnia was not.

Physiologically, fatigue may be described as a lack of energy or inability to participate in an activity. Psychologically, fatigue may be described as a lack of motivation or mental energy. The effects of sleep disruption may be described as drowsiness, or in some sleep disorders as excessive daytime sleepiness which may result in a patient desiring frequent naps or unintentionally falling asleep.[14] One study found increased effort and subsequent energy use in performing tasks was more associated with fatigue rather than disturbed sleep and supported the use of objective sleep studies to distinguish between fatigue and sleep disturbances.[14]

In addition to clinical distinctions, there are also likely pathophysiological distinctions between sleep disturbances and fatigue. Many of the central neurologic structures necessary for appropriate sleep regulation, such as the hypothalamus and midbrain, are at risk for injury during a TBI of any severity. Disruption of these structures may lead to interrupted circadian rhythm and ultimately sleep disorders such as insomnia. In a similar way fatigue may be the result of neuronal injury at multiple structures to include the limbic system and reticular activating system.[15] Slowed processing of various functions such as attention and memory can demand more effort and lead to subjective fatigue as well.[15]

Characterizing sleep disturbances and fatigue is highly subjective and can lead to misdiagnosis and ultimately unnecessary testing and treatments. Unfortunately because of the multiple factors and comorbidities that contribute to these subjective complaints, identification and treatment can be difficult. Both pharmacologic and nonpharmacologic treatment modalities should be considered when approaching sleep disturbances. When considering treatment approaches for fatigue in a patient with co-occurring sleep disturbances after a TBI of any severity, ensure first that the appropriate evaluation has been completed. This includes application of appropriate fatigue and sleep scales and consideration of objective testing with polysomnography, multiple sleep latency testing, and actigraphy as indicated. If specific sleep disorders are identified, treatment can be directed accordingly.[15]

NEUROENDOCRINE DYSFUNCTION AND TBI-RELATED FATIGUE

Fatigue is a common and prevalent symptom of endocrine dysfunction in non-TBI populations, and it has been hypothesized that TBI-associated neuroendocrine dysfunction (NED), most commonly hypopituitarism, may be responsible for certain symptomatology including fatigue.[16]

Hypopituitarism as a result of TBI has been well established, although the actual incidence and prevalence is not entirely certain. The most common reported pituitary deficiency after TBI is growth hormone (GH) deficiency; however, secondary adrenal insufficiency, hypothyroidism, and hypogonadism are also commonly reported, although with considerable variability.[17]

In a prospective cohort study of 70 patients after TBI, 11 patients were identified with GH deficiency or insufficiency and had poorer quality of life scores on the Short Form-36 questionnaire in the areas of energy and fatigue[18] compared to the other patients. One study of 20 male veterans, who sustained an mTBI during combat 8–72 months prior to the start of the study, demonstrated a 25% prevalence of GH deficiency.[19] Another study compared Global Fatigue Index (GFI) and FSS scores with thyroid, adrenal, gonadal, and GH levels following glucagon stimulation in patients with varying degrees of TBI severity at least 1 year after injury.[16] No significant correlations between these hormone levels and fatigue were identified; however, the authors noted a high prevalence of pituitary abnormalities and recommended screening for hypopituitarism. Interestingly there was a direct relationship between higher GH levels and fatigue as compared to prior studies which showed a greater association of fatigue with GH deficiency.[16] A larger study looked at anterior pituitary function and compared it to results from questionnaires on health-related quality of life and fatigue using the Multidimensional Fatigue Inventory (MFI). While overall a very limited relationship was found, an independent relationship between pituitary deficiencies and fatigue in the absence of influencing comorbidities could not be seen.[20]

Recommendations for evaluation of NED vary among studies. The Department of Defense recommends serum screening with morning cortisol, thyroid stimulating hormone (TSH), free thyroxine (T4), insulin-like growth factor (IGF-1), luteinizing hormone (LH), follicle stimulating hormone (FSH), testosterone (males only), and estradiol (females only), when considering NED in patients with various symptoms to include fatigue at least 3 months after mTBI.[21] Additional endocrine evaluation can be considered as clinically indicated.

CHRONIC PAIN AND TBI-RELATED FATIGUE

The correlation between chronic pain and increased fatigue has been well established in the general population,[22] as well as a number of painful conditions such as rheumatoid arthritis.[23] In fact, the relationship between pain and fatigue has been studied much more extensively in cancer and rheumatologic disorders than in TBI, especially mTBI. A longitudinal study of breast cancer survivors found that pain as well as depressive symptoms were significant predictors of posttreatment fatigue.[24] A cross-sectional and longitudinal study of 249 breast cancer survivors also showed an association between pain and chronic and persistent fatigue.[25] A systematic review was conducted to determine which aspects of the rheumatoid arthritis disease process, including pain, are most associated with fatigue. Of all the factors assessed, pain appeared to have the greatest influence, and the authors suggested adequate pain control would also improve fatigue in rheumatoid arthritis.[23]

The type and severity of pain associated with TBI is highly dependent on the mechanism of injury. Where an individual who sustains a sport-related concussion may experience headaches, TBI sustained through a motor vehicle accident or combat-related trauma will also likely experience significant pain in other areas of the body.

Time since injury may also be a factor in pain-related fatigue following TBI. In one longitudinal study investigating the relationship between pain and fatigue, a significant positive correlation was seen between pain ratings and MFI scores at 4 and 8 months after TBI, but not at 12 months.[26] This relationship may be due to the fact that headaches and other forms of pain are greater closer to the time of injury or because individuals adapt to their pain over time.[26]

Ponsford et al. investigated the relationship between pain, as well as other factors, and fatigue following a TBI.[14] Fatigue was measured in a group of 139 patients who suffered mild to severe TBI using the Causes of Fatigue Questionnaire (COF), VAS-F, and FSS. Patients with TBI showed significantly higher pain severity ratings and demonstrated a moderately significant association with fatigue. This study, similar to others, stressed the importance of appropriate assessment and treatment of pain to reduce TBI-related fatigue.

PSYCHIATRIC COMORBIDITY AND TBI-RELATED FATIGUE

Besides physical fatigue, mTBI patients may also exhibit psychological fatigue, which has been proposed as a type of protective mechanism or warning system to prevent further activity and potential exhaustion.[4] There is a clear association between psychological symptoms, such as depression and anxiety, with fatigue; however, the underlying mechanism for the relationship is not known. The degree to which psychological symptoms lead to the subjective experience of fatigue varies considerably between individuals.

One factor that may influence fatigue susceptibility is resilience. Resilience has been defined as a quality that allows an individual to recover faster from adversity. Individuals with resilience appear to have a more positive outlook in negative situations, allowing them to manage those situations more quickly. One study looked at resilience in a group of 74 individuals with mTBI who completed a Resilience Scale at 1, 6, and 12 months post injury.[27] Correlations were found between greater resilience and reduced fatigue, depressive symptoms as well as overall improved quality of life at 6 months. The Barrow Neurological Institute Fatigue Scale (BNI-FSS) was used to assess fatigue in this study. A correlation was also found between greater resilience and reduced traumatic stress at 1 month post injury.[27]

Depressive symptoms should be considered when assessing fatigue. Depression after a TBI of any severity has been reported as high as 53%, but will vary among studies depending on the measurement instrument or scale used. Depression appears to have a higher prevalence than other psychological comorbidities such as anxiety following TBI.[28]

A longitudinal study looking at 118 individuals with mixed severity TBI up to 5 years post injury showed at least a moderate correlation between fatigue, as measured by the FSS, and depressive symptoms. Anxiety was found to be the strongest predictor of depressive symptoms at 1 year post injury, and fatigue did not increase significantly over time. The demonstrated correlation between fatigue and depressive symptoms in this study reinforces the complex interactions between physical and psychological disturbances after TBI.[28]

In one large study of 722 patients with mixed severity TBI, fatigue was the most commonly cited manifestation of major depressive disorder.[29] A similar study of 119 individuals, also with mixed severity TBI and at least 1 year post injury, showed 37% of participants reported mild depression, and one-third reported moderate to severe depression, while 53% reported fatigue on the MAF, and one-third reported fatigue on the FSS. Robust correlation was found between fatigue and depression in this study suggesting inclusion of depression screening for post-TBI fatigue assessment.[30]

Another consideration in the assessment of TBI-related fatigue is co-occurring post-traumatic stress sisorder (PTSD). Compared to depressive symptoms there is a relative lack of information regarding the relationship between PTSD and fatigue following TBI, and this relationship may differ between military and civilian trauma. A study of 84 civilian individuals with mild to moderate TBI, assessed on average 15 months after injury, looked at the relationship between fatigue-related quality of life and event-related stress (i.e., PTSD), as well as situation-dependent stress (i.e., stressors experienced over the previous month). Interestingly fatigue, as measured by the MFIS, was associated with situation-dependent stress, however not significantly associated with event-related stress, suggesting the chronic, or ongoing nature of life stressors may have an overwhelming effect in this population.[31] A study of fatigue using the MFIS in 60 veterans found physical and cognitive fatigue to be significantly related to multiple assessed psychiatric factors including PTSD. Physical fatigue was also found to be significantly predicted by PTSD symptoms and post-traumatic amnesia.[32] The above studies suggest that PTSD plays an important role in fatigue for at least the military/veteran population and that ongoing situational stress may be a contributing factor for fatigue in patients with TBI.

CLINICAL APPROACH FOR TREATMENT OF TBI-RELATED FATIGUE

An algorithm for the clinical assessment and treatment of TBI-related fatigue is provided in Fig. 10.1 and consists of assessment for comorbid disorders as described above, use of a validated fatigue assessment instrument, and then consideration of a number of interventions described below.

PSYCHOEDUCATIONAL INTERVENTIONS

Psychotherapeutic interventions have included education,[33] cognitive-behavioral therapy (CBT), or a combination of both.[34] The VA/DoD Clinical Practice Guidelines for the Management of Mild TBI acknowledge both education and CBT as useful management approaches for post-traumatic fatigue.[35]

One educational intervention that has been studied for chronic symptoms following head injury is an education booklet. In one controlled study of mTBI participants who presented to the ED,[33] participants were assigned in an alternating fashion to either receiving an education booklet listing common symptoms, expected time course, and coping strategies or treatment as usual (TAU). Three months later, individuals in the TAU group reported more sleep disturbance and anxiety on the Post-Concussive Symptom Checklist versus the educational intervention group, but no difference in severity of fatigue symptoms.

In a randomized, blinded, controlled trial of mTBI patients admitted to an inpatient ward, Mittenberg, et al.[34] studied the effect of a CBT intervention supported by an education manual about concussion symptoms. The individuals receiving the intervention each met with a therapist for approximately 1 hour to discuss current symptoms, the reattribution of symptoms to selective attention, anxiety-arousing or depressive self-statements, the role of stress in symptoms, and cognitive behavioral strategies to stop and replace negatively biased thoughts. The control group in this study received standard hospital discharge instructions. The outcome measure for this trial was a structured interview using a symptom checklist administered at baseline and 6 months post injury. Of those who endorsed fatigue immediately following injury, 47% in the intervention group continued to endorse fatigue, versus 82% in the control group ($P < .05$).

EXERCISE THERAPY FOR FATIGUE

Exercise is a commonly used intervention for fatigue in patients with multiple sclerosis, cancer, and rheumatoid arthritis.[36–38] The evidence, however, is insufficient to give clear recommendations for exercise or other types of physical activity to treat fatigue. For example, despite the numerous randomized, controlled trials that have been conducted to determine effect of exercise on cancer-related fatigue, there remains uncertainty regarding the optimal level of exercise to prescribe, and how to tailor exercise to an individual.[38] There is considerably less evidence regarding the use of exercise as an intervention for TBI-related fatigue and more specifically mTBI. Nonetheless, exercise is routinely recommended to patients with fatigue following TBI. There are several reasons for this. The benefits of exercise on cardiovascular and general physical health are well known and support overall physiologic recovery following an injury. The risk of harm from the use of exercise as an intervention is also relatively low.[39] Literature from the study of cerebrovascular disease has shown exercise and physical activity to improve or

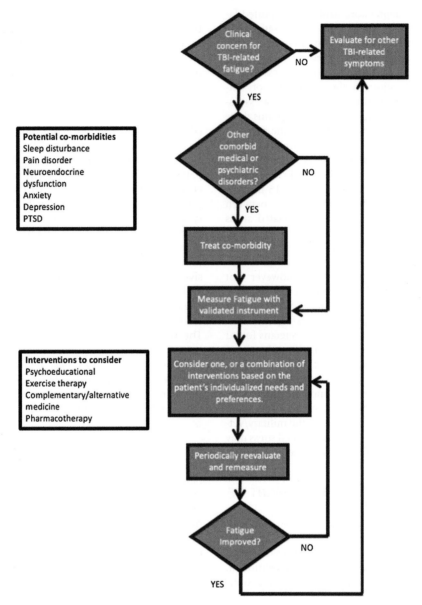

FIG. 10.1 Suggested algorithm for evaluation and treatment of TBI-related fatigue.

accelerate recovery and rehabilitation through several possible mechanisms to include modulating neuroplasticity, reducing inflammatory processes, and stabilizing vasomotor activity.[40] Furthermore, the combination of physical activity and exercise combined with other treatment modalities appears to optimize clinical recovery of cognition following a stroke.[41]

The mechanism by which TBI-related fatigue is reduced through exercise remains unclear. There is growing evidence that exercise may, in a similar mechanism to cerebrovascular disease, decrease neuroinflammation and neuronal apoptosis allowing for greater brain plasticity.[42] Physical activity and exercise has been shown to modulate processes at a cellular level affecting neurotransmitter function and optimizing behavioral health.[43] Studies have yet to determine which type of exercise is most beneficial for the treatment of depression.[44] What is promising, however, is that multiple forms of exercise may be beneficial, allowing for greater individualization and possibly greater adherence to an exercise program.

Similarly, patients with fatigue and comorbid pain may respond well to exercise therapy. The treatment of pain with physical activity and exercise is well established and has shown to be beneficial on multiple metrics of quality of life. While no one particular exercise type is recommended, more recent evidence suggests multimodal exercise programs are effective for reducing pain.[45]

There is debate as to the timing and level of intensity of an exercise routine for treatment of TBI-related fatigue. Multiple texts suggest a home exercise program accommodating an individual's injury and ability to participate in physical activity or exercise. These home exercise programs are often aimed at improving overall physical and cardiovascular health, and not necessarily fatigue as it relates to TBI.[39,46] One study looked specifically at fitness center— versus home-based exercise following a TBI and found that both were equally effective in improving cardiovascular fitness, although fatigue was not assessed.[47] Another smaller study observed individuals with TBI during a 12 week aerobic exercise training program and found not only improved cardiovascular fitness but subjective improvement in fatigue as measured by the FSS, suggesting benefit to a more vigorous aerobic exercise program.[48] This study did not directly compare different types of exercise or physical activity.

A more recent study looked at a graduated exercise program that involved incremental increases in the number of steps taken at home over a 12-week period. There was improvement in fatigue as measured by multiple scales, including the GFI, BNI-FS, and MFI, that persisted for up to 24 weeks after the initial 12-week intervention.[42] This suggests that physical activity as simple and accessible as walking can be used to treat TBI-related fatigue.

Tai Chi is a very mild form of exercise which includes components of mindfulness, and in one study was evaluated as an intervention for multiple symptoms related to TBI. Participants in this study reported more energy following participation in Tai Chi; however, only the immediate and not long-term effects of Tai Chi Chuan were evaluated.[49] Similarly yoga is considered a gentle method of exercise and physical activity. Yoga has been studied for the treatment of fatigue related to cancer and multiple sclerosis demonstrating symptom reduction in at least in the short term following intervention.[50]

The use of physical activity and exercise as a treatment modality for TBI-related fatigue should be individualized and take into account a patient's overall clinical status including comorbid symptoms associated with the TBI.

COMPLEMENTARY AND ALTERNATIVE MEDICINE APPROACHES

Various Complementary and Alternative Medicine (CAM) treatments such as acupuncture, electroencephalography (EEG) biofeedback, transcranial electrotherapy, and light therapy have been used to treat fatigue.

Acupuncture has been studied as a treatment for fatigue related to several disease processes, most extensively in cancer-related fatigue. Multiple systematic reviews of studies looking at acupuncture for cancer-related fatigue suggest that it can be an effective intervention, but also revealed flaws in methodology and the need for better designed randomized controlled trials to determine the true effectiveness.[51,52] Several studies have also looked at acupuncture as a treatment of fatigue in Parkinson's Disease and found that both real and sham acupuncture had clinically meaningful improvements in fatigue.[53,54] No studies have been conducted specifically looking at acupuncture as an intervention for TBI-related fatigue. Several studies of the use of acupuncture in TBI indicate possible improvements in functional outcomes as measured by Glasgow Coma Scale and Barthel Index.[55]

Neurofeedback or neurotherapy, often referred to as EEG biofeedback, is a learning method or type of biofeedback typically mediated through auditory and visual feedback to include EEG. This type of intervention has been studied on various behavioral disorders such as ADHD in addition to TBI. One controlled study looking at neurotherapy for the treatment of TBI found improvement in various forms of fatigue, assessed by the MFI, after 25 treatment sessions compared to controls.[56,57] Two smaller but more recent studies looked at the use of neurotherapy in Vietnam Veterans[58] and OEF/OIF Veterans[59] with mixed TBI/PTSD diagnoses who expressed multiple somatic and behavioral symptoms on the PTSD Symptom Scale (PSS). These studies found reductions in the burden of many chronic symptoms, including fatigue.

Cranial electrotherapy stimulation (CES) is a low-intensity, pulsed current applied to the scalp or earlobes. It is FDA approved for insomnia, depression, and anxiety, although the mechanism of action of

CES is poorly understood. One study looked at the use of CES for the treatment of closed head injuries and found improvement in the fatigue/inertia subscale of the Profile of Mood States after intervention for 45 min daily, 4 days per week for 3 weeks.[56]

Light therapy is an intervention for fatigue and sleepiness that typically involves short wavelength light (such as blue light) inhibiting melatonin production in the brain and stabilizing the circadian rhythm.[60] A recent study showed that blue light therapy may support structural and functional recovery following mTBI as demonstrated by correlations between various white matter diffusion properties on MRI, improvements in daytime sleep onset latency, and delayed memory.[60] Light therapy has shown to significantly reduce fatigue in multiple studies looking at cancer-related fatigue.[61,62] Interventions in these studies lasted 4 weeks and consisted of daily morning exposure to light for 30 min. In addition to reduction of fatigue, one study also saw improvement in secondary outcomes of mood and quality of life.[62] Another study looking at blue light therapy for TBI-related fatigue assessed participants exposed to blue light for 45 min per day over 4 weeks and reported significant reductions in fatigue (measured by the FSS) and secondary outcome measures of daytime sleepiness (measured by the Epworth Sleepiness Scale [ESS], PSQI, and BDI) compared to yellow light exposure controls.[63] Light therapy is typically a low-cost, low-risk, and relatively accessible intervention for fatigue.

CAM treatments may be reasonable to consider as primary or adjunctive therapies depending on accessibility and patient and provider comfort levels given their relatively low cost and risk of harm.

PHARMACOTHERAPY INTERVENTIONS

Stimulants have been used to treat cognitive disturbance following traumatic brain injury, primarily to improve attention and memory.[64] In a systematic review of stimulant use for mTBI symptoms, the highest quality studies of predominantly mTBI patients selected primary outcome measures of improvement in cognitive complaints,[65] mood symptoms,[66] or mental fatigue.[67–69] All of these studies used immediate release methylphenidate as the stimulant arm.

In a crossover study of immediate release methylphenidate, 51 participants (>90% mTBI) underwent treatment with no methylphenidate, low dose (titrated to 15 mg in three divided doses), or normal dose (60 mg titration in three divided doses).[67] The primary outcome measure was change in the Mental Fatigue Scale. Participants reported less fatigue, in a dose dependent manner, with the most robust response at the 60 mg daily dose. The medication was well tolerated, with 44 individuals completing the study. In those who tolerated and chose to continue the medication, the benefit was maintained at 6 months[68] and 2 years.[69]

The effect of modafinil on post-traumatic fatigue has been evaluated in two randomized, double-blind, placebo-controlled trials. In one study of 20 severely injured individuals with persistent post-traumatic fatigue or excessive daytime somnolence, a dose of 100–200 mg each morning improved self-reported daytime somnolence but not fatigue as measured by the FSS.[70] In a 10-week study of 53 individuals of mixed severity (25% mild), individuals taking modafinil reported an improvement in fatigue at week 4 compared to placebo as measured by the MFIS (a secondary outcome), but not in the coadministered FSS selected a priori as the primary outcome. By week 10, there was no difference in either score.[71]

There is limited evidence, largely based on a retrospective case control study,[72] for the use of amantadine 100 mg twice daily to treat postconcussive symptoms. Fatigue was not assessed in this study.

Pharmacotherapy may be a useful treatment option, usually best reserved for cases refractory to the previously discussed modalities.

CONCLUSION

TBI-related fatigue can remain for years following mTBI. A number of factors can contribute to fatigue following mTBI, including sleep disturbance, chronic pain, depression, anxiety, PTSD, and NED. Many of these comorbidities can be distinguished from fatigue by history and ancillary testing, and their treatment can often reduce the patient's experience of fatigue.

A number of nonpharmacologic interventions have been shown to reduce fatigue, including psychoeducational interventions, exercise therapy, and several CAM interventions. Many of these can be safely combined, allowing a multimodality approach to treating refractory fatigue. Much of the robust data for exercise therapy and CAM comes from studies using these approaches to treat fatigue from other medical conditions, but there is a growing body of literature supporting their use in TBI-related fatigue. When indicated, stimulants may be considered for treatment of fatigue; however, there are limited data to support their use.

Determining response to therapy can be difficult without an appropriate outcome measure, particularly a validated scale. A number of unidimensional and multidimensional scales are available and discussed above. Further research is needed to determine which have the best sensitivity for TBI-related fatigue.

Finally, the number of available treatments allows for an individualized approach to care. Working with the patient to find the appropriate plan of care that most suits their lifestyle and preferences can increase the patient's self-efficacy and quality of life. This collaborative approach may itself be helpful in reducing this often troubling and disabling symptom following mTBI.

DISCLAIMER

The views expressed are those of the authors and do not reflect the official views or policy of the Department of Defense or its Components.

REFERENCES

1. Lundin A, de Boussard C, Edman G, Borg J. Symptoms and disability until 3 months after mild TBI. *Brain Inj.* 2006; 20(8):799−806.
2. Prins M, Greco T, Alexander D, Giza CC. The pathophysiology of traumatic brain injury at a glance. *Dis Model Mech.* 2013;6(6):1307−1315.
3. Giza CC, Hovda DA. The new neurometabolic cascade of concussion. *Neurosurgery.* 2014;75(Suppl 4):S24−S33.
4. Wylie GR, Flashman LA. Understanding the interplay between mild traumatic brain injury and cognitive fatigue: models and treatments. *Concussion.* 2017;2(4):CNC50.
5. Whitehead L. The measurement of fatigue in chronic illness: a systematic review of unidimensional and multidimensional fatigue measures. *J Pain Symptom Manag.* 2009;37(1):107−128.
6. Mercier E, Tardif PA, Emond M, et al. Characteristics of patients included and enrolled in studies on the prognostic value of serum biomarkers for prediction of postconcussion symptoms following a mild traumatic brain injury: a systematic review. *BMJ Open.* 2017;7(9):e017848.
7. Bodapati AS, Combs HL, Pastorek NJ, et al. Detection of symptom over-reporting on the Neurobehavioral Symptom Inventory in OEF/OIF/OND veterans with history of mild TBI. *Clin Neuropsychol.* 2018:1−18.
8. Norrie J, Heitger M, Leathem J, Anderson T, Jones R, Flett R. Mild traumatic brain injury and fatigue: a prospective longitudinal study. *Brain Inj.* 2010;24(13−14):1528−1538.
9. Schiehser DM, Delano-Wood L, Jak AJ, et al. Validation of the Modified Fatigue Impact Scale in mild to moderate traumatic brain injury. *J Head Trauma Rehabil.* 2015; 30(2):116−121.
10. Ziino C, Ponsford J. Selective attention deficits and subjective fatigue following traumatic brain injury. *Neuropsychology.* 2006;20(3):383−390.
11. Viola-Saltzman M, Musleh C. Traumatic brain injury-induced sleep disorders. *Neuropsychiatric Dis Treat.* 2016; 12:339−348.
12. Bushnik T, Englander J, Wright J. The experience of fatigue in the first 2 years after moderate-to-severe traumatic brain injury: a preliminary report. *J Head Trauma Rehabil.* 2008; 23(1):17−24.
13. Cantor JB, Bushnik T, Cicerone K, et al. Insomnia, fatigue, and sleepiness in the first 2 years after traumatic brain injury: an NIDRR TBI model system module study. *J Head Trauma Rehabil.* 2012;27(6):E1−E14.
14. Ponsford JL, Ziino C, Parcell DL, et al. Fatigue and sleep disturbance following traumatic brain injury–their nature, causes, and potential treatments. *J Head Trauma Rehabil.* 2012;27(3):224−233.
15. Ponsford JL, Sinclair KL. Sleep and fatigue following traumatic brain injury. *Psychiatr Clin.* 2014;37(1):77−89.
16. Bushnik T, Englander J, Katznelson L. Fatigue after TBI: association with neuroendocrine abnormalities. *Brain Inj.* 2007;21(6):559−566.
17. Fernandez-Rodriguez E, Bernabeu I, Castro AI, Casanueva FF. Hypopituitarism after traumatic brain injury. *Endocrinol Metab Clin N Am.* 2015;44(1):151−159.
18. Bavisetty S, Bavisetty S, McArthur DL, et al. Chronic hypopituitarism after traumatic brain injury: risk assessment and relationship to outcome. *Neurosurgery.* 2008;62(5): 1080−1093. discussion 1093−1084.
19. Ioachimescu AG, Hampstead BM, Moore A, Burgess E, Phillips LS. Growth hormone deficiency after mild combat-related traumatic brain injury. *Pituitary.* 2015; 18(4):535−541.
20. Klose M, Stochholm K, Janukonyte J, et al. Patient reported outcome in posttraumatic pituitary deficiency: results from the Danish National Study on posttraumatic hypopituitarism. *Eur J Endocrinol.* 2015;172(6):753−762.
21. DVBIC. *DoD Clinical Recommendation: Indications and Conditions for Neuroendocrine Dysfunction Screening Post Mild Traumatic Brain Injury.* Maryland: D. o. Defense. Silver Spring; 2018.
22. Crowe M, Jordan J, Gillon D, McCall C, Frampton C, Jamieson H. The prevalence of pain and its relationship to falls, fatigue, and depression in a cohort of older people living in the community. *J Adv Nurs.* 2017;73(11): 2642−2651.
23. Madsen SG, Danneskiold-Samsoe B, Stockmarr A, Bartels EM. Correlations between fatigue and disease duration, disease activity, and pain in patients with rheumatoid arthritis: a systematic review. *Scand J Rheumatol.* 2016; 45(4):255−261.
24. Bower JE, Ganz PA, Desmond KA, et al. Fatigue in long-term breast carcinoma survivors: a longitudinal investigation. *Cancer.* 2006;106(4):751−758.
25. Reinertsen KV, Cvancarova M, Loge JH, Edvardsen H, Wist E, Fossa SD. Predictors and course of chronic fatigue in long-term breast cancer survivors. *J Cancer Surviv.* 2010; 4(4):405−414.
26. Beaulieu-Bonneau S, Ouellet MC. Fatigue in the first year after traumatic brain injury: course, relationship with injury severity, and correlates. *Neuropsychol Rehabil.* 2017; 27(7):983−1001.

27. Losoi H, Waljas M, Turunen S, et al. Resilience is associated with fatigue after mild traumatic brain injury. *J Head Trauma Rehabil.* 2015;30(3):E24–E32.

28. Sigurdardottir S, Andelic N, Roe C, Schanke AK. Depressive symptoms and psychological distress during the first five years after traumatic brain injury: relationship with psychosocial stressors, fatigue and pain. *J Rehabil Med.* 2013; 45(8):808–814.

29. Kreutzer JS, Seel RT, Gourley E. The prevalence and symptom rates of depression after traumatic brain injury: a comprehensive examination. *Brain Inj.* 2001;15(7): 563–576.

30. Englander J, Bushnik T, Oggins J, Katznelson L. Fatigue after traumatic brain injury: association with neuroendocrine, sleep, depression and other factors. *Brain Inj.* 2010; 24(12):1379–1388.

31. Bay E, de-Leon MB. Chronic stress and fatigue-related quality of life after mild to moderate traumatic brain injury. *J Head Trauma Rehabil.* 2011;26(5):355–363.

32. Schiehser DM, Delano-Wood L, Jak AJ, et al. Predictors of cognitive and physical fatigue in post-acute mild-moderate traumatic brain injury. *Neuropsychol Rehabil.* 2017;27(7): 1031–1046.

33. Ponsford J, Willmott C, Rothwell A, et al. Impact of early intervention on outcome following mild head injury in adults. *J Neurol Neurosurg Psychiatry.* 2002;73(3):330–332.

34. Mittenberg W, Tremont G, Zielinski RE, Fichera S, Rayls KR. Cognitive-behavioral prevention of postconcussion syndrome. *Arch Clin Neuropsychol.* 1996;11(2): 139–145.

35. VA/DOD. *VA/DoD Clinical Practice Guideline for the Management of Concussion-Mild Traumatic Brain Injury.* 2nd Version 2016.

36. Tomlinson D, Diorio C, Beyene J, Sung L. Effect of exercise on cancer-related fatigue: a meta-analysis. *Am J Phys Med Rehabil.* 2014;93(8):675–686.

37. Rongen-van Dartel SA, Repping-Wuts H, Flendrie M, et al. Effect of aerobic exercise training on fatigue in rheumatoid arthritis: a meta-analysis. *Arthritis Care Res.* 2015;67(8): 1054–1062.

38. Mikulakova W, Klimova E, Kendrova L, Gajdos M, Chmelik M. Effect of rehabilitation on fatigue level in patients with multiple sclerosis. *Med Sci Mon Int Med J Exp Clin Res.* 2018;24:5761–5770.

39. Henrie M, EP E. Fatigue assessment and treatment. In: Zasler N, Katz D, Zafonte R, eds. *Brain Injury Medicine Principles and Practice.* New York: Demos; 2013.

40. Billinger SA, Arena R, Bernhardt J, et al. Physical activity and exercise recommendations for stroke survivors: a statement for healthcare professionals from the American Heart Association/American Stroke Association. *Stroke.* 2014;45(8):2532–2553.

41. Constans A, Pin-Barre C, Temprado JJ, Decherchi P, Laurin J. Influence of aerobic training and combinations of interventions on cognition and neuroplasticity after stroke. *Front Aging Neurosci.* 2016;8:164.

42. Kolakowsky-Hayner SA, Bellon K, Toda K, et al. A randomised control trial of walking to ameliorate brain injury fatigue: a NIDRR TBI model system centre-based study. *Neuropsychol Rehabil.* 2016:1–17.

43. Phillips C, Fahimi A. Immune and neuroprotective effects of physical activity on the brain in depression. *Front Neurosci.* 2018;12:498.

44. Carek PJ, Laibstain SE, Carek SM. Exercise for the treatment of depression and anxiety. *Int J Psychiatry Med.* 2011;41(1): 15–28.

45. Ambrose KR, Golightly YM. Physical exercise as non-pharmacological treatment of chronic pain: why and when. *Best Pract Res Clin Rheumatol.* 2015;29(1):120–130.

46. Henrie M, Elovic E. Selected somatic disorders associated with mild traumatic brain injury: fatigue, dizziness, and balance impairment, and whiplash injury. In: Zollman F, ed. *Manual of Traumatic Brain Injury Assessment and Management.* New York: Demos; 2016.

47. Hassett LM, Moseley AM, Tate RL, Harmer AR, Fairbairn TJ, Leung J. Efficacy of a fitness centre-based exercise programme compared with a home-based exercise programme in traumatic brain injury: a randomized controlled trial. *J Rehabil Med.* 2009;41(4):247–255.

48. Chin LM, Chan L, Woolstenhulme JG, Christensen EJ, Shenouda CN, Keyser RE. Improved cardiorespiratory fitness with aerobic exercise training in individuals with traumatic brain injury. *J Head Trauma Rehabil.* 2015; 30(6):382–390.

49. Gemmell C, Leathem JM. A study investigating the effects of Tai Chi Chuan: individuals with traumatic brain injury compared to controls. *Brain Inj.* 2006;20(2):151–156.

50. Sadja J, Mills PJ. Effects of yoga interventions on fatigue in cancer patients and survivors: a systematic review of randomized controlled trials. *Explore.* 2013;9(4):232–243.

51. Zeng Y, Luo T, Finnegan-John J, Cheng AS. Meta-Analysis of randomized controlled trials of acupuncture for cancer-related fatigue. *Integr Cancer Ther.* 2014;13(3): 193–200.

52. Zhang Y, Lin L, Li H, Hu Y, Tian L. Effects of acupuncture on cancer-related fatigue: a meta-analysis. *Support Care Canc.* 2018;26(2):415–425.

53. Kluger BM, Rakowski D, Christian M, et al. Randomized, controlled trial of acupuncture for fatigue in Parkinson's disease. *Mov Disord.* 2016;31(7):1027–1032.

54. Kong KH, Ng HL, Li W, et al. Acupuncture in the treatment of fatigue in Parkinson's disease: a pilot, randomized, controlled, study. *Brain Behav.* 2018;8(1):e00897.

55. Wong V, Cheuk DK, Lee S, Chu V. Acupuncture for acute management and rehabilitation of traumatic brain injury. *Cochrane Database Syst Rev.* 2013;3:CD007700.

56. Smith RB, Tiberi A, Marshall J. The use of cranial electrotherapy stimulation in the treatment of closed-head-injured patients. *Brain Inj.* 1994;8(4):357–361.

57. Schoenberger NE, Shif SC, Esty ML, Ochs L, Matheis RJ. Flexyx Neurotherapy System in the treatment of traumatic brain injury: an initial evaluation. *J Head Trauma Rehabil.* 2001;16(3):260–274.

58. Nelson DV, Esty ML. Neurotherapy of traumatic brain injury/post-traumatic stress symptoms in Vietnam veterans. *Mil Med.* 2015;180(10):e1111–1114.

59. Nelson DV, Esty ML. Neurotherapy of traumatic brain injury/posttraumatic stress symptoms in OEF/OIF veterans. *J Neuropsychiatry Clin Neurosci.* 2012;24(2):237–240.

60. Bajaj S, Vanuk JR, Smith R, Dailey NS, Killgore WDS. Blue-light therapy following mild traumatic brain injury: effects on white matter water diffusion in the brain. *Front Neurol.* 2017;8:616.

61. Redd WH, Valdimarsdottir H, Wu LM, et al. Systematic light exposure in the treatment of cancer-related fatigue: a preliminary study. *Psycho Oncol.* 2014;23(12):1431–1434.

62. Johnson JA, Garland SN, Carlson LE, et al. Bright light therapy improves cancer-related fatigue in cancer survivors: a randomized controlled trial. *J Cancer Surviv.* 2018;12(2):206–215.

63. Sinclair KL, Ponsford JL, Taffe J, Lockley SW, Rajaratnam SM. Randomized controlled trial of light therapy for fatigue following traumatic brain injury. *Neurorehabilitation Neural Repair.* 2014;28(4):303–313.

64. Arciniegas DB, Silver JM. Pharmacotherapy of posttraumatic cognitive impairments. *Behav Neurol.* 2006;17(1):25–42.

65. McAllister TW, Zafonte R, Jain S, et al. Randomized placebo-controlled trial of methylphenidate or galantamine for persistent emotional and cognitive symptoms associated with PTSD and/or traumatic brain injury. *Neuropsychopharmacology.* 2016;41(5):1191–1198.

66. Lee H, Kim SW, Kim JM, Shin IS, Yang SJ, Yoon JS. Comparing effects of methylphenidate, sertraline and placebo on neuropsychiatric sequelae in patients with traumatic brain injury. *Hum Psychopharmacol.* 2005;20(2):97–104.

67. Johansson B, Wentzel AP, Andrell P, Mannheimer C, Ronnback L. Methylphenidate reduces mental fatigue and improves processing speed in persons suffered a traumatic brain injury. *Brain Inj.* 2015;29(6):758–765.

68. Johansson B, Wentzel AP, Andrell P, Ronnback L, Mannheimer C. Long-term treatment with methylphenidate for fatigue after traumatic brain injury. *Acta Neurol Scand.* 2017;135(1):100–107.

69. Johansson B, Wentzel AP, Andrell P, Ronnback L, Mannheimer C. Two-year methylphenidate treatment of mental fatigue and cognitive function after a traumatic brain injury: a clinical prospective study. *J Clin Psychopharmacol.* 2018;38(2):164–165.

70. Kaiser PR, Valko PO, Werth E, et al. Modafinil ameliorates excessive daytime sleepiness after traumatic brain injury. *Neurology.* 2010;75(20):1780–1785.

71. Jha A, Weintraub A, Allshouse A, et al. A randomized trial of modafinil for the treatment of fatigue and excessive daytime sleepiness in individuals with chronic traumatic brain injury. *J Head Trauma Rehabil.* 2008;23(1):52–63.

72. Reddy CC, Collins M, Lovell M, Kontos AP. Efficacy of amantadine treatment on symptoms and neurocognitive performance among adolescents following sports-related concussion. *J Head Trauma Rehabil.* 2013;28(4):260–265.

CHAPTER 11

Management of Adult Sports Concussion

KATHERINE L. DEC, MD, FAAPMR, FAMSSM • KASSANDRA C. KELLY, MS, ATC • JARED B. GILMAN, MD

INTRODUCTION

Sports-related concussions (SRCs) receive significant attention in youth, secondary school, and college athletics. SRCs encompass both those in recreational sports without formal team dynamics, i.e., hiking, and in formal team settings with established policies and sideline medical assistance. In the adult setting, classified here as over age 21 years old (see Chapter 12 for younger athletes), most often these injuries occur in solo activities such as fitness, recreational leagues, mass events, and weekend pursuits where there are no medical assistance or established protocols. The professional sporting arena overlaps these adult SRC demographics. Their high level of medical management and protocols for treatment are similar to collegiate athletics. Each professional league establishes their policies and protocols (National Basketball Association [NBA], National Hockey League [NHL], National Football League [NFL], etc.). However, it is clear there is no significant research in best practice guidelines, injury pathophysiology, and neuroregenerative and physiologic recovery in SRC. Most information is gleaned from populations with various mechanisms of concussive event, age differences, and comorbidities that can affect recovery and neuroplasticity.

Definitions

Traumatic brain injury (TBI) is defined as an alteration to the brain's function caused by an external force. In SRC, the most common definition is derived from the Concussion in Sports Group consensus statements: "a complex pathophysiological process affecting the brain, induced by traumatic biomechanical forces."[1] The World Health Organization defines mild TBI (mTBI) as "MTBI is an acute brain injury resulting from mechanical energy to the head from external physical forces. Operational criteria for clinical identification include: (1) one or more of the following: confusion or disorientation, loss of consciousness for 30 minutes or less, post-traumatic amnesia for less than 24 hours, and/or other transient neurological abnormalities such as focal signs, seizure, and intracranial lesion not requiring surgery; and (2) Glasgow Coma Scale (GCS) score of 13−15 after 30 minutes post-injury or later upon presentation for healthcare."[2] Both definitions note symptoms cannot be due to drugs, alcohol, or other injures, medications, or coexisting conditions. Yet, as noted, even these two definitions are not consistent in description of neurophysiology, symptom manifestation, or clinical findings for "concussion." Most SRCs have a normal Glasgow Coma Scale (GCS) score of "15" but "mild" can be in the range of "13−15" for "mild" quantification.[3] In predicting recovery for return to play, paramount in SRC, no one objective test is satisfactory.

EPIDEMIOLOGY

Fifty percent of the world's population will have a TBI injury in their lifetime, with a study in New Zealand showing 31% of the population will experience at least one TBI by the age of 25 years old.[4,5] In the United States, upwards of 213 million people ages six years and older participated in sports and fitness activities in 2015.[6] With such a large portion of the population physically active, further investigation into the injury risk and trends of SRC is warranted.

It is estimated that between 1.6 and 3.8 million SRCs occur annually in the United States.[7] These estimates are hypothesized to be low as many injuries will go unrecognized and unreported, leaving the true rates of SRC occurrence unknown.[7−10] In recent years, injury surveillance systems are a popular way to track SRC in collegiate and professional sports settings. These systems

Concussion. https://doi.org/10.1016/B978-0-323-65384-8.00011-0
Copyright © 2020 Elsevier Inc. All rights reserved.

allow for comprehensive tracking and help identify important injury estimates with detailed analysis of the injury assisting with rule changes, practice strategies, and risk minimization[11] (Table 11.1[12–15]; and Table 11.2).[16–20] As emphasis is placed on rule changes in sports to reduce brain injury, these surveillance systems can also monitor resultant changes in SRC incidence.

Outside of structured team sports, mTBIs are tracked through prevalence of emergency room visits and their corresponding diagnosis codes. These studies are helpful in understanding injury rate in the recreationally active population; however, evidence suggests tracking ICD9 (now ICD10) codes may not be ideal. One study analyzing the accuracy of ICD9 codes used to track injury revealed 98% specificity but only 46% sensitivity for concussion.[21] As coding practices change and databases such as the National Trauma Data Bank become more easily accessible, recent studies are beginning to show the SRC burden of adults in the general population. One recent study analyzing data from US trauma centers over a 10-year period showed 18,310 sports-related TBIs being seen in these facilities with 85.6% being classified as mTBI or concussion.[22] The highest incidence rate of SRC in adults corresponded to equestrian sports (45.2%) followed by fall or interpersonal contact (20.3%), roller sports (19%), skiing/snowboarding (12.0%), and aquatic sports (3.5%).[22] Young adults 18–29 years old accounted for 44% of all SRC, but, interestingly 71% equestrian SRC was in athletes 60 years and older.[22]

Detailed analysis of epidemiological trends in SRC reveal injury trends related to gender, with females demonstrating greater incidence of concussion injuries, and different symptom clusters, than their male counterparts.[6,23–28] Specific issues in females with concussion are reviewed in Chapter 14.

TABLE 11.1
NCAA Injury Rate/1000 Athlete-Exposures (95% Confidence Interval).

Sport	Gender	Practice	Competition
Volleyball[12]		0.19 (0.15,0.23)	0.33 (0.24, 0.41)
Soccer[13]	Women's	0.23 (0.19,0.27)	1.91 (1.71, 2.11)
	Men's	0.17 (0.14,0.21)	1.24 (1.06, 1.41)
Wrestling[14]		0.48 (0.32, 0.65)	4.31 (2.88, 5.74)
Men's football[15]		0.40 (0.38, 0.42)	3.01 (2.80, 3.21)
Ice hockey[14]	Women's	0.33 (0.19, 0.47) 60	2.75 (2.04, 3.47)
	Men's	0.10 (0.08, 0.12)	1.49 (1.34, 1.63) 61
Softball[14]		0.18 (0.09, 0.26)	0.42 (0.25, 0.59)
Baseball[14]		0.04 (0.00, 0.08)	0.16 (0.06, 0.27)

TABLE 11.2
Professional Sports Injury Rate in Competition.

Sport	Competition
Major league baseball (MLB)[16]	0.26 per 1000 A-E
Minor league baseball[16]	0.46 per 1000 A-E
National football league (NFL)[17]	6.61 per 1000 player hours
National hockey league (NHL)[18]	1.8 concussions per 1000 player-hours
Australian rule's football[19]	9.53 per 1000 A-E

A-E, Athlete-Exposure.

ASSESSMENT

Emphasis is on timely, accurate diagnosis to mitigate the effects of SRC. Sports medicine clinicians must navigate a myriad of unique challenges to perform a competent, multidimensional assessment within the time constraints created by competition. The addition of game play decision with concurrent SRC assessment necessitates awareness of how factors such as dehydration, heat illness, athlete prioritization to return to play, and the external pressures in close competition may influence clinical injury presentation and decision-making.[29–33] Further complicating clinical assessment is the unpredictable evolution of SRC symptoms: some athletes experience a rapid onset of symptoms, others experience symptom evolution over minutes to hours.[1] No ideal test or biomarker exists to immediately and accurately recognize and diagnose SRC. Recent consensus statements emphasize a multifaceted approach to assessment.[1,29,34]

The primary objective of acute sideline concussion assessment is to rapidly triage a player for possible injuries to the brain, skull, neck, or spine, determining if continuing activity is safe.[1,32] The evaluation of an SRC begins when an athlete sustains a forcible impact to the head or body that results in visible signs or reported symptoms of injury, and/or other clinical suspicion recognized by the observing staff.[35] Recently, professional leagues have begun utilizing different strategies to help report suspected concussive events and commence assessments for determining safety of continued play.[35,36] In addition to game officials being able to report possible concussions to medical staff, concussion "spotters" and video surveillance of competition have emerged to aid in recognition of possible SRC.[35,36] The AFL, NFL, NHL and rugby union all utilize video to aid sideline medical personnel with SRC assessment.[35] With the ability to replay game play at multiple angles and in slow motion, video review improves the sensitivity of SRC recognition.[35,37] Video definitions and guidelines to inform sideline personnel of potential injury are emerging as video review becomes widely used.[36] Currently there are no guidelines for the best implementation of video review for SRC and current utilization has been variable.[38] Nevertheless, these tools may provide sufficient information to aid clinicians to confidently remove an athlete from play until undergoing a formalized assessment.[36]

Lack of a gold standard in assessment has led to a variety of practice patterns employed by sideline clinicians.[39–41] Evidence has also emerged that clinicians are inconsistent in employing a multimodal approach of the various concussion domains impacted by injury despite guidelines.[39–41] Multifactorial testing batteries have shown increased sensitivity rates in concussion recognition when compared to the sensitivity of any individual domain alone and may limit the clinician's ability to accurately diagnose SRC.[42,43] A primary assessment should be completed first after suspected injury to rule out cervical spine injury and/ or a more serious injury that would require the initiation of an emergency action plan.[29,44,45] Once the possibility of more severe injury has been excluded, the athlete should be removed from play and undergo a formalized assessment.[29]

SRC examination includes a detailed injury history, symptom assessment, observation of the patient, tests for mental status, motor control, and a physical examination to rule out other orthopedic/neurologic injury.[29,46,47] One commonly recommended standardized sideline evaluation tool that assesses multiple domains is the Sport Concussion Assessment Tool (SCAT5). This simple and brief assessment tool has been recognized as the standard for acute sideline concussion assessment by several professional sporting organizations including the NFL, NBA, MLB, and NHL.[48] The recently developed SCAT5 expands the components of the previously utilized SCAT3; it includes a brief interview of clinical concussion history and demographics, the GCS, Maddocks questions, a symptom checklist, a brief neck examination, a balance assessment (modified Balance Error Scoring System [BESS] and/or Tandem gait), coordination assessment, and a brief cognition assessment (Standard Assessment of Concussion).[1,49] Recent evidence suggests that acute evaluation models containing the Standardized Assessment of Concussion (SAC), SCAT, and BESS are sensitive to the effects of concussion.[50]

Domains the SCAT5 does not assess in detail are the vestibular and ocular motor systems. Dizziness, which may include impairments to these systems, is reported by 50% of concussed athletes and carries a 6.4 times greater risk, compared to any other single reported acute symptom, in predicting prolonged recovery.[51,52] As such, clinicians should be sure to incorporate brief ocular motor and vestibular screens into their sideline testing battery. The Vestibular Ocular-Motor Screening (VOMS) is a simple, brief assessment that has been shown to be sensitive in screening these concussion symptoms.[53]

In recreational sports arenas, adults may continue to play or be undiagnosed at the initial injury. When adult athletes do seek medical attention in an outpatient office, they should be provided education regarding the common symptoms, functional components in work and daily living, and typical recovery process.[54] One caveat: if the injury sustained was unwitnessed, i.e., falling while hiking, and a predisposition to bleeding is present, further evaluation of the athlete in a hospital setting is required. One study noted that patients with a GCS of 15 and no symptoms have a low risk of adverse outcomes (2.7%) regardless of INR.[55]

MANAGEMENT

Sideline management should not replace a comprehensive medical evaluation and thus it is recommended a follow-up appointment occur within 72 hours of injury.[56] The evaluation includes history of current and prior concussive injuries, history of attention deficit hyperactivity disorder, mood disorder, other learning impairment, and sleep assessment. Testing options and imaging are covered in Chapter 1 for acute management and further in Chapter 16. While biomarkers may have application in the future for prognosis and clinical management applications, their current role in determining return to play and full recovery have not been established.[57–59]

The physical examination includes vital signs as SRC has been shown to cause large acute effects on resting systolic blood pressure, orthostatic systolic blood pressure changes, and heart rate within the acute stages of injury.[60] These changes suggest the onset of cardiac autonomic dysregulation after injury.[60,61] After concussion, autonomic nervous system (ANS) regulation is believed to be altered due to changes in the autonomic centers of the brain and/or an uncoupling of the connections between the central ANS, arterial baroreceptors, and the heart.[62] This dysregulation may manifest as exercise intolerance in a patient with SRC, a finding that can help distinguish concussion from other injury.[61,63]

The neurological assessment of cranial nerves, postural control, and motor coordination is key. Chapter 9 has further details on specific neurosensory testing/management. While the BESS/modified BESS may be appropriately incorporated into sideline SRC assessments, the test loses its ability to discriminate continued SRC-related balance issues 72 hours after injury. Clinicians may find single and dual task tandem gait to be a useful alternative assessment. Both tests have been shown to be more sensitive to the subtle changes following SRC and are more accurate detecting deficits further removed from onset of injury.[64] Tandem gait is cost-efficient and quick when monitoring athlete's recovery. Subacute neck injuries can present similar symptoms to SRC, including headaches, visual disturbances, poor postural control, and dizziness.[61,65,66] Physical examination of the cervical spine should be performed to identify any musculoskeletal neck and/or neurological injury.[65] The professional team's medical protocols will govern the process for these individual athletes. Please refer to respective league policies.[67,68]

Rehabilitation Considerations

Symptoms after SRC can require modifications in work and leisure tasks for optimal minimization of potential triggers of concussion symptoms. The psychological stress response in the athlete needs to be addressed as one study noted heightening of the stress response in rats during the first couple weeks post brain injury that may have further physiologic implications in the recovery after mTBI.[69] Yoga utilized to improve quality of life had positive effects in a small subset of TBI and could be considered in treatment during the acute phase to integrate movement, improve rest, and decrease stress emotions.[70]

Physical stressors include limiting liquid crystal display (LCD) screen usage due to the high flicker frequency that may exacerbate light sensitivity and lead to difficulty concentrating, headache, or eye strain. LCD screen use could be limited to mitigate long-term concussive symptoms.[71] Some options to avoid screen use include audiobooks, timed usage of computer for work or college, filter screens for monitors if electronics must be used during recovery.

Recovery from SRC signs and symptoms usually occurs within the first 2 weeks after injury for the majority of adult athletes. The return-to-play protocol may begin as early as 24–48 hours following the initial injury if athlete is asymptomatic and has a normal clinical examination (Fig. 11.1). To note, absolute rest beyond the first 3 days may put the individual at increased risk for exacerbation or prolonged concussion-like symptoms.[72]

There are currently no standardized guidelines for adult athletes regarding return to cognitive activities in

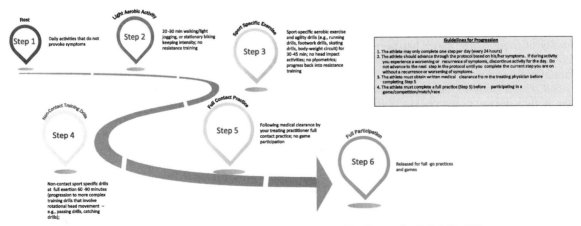

FIG. 11.1 Return-to-play protocol. Illustration created by Kassandra Kelly MS, ATC.

the graduate school or occupational settings. However, a stepwise pattern of increasing cognitive and physical stressors is encouraged. The SAC may be elected for assessing cognitive change; however, research has shown its accuracy decreases after 48 hours post injury. In fact the entire test battery of the SCAT3, which includes SAC and BESS, loses its clinical utility 3–5 days post injury.[73] Additionally, various popular computerized neurocognitive assessments have evidence questioning their validity and reliability following injury. Despite the shortcomings of these assessment tools, they are still commonly utilized to track injury recovery in SRC. In Chapter 2, neuropsychological consultation is discussed and offers the clinician greater information to assist in determining return-to-work or sports-specific skill acquisition when cognitive impairment is present.

Exercise is beneficial with slowing the neurodegenerative process of other disorders, and it has positive effects on cognition and neuroplasticity.[74] Studies in rat models noted performance improvement when exercise is a component of treatment. A retrospective study of 95 collegiate athletes who suffered SRC was randomly assigned to one of five groups based on post injury activity intensity scale (AIS). Best outcomes on neurocognitive tests and lowest symptom scores were reported in those doing moderate activity (AIS 2).[75] Management choices can affect multiple SRC domains in neuroregenerative process.

Vestibular dysfunction with dizziness and imbalance can benefit from visual static and dynamic postural stability exercises and training of somatosensory cues. Visual issues with perception, processing, and tracking/fixation can be present in concussion. Primary studies have shown favorable outcomes with vestibular rehabilitation; however, systematic reviews note evidence is limited due to small sample sizes and lack of controls. Clinicians can provide postural education such as maintaining a neutral cervical spine position to help athlete's dizziness and cervicogenic issues. One double-blinded RCT demonstrated that sustained natural apophyseal glides provided significant and sustained reduction of cervicogenic dizziness.[76] Appropriate assessment and treatment of the cervical spine with vestibular dysfunction may facilitate improved function and shorten recovery time.

Headaches are a common symptom reported and managed in adult SRC. Accompanying photophobia and hyperacusis, nausea, in addition to the headache, can be cervicogenic in etiology. Acetaminophen can be used safely in most athletes as well as low light and/or a quiet environment in the case of hypersensitivity. Cervicogenic musculoskeletal component of headaches can

occur if mechanism of injury involves a "whiplash" movement. Management of these symptoms may consist of imaging the cervical spine and/or electrodiagnostic studies. Assessing treatment of cervicogenic headaches, one study demonstrated neck pain improvement with an exercise program combined with manipulation, proprioceptive neuromuscular facilitation, acupressure on trigger points, and range of motion exercises.[77] Headaches are discussed in Chapter 6.

Adequate sleep is important to address mental and physical fatigue during recovery. Insomnia may also contribute to daytime fatigue. There are ongoing studies that have shown exposure to short wavelength light (~430–475 nm, blue light therapy) in the morning hours can improve daytime alertness, concentration, and sleep quality. The underlying mechanism of light therapy is in suppressing melatonin production which contributes to stabilizing the circadian rhythm.[78,79] If athletes complain of sleep difficulties within the first few days, providers should encourage good sleep hygiene as there is no evidence in support of a stimulant or sleep-promoting medications in the acute setting.[34] Avoiding caffeine, nicotine, and alcohol are also important. If sleep difficulties continue, other options, including melatonin, may be considered.

Pharmacology

Individual chapters of this textbook assess the pharmacologic components of specific concussion domains. In SRC, there is overlap of self-prescribed supplements and nutraceuticals adult athletes select for performance with no clear understanding of effect on SRC. Lack of regulations on product purity, individual's dosage patterns preinjury, and *potential* effects on neurophysiologic recovery are theoretical and minimal randomized control trials are available. Additionally, there is no convincing evidence that a particular medication is effective in treating the acute symptoms of SRC (see list 1 for summary).

1. Avoid any medications that might alter mental status during the first 10 hours following injury
2. Treatment should be based on common approaches to each specific symptom
3. There is no established role for stimulant medication in treating acute attention difficulties or for excessive daytime somnolence
4. There is no established role for sleep aid medication in treating sleep disturbances
5. There is no established role for mood disturbances in the acute setting, but if symptoms persist >6 weeks then medications can be considered

LIST 1. POINTS TO CONSIDER IN SRC PHARMACOLOGY[34]

Omega-3 fish oil such as docosahexaenoic acid (DHA) or eicosapentaenoic acid (EPA) is important in brain development and function; supplementation has been shown to decrease inflammatory cytokines and reduce reactive oxidative production. There have been animal studies demonstrating supplementation before and after TBI reduces the post-traumatic elevations in protein oxidation and limits axon and neuronal apoptosis.[80] Despite the lack of human data, considering supplementation with DHA at a dose of 10 mg/kg per day or 2 g/day to begin within 24 hours postconcussion is safe as it has no serious adverse effects.

Melatonin is a hormone secreted by the pineal gland that helps regulate sleep/wake cycles and has demonstrated antioxidative, neuroprotective, and anti-inflammatory properties as well. Historically melatonin has been used to alleviate jet lag and help nighttime workers adjust to their nocturnal regimen. In regards to adult SRC, very limited clinical evidence exists for sleep improvement; however, it has been used in adults after concussion for delayed sleep phase. The recommended dose is 0.5−5 mg given in the early evening initially, then maintenance dosing prior to normal bedtime.[81]

Vitamin supplementation with C, D, and E has theoretical benefit from prior animal studies. Vitamins C and E have been shown to decrease functional neurological deficits, decrease amyloid accumulation, and inhibit lipid peroxidation in one animal trial.[82] Vitamin D has been found to modulate gene transcription for neuronal proliferation and maintain calcium homeostasis. Some data suggest vitamin D deficiency may increase inflammatory damage and behavioral impairment after brain injury. There is some evidence vitamin D supplementation improves functional outcomes in humans with severe TBI, but there are no studies in SRC. This same study also noted use of progesterone + vitamin D supplementation had the best outcomes.[83] Currently there is no recommendation for vitamin D supplementation after SRC, but replacement therapy for athletes who are deficient is recommended.

Creatine is a supplement frequently used by athletes to aid in improving muscle mass. Creatine is used by skeletal muscle and the central nervous system as an energy source. In one small study of 11 athletes with SRC, the levels of creatine decreased in the brain as seen on proton magnetic resonance spectroscopy.[84] Animal research has documented a neuroprotective benefit with creatine-enriched diets prior to brain injury. Two randomized control trials in moderate to severe TBI pediatric patients evaluated the use of creatine supplementation with improvements in the short term (less time intubated, less ICU time) and long term (cognition, communication, and self-care) noted. However, SRCs are mild, resolve quickly, and application across age group and TBI severity is unfounded. A dosage of up to 5 g/day is considered safe and may have neuroprotective properties against concussions.[85]

Branched chain amino acids (BCAAs) are another supplement used by athletes in strength building. They are also needed for the synthesis of glutamate and gamma aminobutyric acid (GABA). Following a mild brain injury, BCAA levels are decreased when compared to controls. One human study of severe TBI patients demonstrated cognitive benefits with BCAA supplementation.[86] However, no studies assessed SRC, and there is currently insufficient evidence to recommend BCAA supplementation.

Caffeine intake is very common in the adult population. Its main effect is inhibition of the adenosine (A1 and A2A) receptors leading to increased glutamate release and increased inflammatory cytokines. By blocking adenosine, it inhibits the neuroprotective effects and can also impair the awareness of fatigue. We do know in healthy individuals caffeine ingestion prior to testing can improve memory, visual processing speed, and reaction which may be helpful in SRC. However, there is no currently recommended intake of caffeine in acute SRC recovery. Methylphenidate, often used in helping with processing and attention in the more severely brain injured patient, also has not been evaluated in the SRC population.

Consideration that athletes need to regain high-level sports-specific skills prior to returning to play is necessary. Visually guided motor tasks of sports-specific skills need to be incorporated. Studies have found some impairment of the transformation of visual information into programmed motor outputs.[87] Proprioception training is a component in skill rehabilitation; proprioceptive process connects information about motion and body orientation from central processes, with stretch receptors in the muscles and joint-related soft tissue (i.e., ligaments). While the exact pathway has not been discovered, complex balance and proprioceptive processes are both conscious and unconscious (mediated by posterior column medial lemniscus pathway, dorsal spinocerebellar tract, and ventral spinocerebellar tract, respectively in humans).[88] Integration of movement therapies, such as Alexander Technique, Feldenkrais method, T'ai Chi Ch'uan, and yoga, have been successful in reintegrating movement and proprioceptive components of balance.[89] While research is sparse, athletes may benefit from integration of movement therapies. Lastly, management includes education and knowing the benefit of helmet use can help attenuate impact or reduce brain injury[90,91]

In summary, adult SRC management to date has followed a combination of research applied across younger athletes and all types of concussive injury. In the adult athlete, the best treatment approach is still evolving. This lack of information creates debate in decisions of medical retirement from sports after SRC. One article offers a practical evaluation for these decisions,[92] but it remains an individualized discussion between medical professionals and athletes. There is no absolute number of concussions or objective test that can define social or occupational factors influencing the future risk of injury.

REFERENCES

1. McCrory P, Meeuwisse W, Dvorak J, et al. Consensus statement on concussion in sport-the 5(th) international conference on concussion in sport held in Berlin, October 2016. *Br J Sports Med.* 2017;51(11):838−847.
2. Carroll LJ, Cassidy JD, Holm L, Kraus J, Coronado VG, Injury WHOCCTFoMTB. Methodological issues and research recommendations for mild traumatic brain injury: the WHO Collaborating Centre task force on mild traumatic brain injury. *J Rehabil Med.* 2004;(43 suppl): 113−125.
3. Teasdale G, Jennett B. Assessment of coma and impaired consciousness. A practical scale. *Lancet.* 1974;2(7872): 81−84.
4. Corrigan JD, Selassie AW, Orman JA. The epidemiology of traumatic brain injury. *J Head Trauma Rehabil.* 2010;25(2): 72−80.
5. Maas AIR, Menon DK, Adelson PD, et al. Traumatic brain injury: integrated approaches to improve prevention, clinical care, and research. *Lancet Neurol.* 2017;16(12):987−1048.
6. Covassin T, Moran R, Elbin RJ. Sex differences in reported concussion injury rates and time loss from participation: an update of the National Collegiate Athletic Association injury surveillance program from 2004-2005 through 2008-2009. *J Athl Train.* 2016;51(3):189−194.
7. Langlois JA, Rutland-Brown W, Wald MM. The epidemiology and impact of traumatic brain injury: a brief overview. *J Head Trauma Rehabil.* 2006;21(5):375−378.
8. Beidler E, Bretzin AC, Hanock C, Covassin T. Sport-related concussion: knowledge and reporting behaviors among collegiate club-sport athletes. *J Athl Train.* 2018;53(9): 866−872.
9. Delaney JS, Caron JG, Correa JA, Bloom GA. Why professional football players chose not to reveal their concussion symptoms during a practice or game. *Clin J Sport Med.* 2018;28(1):1−12.
10. Delaney JS, Lamfookon C, Bloom GA, Al-Kashmiri A, Correa JA. Why university athletes choose not to reveal their concussion symptoms during a practice or game. *Clin J Sport Med.* 2015;25(2):113−125.
11. Kerr ZY, Zuckerman SL, Register-Mihalik JK, et al. Estimating concussion incidence using sports injury surveillance systems: complexities and potential pitfalls. *Neurol Clin.* 2017;35(3):409−434.
12. Kerr ZY, Gregory AJ, Wosmek J, et al. The first decade of web-based sports injury surveillance: descriptive epidemiology of injuries in US High School Girls' Volleyball (2005-2006 through 2013-2014) and National Collegiate Athletic Association Women's Volleyball (2004-2005 through 2013-2014). *J Athl Train.* 2018;53(10): 926−937.
13. Kerr ZY, Putukian M, Chang CJ, et al. The first decade of web-based sports injury surveillance: descriptive epidemiology of injuries in US High School Boys' Soccer (2005-2006 through 2013-2014) and National Collegiate Athletic Association Men's Soccer (2004-2005 through 2013-2014). *J Athl Train.* 2018;53(9):893−905.
14. Kerr ZY, Roos KG, Djoko A, et al. Epidemiologic measures for quantifying the incidence of concussion in National Collegiate Athletic Association sports. *J Athl Train.* 2017; 52(3):167−174.
15. Kerr ZY, Wilkerson GB, Caswell SV, et al. The first decade of web-based sports injury surveillance: descriptive epidemiology of injuries in United States High School Football (2005-2006 through 2013-2014) and National Collegiate Athletic Association football (2004-2005 through 2013-2014). *J Athl Train.* 2018;53(8):738−751.
16. Green GA, Pollack KM, D'Angelo J, et al. Mild traumatic brain injury in major and Minor League Baseball players. *Am J Sports Med.* 2015;43(5):1118−1126.
17. Nathanson JT, Connolly JG, Yuk F, et al. Concussion incidence in professional football: position-specific analysis with use of a novel metric. *Orthop J Sports Med.* 2016; 4(1). https://doi.org/10.1177/2325967115622621.
18. Benson BW, Meeuwisse WH, Rizos J, Kang J, Burke CJ. A prospective study of concussions among National Hockey League players during regular season games: the NHL-NHLPA Concussion Program. *CMAJ.* 2011;183(8): 905−911.
19. Costello DM, Ernest J, Kaye AH, O'Brien TJ, Shultz SR. Concussion incidence in amateur Australian rules footballers. *J Clin Neurosci.* 2018;56:88−89.
20. Eirale C, Tol JL, Targett S, Holmich P, Chalabi H. Concussion surveillance: do low concussion rates in the Qatar Professional Football League reflect a true difference or emphasize challenges in knowledge translation? *Clin J Sport Med.* 2015;25(1):73−74.
21. Bazarian JJ, Veazie P, Mookerjee S, Lerner EB. Accuracy of mild traumatic brain injury case ascertainment using ICD-9 codes. *Acad Emerg Med.* 2006;13(1):31−38.
22. Winkler EA, Yue JK, Burke JF, et al. Adult sports-related traumatic brain injury in United States trauma centers. *Neurosurg Focus.* 2016;40(4):E4.

23. Covassin T, Swanik CB, Sachs ML. Sex differences and the incidence of concussions among collegiate athletes. *J Athl Train*. 2003;38(3):238−244.

24. Broshek DK, Kaushik T, Freeman JR, Erlanger D, Webbe F, Barth JT. Sex differences in outcome following sports-related concussion. *J Neurosurg*. 2005;102(5):856−863.

25. Covassin T, Elbin R, Kontos A, Larson E. Investigating baseline neurocognitive performance between male and female athletes with a history of multiple concussion. *J Neurol Neurosurg Psychiatry*. 2010;81(6):597−601.

26. Covassin T, Schatz P, Swanik CB. Sex differences in neuro-psychological function and post-concussion symptoms of concussed collegiate athletes. *Neurosurgery*. 2007;61(2): 345−350. discussion 350-341.

27. Covassin T, Swanik CB, Sachs M, et al. Sex differences in baseline neuropsychological function and concussion symptoms of collegiate athletes. *Br J Sports Med*. 2006; 40(11):923−927. discussion 927.

28. Sicard V, Moore RD, Ellemberg D. Long-term cognitive outcomes in male and female athletes following sport-related concussions. *Int J Psychophysiol*. 2018;132(Pt A): 3−8.

29. Broglio SP, Cantu RC, Gioia GA, et al. National Athletic Trainers' Association position statement: management of sport concussion. *J Athl Train*. 2014;49(2):245−265.

30. Kroshus E, Baugh CM, Daneshvar DH, Stamm JM, Laursen RM, Austin SB. Pressure on sports medicine clinicians to prematurely return collegiate athletes to play after concussion. *J Athl Train*. 2015;50(9):944−951.

31. Mihalik JP, Sumrall AZ, Yeargin SW, et al. Environmental and physiological factors affect football head impact biomechanics. *Med Sci Sports Exerc*. 2017;49(10): 2093−2101.

32. Podell K, Presley C, Derman H. Sideline sports concussion assessment. *Neurol Clin*. 2017;35(3):435−450.

33. Weber AF, Mihalik JP, Register-Mihalik JK, Mays S, Prentice WE, Guskiewicz KM. Dehydration and performance on clinical concussion measures in collegiate wrestlers. *J Athl Train*. 2013;48(2):153−160.

34. Harmon KG, Clugston JR, Dec K, et al. American Medical Society for Sports Medicine position statement on concussion in sport. *Br J Sports Med*. 2019.

35. Patricios JS, Ardern CL, Hislop MD, et al. Implementation of the 2017 Berlin Concussion in Sport Group Consensus Statement in contact and collision sports: a joint position statement from 11 national and international sports organisations. *Br J Sports Med*. 2018;52(10):635−641.

36. Davis G, Makdissi M. Use of video to facilitate sideline concussion diagnosis and management decision-making. *J Sci Med Sport*. 2016;19(11):898−902.

37. Fuller GW, Kemp SP, Raftery M. The accuracy and repro-ducibility of video assessment in the pitch-side management of concussion in elite rugby. *J Sci Med Sport*. 2017; 20(3):246−249.

38. Davis GA, Makdissi M, Bloomfield P, et al. International study of video review of concussion in professional sports. *Br J Sports Med*. 2018.

39. Baugh CM, Kroshus E, Stamm JM, Daneshvar DH, Pepin MJ, Meehan 3rd WP. Clinical practices in collegiate concussion management. *Am J Sports Med*. 2016;44(6): 1391−1399.

40. Buckley TA, Burdette G, Kelly K. Concussion-management practice patterns of National Collegiate Athletic Association division II and III athletic trainers: how the other half lives. *J Athl Train*. 2015;50(8):879−888.

41. Kelly KC, Jordan EM, Joyner AB, Burdette GT, Buckley TA. National Collegiate Athletic Association Division I athletic trainers' concussion-management practice patterns. *J Athl Train*. 2014;49(5):665−673.

42. Broglio SP, Macciocchi SN, Ferrara MS. Sensitivity of the concussion assessment battery. *Neurosurgery*. 2007;60(6): 1050−1057. discussion 1057-1058.

43. Register-Mihalik JK, Guskiewicz KM, Mihalik JP, Schmidt JD, Kerr ZY, McCrea MA. Reliable change, sensitivity, and specificity of a multidimensional concussion assessment battery: implications for caution in clinical practice. *J Head Trauma Rehabil*. 2013;28(4):274−283.

44. McCrea M, Iverson GL, Echemendia RJ, Makdissi M, Raftery M. Day of injury assessment of sport-related concussion. *Br J Sports Med*. 2013;47(5):272−284.

45. Putukian M, Raftery M, Guskiewicz K, et al. Onfield assessment of concussion in the adult athlete. *Br J Sports Med*. 2013;47(5):285−288.

46. Broglio SP, Guskiewicz KM. Concussion in sports: the sideline assessment. *Sport Health*. 2009;1(5):361−369.

47. Guskiewicz KM, Broglio SP. Sport-related concussion: on-field and sideline assessment. *Phys Med Rehabil Clin*. 2011; 22(4):603−617. vii.

48. Cochrane GD, Owen M, Ackerson JD, Hale MH, Gould S. Exploration of US men's professional sport organization concussion policies. *Physician Sportsmed*. 2017;45(2): 178−183.

49. Echemendia RJ, Meeuwisse W, McCrory P, et al. The sport concussion assessment tool 5th edition (SCAT5): background and rationale. *Br J Sports Med*. 2017;51(11): 848−850.

50. Garcia GP, Broglio SP, Lavieri MS, McCrea M, McAllister T, Investigators CC. Quantifying the value of multidimensional assessment models for acute concussion: an analysis of data from the NCAA-DoD care consortium. *Sports Med*. 2018;48(7):1739−1749.

51. Kontos AP, Elbin RJ, Schatz P, et al. A revised factor structure for the post-concussion symptom scale: baseline and postconcussion factors. *Am J Sports Med*. 2012;40(10): 2375−2384.

52. Lau BC, Kontos AP, Collins MW, Mucha A, Lovell MR. Which on-field signs/symptoms predict protracted recovery from sport-related concussion among high school football players? *Am J Sports Med*. 2011;39(11): 2311−2318.

53. Mucha A, Collins MW, Elbin RJ, et al. A Brief Vestibular/Ocular Motor Screening (VOMS) assessment to evaluate concussions: preliminary findings. *Am J Sports Med*. 2014; 42(10):2479−2486.

54. Ponsford J, Willmott C, Rothwell A, et al. Impact of early intervention on outcome following mild head injury in adults. *J Neurol Neurosurg Psychiatry.* 2002;73(3):330−332.

55. Mason S, Kuczawski M, Teare MD, et al. AHEAD Study: an observational study of the management of anticoagulated patients who suffer head injury. *BMJ Open.* 2017;7(1): e014324.

56. Shirley E, Hudspeth LJ, Maynard JR. Managing sports-related concussions from time of injury through return to play. *J Am Acad Orthop Surg.* 2018;26(13):e279−e286.

57. Shahim P, Tegner Y, Wilson DH, et al. Blood biomarkers for brain injury in concussed professional ice hockey players. *JAMA Neurol.* 2014;71(6):684−692.

58. Asken BM, Bauer RM, DeKosky ST, et al. Concussion biomarkers assessed in collegiate Student-athletes (BASICS) I: normative study. *Neurology.* 2018;91(23):e2109−e2122.

59. McCrea M, Meier T, Huber D, et al. Role of advanced neuroimaging, fluid biomarkers and genetic testing in the assessment of sport-related concussion: a systematic review. *Br J Sports Med.* 2017;51(12):919−929.

60. Dobson JL, Yarbrough MB, Perez J, Evans K, Buckley T. Sport-related concussion induces transient cardiovascular autonomic dysfunction. *Am J Physiol Regul Integr Comp Physiol.* 2017;312(4):R575−R584.

61. Haider MN, Leddy JJ, Du W, Macfarlane JA, Viera KB, Willer BS. Practical management: brief physical examination for sport-related concussion in the outpatient setting. *Clin J Sport Med.* 2018.

62. Leddy JJ, Haider MN, Ellis M, Willer BS. Exercise is medicine for concussion. *Curr Sports Med Rep.* 2018;17(8): 262−270.

63. Baker JG, Freitas MS, Leddy JJ, Kozlowski KF, Willer BS. Return to full functioning after graded exercise assessment and progressive exercise treatment of postconcussion syndrome. *Rehabil Res Pract.* 2012;2012:705309.

64. Oldham JR, Difabio MS, Kaminski TW, Dewolf RM, Howell DR, Buckley TA. Efficacy of tandem gait to identify impaired postural control after concussion. *Med Sci Sports Exerc.* 2018;50(6):1162−1168.

65. Leddy JJ, Baker JG, Merchant A, et al. Brain or strain? Symptoms alone do not distinguish physiologic concussion from cervical/vestibular injury. *Clin J Sport Med.* 2015; 25(3):237−242.

66. Matuszak JM, McVige J, McPherson J, Willer B, Leddy J. A practical concussion physical examination toolbox. *Sport Health.* 2016;8(3):260−269.

67. National Basketball Associatoin. *2017-18 Concussion Policy - NBA Official.* National Basketball Association Website; 2017. http://official.nba.com/wp-content/.../4/2017/.../Concussion-Program-Summary-2017-18.pdf.

68. National Hockey League. *Concussion Evaluation and Management Protocol NHL. 2016/2017 Season.* National Hockey League Website; October 5, 2016. https://nhl.bamcontent.com/images/assets/binary/282574512/binary-file/file.pdf.

69. Griesbach GS, Hovda DA, Tio DL, Taylor AN. Heightening of the stress response during the first weeks after a mild traumatic brain injury. *Neuroscience.* 2011;178: 147−158.

70. Donnelly KZ, Linnea K, Grant DA, Lichtenstein J. The feasibility and impact of a yoga pilot programme on the quality-of-life of adults with acquired brain injury. *Brain Inj.* 2017;31(2):208−214.

71. Mansur A, Hauer TM, Hussain MW, et al. A nonliquid crystal display screen computer for treatment of photosensitivity and computer screen intolerance in postconcussion syndrome. *J Neurotrauma.* 2018;35(16): 1886−1894.

72. Silverberg ND, Iverson GL. Is rest after concussion "the best medicine?": recommendations for activity resumption following concussion in athletes, civilians, and military service members. *J Head Trauma Rehabil.* 2013;28(4): 250−259.

73. Downey RI, Hutchison MG, Comper P. Determining sensitivity and specificity of the Sport Concussion Assessment Tool 3 (SCAT3) components in university athletes. *Brain Inj.* 2018;32(11):1345−1352.

74. van Praag H. Neurogenesis and exercise: past and future directions. *NeuroMolecular Med.* 2008;10(2):128−140.

75. Majerske CW, Mihalik JP, Ren D, et al. Concussion in sports: postconcussive activity levels, symptoms, and neurocognitive performance. *J Athl Train.* 2008;43(3): 265−274.

76. Reid SA, Rivett DA, Katekar MG, Callister R. Sustained natural apophyseal glides (SNAGs) are an effective treatment for cervicogenic dizziness. *Man Ther.* 2008;13(4): 357−366.

77. Kristjansson E, Treleaven J. Sensorimotor function and dizziness in neck pain: implications for assessment and management. *J Orthop Sport Phys Ther.* 2009;39(5):364−377.

78. Chellappa SL, Steiner R, Blattner P, Oelhafen P, Gotz T, Cajochen C. Non-visual effects of light on melatonin, alertness and cognitive performance: can blue-enriched light keep us alert? *PLoS One.* 2011;6(1):e16429.

79. Wright HR, Lack LC, Kennaway DJ. Differential effects of light wavelength in phase advancing the melatonin rhythm. *J Pineal Res.* 2004;36(2):140−144.

80. Trojian TH, Jackson E. Omega-3 polyunsaturated fatty acids and concussions: treatment or not? *Curr Sports Med Rep.* 2011;10(4):180−185.

81. Arendt J, Van Someren EJ, Appleton R, Skene DJ, Akerstedt T. Clinical update: melatonin and sleep disorders. *Clin Med.* 2008;8(4):381−383.

82. Conte V, Uryu K, Fujimoto S, et al. Vitamin E reduces amyloidosis and improves cognitive function in Tg2576 mice following repetitive concussive brain injury. *J Neurochem.* 2004;90(3):758−764.

83. Tang H, Hua F, Wang J, et al. Progesterone and vitamin D combination therapy modulates inflammatory response after traumatic brain injury. *Brain Inj.* 2015:1−10.

84. Vagnozzi R, Signoretti S, Floris R, et al. Decrease in N-acetylaspartate following concussion may be coupled to decrease in creatine. *J Head Trauma Rehabil.* 2013;28(4): 284−292.

85. Scheff SW, Dhillon HS. Creatine-enhanced diet alters levels of lactate and free fatty acids after experimental brain injury. *Neurochem Res.* 2004;29(2):469−479.

86. Aquilani R, Boselli M, Boschi F, et al. Branched-chain amino acids may improve recovery from a vegetative or minimally conscious state in patients with traumatic brain injury: a pilot study. *Arch Phys Med Rehabil.* 2008;89(9): 1642−1647.

87. Brown JA, Dalecki M, Hughes C, Macpherson AK, Sergio LE. Cognitive-motor integration deficits in young adult athletes following concussion. *BMC Sports Sci Med Rehabil.* 2015;7:25.

88. Sherrington CS. On the proprioceptive system, especially its reflex aspect. *Brain.* 1907;29(4):467−485.

89. Connors KA, Galea MP, Said CM. Feldenkrais method balance classes improve balance in older adults: a controlled trial. *Evid Based Complement Alternat Med.* 2011;2011: 873672.

90. Hagel BE, Pless IB, Goulet C, Platt RW, Robitaille Y. Effectiveness of helmets in skiers and snowboarders: case-control and case crossover study. *BMJ.* 2005;330(7486): 281.

91. Thompson DC, Rivara FP, Thompson R. Helmets for preventing head and facial injuries in bicyclists. *Cochrane Database Syst Rev.* 2000;2:CD001855.

92. Davis-Hayes C, Baker DR, Bottiglieri TS, et al. Medical retirement from sport after concussions: a practical guide for a difficult discussion. *Neurol Clin Pract.* 2018;8(1): 40−47.

FURTHER READING

1. Leddy JJ, Hinds AL, Miecznikowski J, et al. Safety and prognostic utility of provocative exercise testing in acutely concussed adolescents: a randomized trial. *Clin J Sport Med.* 2018;28(1):13−20.

CHAPTER 12

Assessment, Management, and Rehabilitation of Pediatric Concussions

CHRISTINA L. MASTER, MD, CAQSM, FACSM • EILEEN P. STOREY, AB

INTRODUCTION

Concussion is a common injury in childhood, and clinicians caring for children and youth through early adulthood need to be able to diagnose and manage concussions in order to minimize the potential negative impact on quality of life and optimize recovery and outcomes. An estimated 1.9 million children sustain sports- and recreation-related concussions annually.[1] While significant attention has been paid to sports-related concussion recently, it is important to remember that concussions also occur outside of sports in everyday life activities, such as falls. Non—sports-related concussions are particularly common among younger children[2] who deserve special attention in concussion due to issues related to their developmental stage. It is also important to consider that an unknown additional number of children sustain concussion and do not seek medical care.

Of those children who do seek medical care, age often influences where they initially seek care for concussion.[3] Younger children, who tend to have a non—sports- and recreation-related mechanism of injury, often seek initial care in the emergency setting, likely due to increased concern for more serious injury and greater challenges in assessing the child due to developmental limitations.[2] As children enter school age, they are more likely to sustain sports- and recreation-related concussions coincident with increased participation in organized sports, and are more likely to seek initial injury care with their primary care physician[2] As older children and adolescents begin to participate in interscholastic sports, an important point of care becomes the school athletic trainer[1] on the sidelines, who represents yet another important role where a comprehensive understanding of the diagnosis and management of concussion is essential. Throughout this discussion, specific issues related to the various developmental stages of children and their interplay with concussion injury and recovery will be addressed.

As a form of mild traumatic brain injury, the nomenclature of concussion can be confusing for patients and families, who may expect a short-lived, spontaneous recovery from a mild injury. Patients and families may be surprised by the impact that a concussion can have on not only the child and their school and everyday life activities but also the entire family. Even in a straightforward recovery, concussion symptomatology causes an acute disruption in school and life routines. This acute postinjury period often requires clinicians, as well as school and athletic personnel, to partner with the patient and family to make adjustments needed to optimize recovery.[4] It is important for clinicians to frame the conversation surrounding the concussion diagnosis with the patient and family in order to help set appropriate expectations for recovery. While some children may recover within days to weeks, there is evidence that routine recovery from concussion in an adolescent may take up to 4 weeks.[5,6] For the substantial minority of patients who take greater than 4 weeks to recover, approximately 30% of children,[7] special considerations should be made to support patients and families through the management of a prolonged recovery with persistent symptoms.

Since the diagnosis of concussion remains a clinical one, it is important for clinicians to be aware of the current approaches to the diagnosis of concussion, including a concussion-specific history and physical examination. It is essential for clinicians to be familiar with the most common symptoms occurring after concussion, such as headache and dizziness, as well as some of the less common, yet potentially significant symptoms, such as visual problems or feeling more emotional.[8] Clinicians should also look for balance and visiovestibular deficits on physical examination, as they are often seen after concussion and early

Concussion. https://doi.org/10.1016/B978-0-323-65384-8.00012-2
Copyright © 2020 Elsevier Inc. All rights reserved.

identification of these deficits can help direct initial care for the concussion.[3,9]

A basic understanding of the pathophysiology of concussion and the metabolic cascade that occurs after injury will also help clinicians provide guidance to patients and families initially after the injury.[10] Concussion results in a metabolic mismatch with associated symptomatology due to the increased metabolic needs of the brain and the relatively insufficient cerebral blood flow following concussion injury. This can be managed with appropriate symptom-limited physical and cognitive activity modifications.[11] As the altered physiology recovers and symptoms improve, it is important for patients and families to be educated on the importance of gradually returning to their activities rather than abruptly resuming full activities. This gradual approach will help minimize symptom exacerbation during the return to learn and return to play processes.[10,12,13] Clinicians managing concussion need to recognize that multiple partners, including family members as well as medical, school, and athletic personnel, need to be engaged to support a child during this period of activity modification acutely after injury.

For those children with symptoms persisting beyond 4 weeks, there is increasing evidence that active management with targeted rehabilitation therapies has a salutary effect, as it can help address physiologic issues that may be contributing to the prolonged recovery, such as visiovestibular deficits and exercise intolerance.[14–18] Identifying the specific domains causing a child's persistent symptoms is important for determining appropriate active therapy recommendations and developing a personalized treatment approach for each child with concussion. Instead of taking a passive "wait-and-see" stance, active management may improve recovery time for those with prolonged symptoms, thereby improving quality of life and enhancing return to full life activities.

DIAGNOSIS

Concussion remains a clinical diagnosis, with no specific laboratory or imaging testing required to make the diagnosis. While there have been advances in the investigative use of advanced imaging for concussion,[19] currently the only indication for imaging in children with head injury is computed tomography (CT) when there is concern for more serious injury, such as intracranial hemorrhage. Extensive work has been done to minimize unnecessary radiation exposure for children who sustain head injury, and clinical prediction rules have been developed to guide clinicians in

decision-making to identify those at highest risk for intracranial bleeding requiring neurosurgical intervention. One commonly used guideline was developed by the Pediatric Emergency Care Applied Research Network and determined that children over 2 years of age with no mental status changes, no history of loss of consciousness, no vomiting, no signs of basilar skull fracture, no severe headache, and a nonsevere mechanism of injury have a low risk for clinically important traumatic brain injury, and thus, may be observed for 4–6 hours after injury for any neurologic deterioration, and if stable, discharged without imaging.[20]

In the realm of serum biomarkers, a blood test has been approved by the FDA to aid in the diagnosis and acute management of concussion in adults ages 18 years or older. Two serum biomarkers, glial fibrillary acidic protein (GFAP) and ubiquitin C-terminal hydrolase L1 (UCH-L1), have been shown to correlate with the presence of intracranial hemorrhage on CT scan with 97.5% accuracy.[21] However, it is important to note the limitations of this blood test in the context of concussion. While it may be useful immediately following head injury to help decide whether a head CT scan is needed to identify intracranial hemorrhage potentially requiring neurosurgical intervention, it is less useful for concussion since most patients with concussion do not have findings on head CT and thus will have a negative test. As such, it is not, strictly speaking, a blood test for concussion, but rather a blood test for head CT findings after head trauma.

Once a more serious intracranial injury has been excluded and the index of suspicion for concussion remains high, a comprehensive history and examination are essential for diagnosing concussion. The history should include details of the mechanism of injury, including any brief loss of consciousness, alteration in mental status, amnesia, either retrograde or anterograde, and associated events, such as impact seizure. If the injury was sports- or recreation-related, it is useful to determine if the injured athlete continued to play or was removed from play after injury, as continued participation in athletic activity after an injury is associated with prolonged recovery compared to athletes who were immediately removed from play.[22,23] A history of any immediate-onset symptoms should be obtained, including headache, dizziness, and vomiting, among others, followed by a history of progression of symptoms since injury. Standardized concussion symptom questionnaires may be useful in this context. Initial management of the concussion by parents and others should be ascertained, as well as any evaluations by other clinical personnel since the injury. The patient's past medical history should be reviewed, including attention to timing and recovery course of any previous concussions. In addition, any history of premorbid medical conditions that may affect return to activities after concussion or prolong recovery from concussion should be solicited, including a history of migraines, learning disabilities, mood disorders, or motion sickness.[4,24]

The history in young children deserves special attention in that they may have limited semantics to describe their experience with concussion so most symptomatology will likely be reported by parents. Under these circumstances, it becomes even more important to listen to parents' reports about observed changes in behavior and temperament of their injured child. Simple direct questioning should also be utilized, as it may yield helpful candid observations made by younger children. There are validated concussion symptom scales for younger children, as well as parent-reported symptom scales, which may be used to help obtain accurate and complete symptom reports for younger children.[25]

An important component of the initial assessment for pediatric concussion is the physical examination. In the past, standard neurological examinations were often normal in children with concussion. With further investigation, more recent research has identified specific deficits in balance, vision, and vestibular function that are often observed following concussion.[3,26] As such, it is important that clinicians specifically assess these various domains in order to support the diagnosis of concussion; otherwise, the diagnosis is purely subjective and symptom-based without the addition of any physical examination findings.

Brief visiovestibular screens[3,27] are useful for identifying deficits in vestibular function and balance, as they include assessments of tandem gait (eyes open/closed) as well as the vestibular-ocular reflex, visual motion sensitivity, convergence, and accommodation. Visual assessment should involve more than a simple evaluation for visual acuity since that is usually normal in concussion. Oculomotor screening of smooth pursuits and saccades, as well as an assessment of binocular near point of convergence and monocular accommodation will often identify deficits in children with concussion.[3] Visual and vestibular deficits detected on physical examination can help clinicians make tailored recommendations, with a particular focus on successfully returning children to the learning setting where these deficits can have a substantial negative effect.

The physical examination of a younger child with concussion, including a standard neurologic examination, as well as a visiovestibular screen, may be more challenging. In these cases, attempts to evaluate the visual and vestibular systems should still be made, but with modifications accounting for the developmental stage. Children under 5 years may have difficulty with tandem gait under normal circumstances, but gait may still be evaluated. Children who are 8 years of age or older have been shown to reliably perform the tasks required to conduct a visiovestibular screen,[9] and attempts to perform portions of this screening examination in even younger children may yield useful information, such as the manifestations of difficulty performing a task or symptom provocation that a younger child may demonstrate while tracking an object of interest with smooth pursuits.

Brief neurocognitive assessments may be performed both on the sideline of athletic events or in the clinical setting. These assessments may involve paper and pencil testing, such as the Sideline Concussion Assessment Test 5 (SCAT 5), or computerized platforms.[10,31] SCAT 5 has a tool for use under the age of 12 years[28] and most computerized neurocognitive testing platforms are intended for use starting at age 12 years or above; however, some are approved for use in school-aged children as young as 6 years of age.[29,30] Acute comprehensive neuropsychological testing is neither indicated nor necessary given the extensive time and labor commitment involved, so brief neurocognitive screening assessments are commonly used instead. Pre-injury baseline testing of athletes has become common, trickling down from the professional level to the youth sports community. To date, there remains insufficient evidence to mandate such testing even in high-risk collision sports, such as football or ice hockey.[31] Despite that fact, many schools and athletic clubs provide preinjury baseline testing to their student athletes. If patients had this testing performed prior to their injury, it may be used along with other data collected from the history and physical examination to inform a management plan, but it is not necessary.

MANAGEMENT

Initial management of concussion, especially if sport- or recreation-related, is removal from play.[31] In the interscholastic high school and collegiate setting, athletic training staff may be involved in this decision, while in youth club and some interscholastic sports, volunteer coaches and parents may be the primary adults responsible. Awareness of the available sideline screening tools, such as the SCAT 5, as well as a basic understanding of the principles of early concussion identification and management, is essential. Immediate removal from play is critical as continued sports participation carries with it the ongoing exposure risk for an additional head injury. In addition, there are emerging data that support early removal from play, which is associated with sooner return to sport than those continuing to play.[22,23]

After acute assessment, either on the sideline or in the clinical setting, initial management focuses on activity modification. Early interpretations of the concepts of physical and cognitive rest in elite sports were inaccurately translated to the pediatric setting, resulting in inappropriate, excessive, and prolonged restrictions on activity in children after concussion. These recommendations have been refined to more appropriately encompass activity modification focused on limiting severe symptom exacerbation rather than strict physical bed rest or attempts to eliminate all cognitive activity (i.e., cocooning). Prolonged restriction of activities is likely to have negative effects on children and young adults recovering from concussion,[32] so a moderated approach to activity modification is more appropriate. Current recommendations include 48–72 hours of more substantial activity modification to allow concussion symptoms to decrease.[31] It is important to pay close attention to sleep in the postinjury period as sleep is often disrupted after concussion, with patients experiencing trouble falling asleep, trouble staying asleep, and poorer sleep quality compared to prior to the injury. During the first few days after injury, children may sleep more than usual; however, children should gradually return to as normal a sleep routine as possible to prevent lingering problems with sleep developing from both the injury and the response to injury.[33] Once symptoms have improved, a gradual return to activities is recommended since an abrupt return to full activities may cause symptoms to recrudesce. During this period of gradual return, activity modification remains the driving principle of concussion management.

Return to the academic setting is of utmost importance and has been referred to variously as return to school and return to learn.[4] For the purposes of this discussion, the term "return to school" will refer to managing the return to the physical space of school while the term "return to learn" will refer to managing the return to cognitive academic activity. A physical return to school should be facilitated as soon as a child can tolerate it from a symptom perspective. Initial barriers may include challenges with waking the student in time to make transportation to school or loud noisy buses that provoke symptoms, such as headache, dizziness, and motion sickness. Potential solutions could include parents driving the student to school at a later

time. Issues that may affect children in their physical return to school, including deficits in balance and vestibular function, may require provisions, such as extra time in hallways or early dismissal from classes to avoid loud and busy hallways. Bright institutional lights may need to be accounted for and temporary use of hats and sunglasses may need to be permitted. Noisy assemblies and classes, such as music, band, or choir, may need to be excused due to sound sensitivity. Physical education classes should be excused, for the time being, to remove risk of reinjury, and adding cognitive workload in place of physical education should not occur. Depending on symptom burden, a return to school for partial days may be indicated with a gradual return to full days of school.[4,10]

With regard to return to learn, it is critical to remember the pathophysiology of metabolic mismatch to understand that cognitive stamina is substantially reduced acutely after concussion. As such, an immediate return to full academic workload is not advisable and efforts should be made to prioritize only essential, foundational work and medically excuse any nonessential work. Even with these adjustments, additional measures, including extra time for completing assignments and multiple breaks for cognitive pacing, will still likely be necessary. Upon initial return to school, there may not be much immediate return to learning. Many students may need a few days to adjust to the demands of being physically present in school even without much academic workload, using the time to simply listen to and absorb what is occurring in the classroom, without having to visually engage by taking notes or cognitively engage by trying to retain information. Once academic work is reinitiated, any visiovestibular deficits that may affect reading, note-taking, or looking up and down or side to side may need to be accounted for. Additional adjustments, such as providing preprinted notes and potentially using large font, may be necessary for students with visual deficits. Postponing testing during the early return from concussion is indicated and should continue until adjustment back to the school setting with gradual increase in resumption of academic cognitive work has been completed. Students may need extra time to prepare for testing and may need extra time, breaks, or testing over multiple sessions when initially resuming testing. Early front-loading of such academic adjustments is essential for a smooth transition back to school and learning, and will help minimize undue stress to the student recovering from concussion. Recognizing the support needed for concussed students returning to school and learning will help improve the student's symptom management and experience while in school, potentially decreasing the need for longer-term academic accommodations. Younger children with concussion may be able to return to full school days more quickly than older children due to the more forgiving nature of their school schedule and more easily modifiable cognitive workload. In contrast, younger children may have more difficulty with self-awareness of symptom provocation. In these instances, scheduled cognitive pacing breaks every few hours may be more beneficial than waiting for the younger child to experience and identify symptom exacerbation and then make effort to request a break.[4,10]

In terms of return to activity, most of the emphasis has centered around return to play, defined as a return to organized sports, rather than a return to free recreational play as the phrase might be interpreted. For this discussion, we will use return to activity as the terminology for return to life activities, including free recreational play. We will identify the elements involved in the return-to-play process, and we will also provide some guidance on return to driving and return to work as special situations.

For organized sports, a standardized return-to-play protocol has been developed that returns an athlete to full sports participation in a stepwise fashion.[31] If an athlete becomes symptom free after a brief period of physical rest, gradual return to physical activity beginning with light aerobic activity and advancing to heavier aerobic and sport-specific training may commence. Each step is intended to take at least 24 hours and the athlete must complete each step without symptom provocation in order to advance to the next step. The final step is clearance for full contact sports participation, indicating that full clinical recovery from the concussion has occurred. In cases where the concussion symptoms resolve quickly over the span of a few days, the return to play process generally takes approximately 1 week.[31] In many instances, however, the return to play process may be stretched out over a longer period of time and athletes may remain at a step for a few days before advancing. In either case, there is evidence that this symptom-free waiting period has the added benefit of providing additional time for physiologic neurologic recovery that may continue after apparent clinical recovery (i.e., symptom recovery) and appears to reduce the rate of repeat concussion within a short time frame after apparent clinical recovery.[23]

The formal return-to-play process for youth athletes participating in organized interscholastic or collegiate sports may occur under the supervision of a qualified physician or other clinician in conjunction with an athletic trainer. For younger athletes participating in club sports where there may not be any athletic training support, the physician or clinician will need to take a more direct role with the patients and parents in the stepwise process. For children who are returning to noncontact sports, such as running, swimming, or recreational play, the return-to-play process follows the same approach based on the fundamental principle of limiting risk for repeat injury while gradually increasing participation in physical activities. A return-to-activity process may be undertaken at a slower pace than a formal return-to-play process and may be conducted under the direction of a qualified clinician.

Return to work may be an additional challenge for some adolescents and young adults in college. It is important to consider the patient's type of work, whether it is primarily cognitive and computer- and desk-based or physical and manual labor-based. Risk for reinjury should always be factored into any plan for return to work and should not be permitted until the patient has fully recovered from their concussion similar to the process followed by someone returning to a risk-bearing sport. Both physical and cognitive stamina will present issues for those returning to work, so a gradual return to work is recommended. Since cognitive stamina difficulties may be exacerbated by visiovestibular issues, allowing breaks as needed for symptom management as well as accommodations for visual tasks may be helpful. Physical work will also require breaks for physical and cognitive stamina issues. The pacing principles discussed in the return to school section apply to the work setting as well.[2]

Returning an adolescent or young adult to driving also deserves special attention as some teenagers may still have limited licensure and supervision requirements. While there are little data on driving and concussions to support these recommendations, lessons learned from research on teen driving are notably applicable to this situation. Young teen drivers have less experience than older drivers. Although they may have better reaction times than older drivers, reaction time is known to be slowed following concussion,[34] posing a substantial risk for teen drivers and those around them. General recommendations for driving after concussion include not driving while acutely injured or symptomatic, only returning to driving after symptoms have improved and then returning in a gradual fashion, taking shorter trips, and temporarily avoiding long trips at night or in bad weather. Some computerized neurocognitive programs provide a measure of reaction time that may provide clinicians with additional data in their decision-making regarding returning to driving.

PERSISTENT CONCUSSION SYMPTOMS

Postconcussion syndrome is a term that is used very broadly and imprecisely with definitions varying between ICD-10 and DSM-V.[19] In this discussion, we will instead use the term persistent concussion symptoms, defined here as symptoms lasting longer than 4 weeks after injury in children. Up to 1/3 of children may experience such prolonged recoveries,[7] and their clinical management warrants special attention. Currently there is not an accurate means of predicting which children will go on to experience persistent concussion symptoms; however, recent progress has been made with the development of a clinical risk prediction score. Based on this prediction score, females, age 13 years or older, history of physician-diagnosed migraine, prior concussion with symptoms lasting longer than 1 week, headache, sensitivity to noise, fatigue, answering questions slowly, and four or more errors on the BESS tandem stance upon presentation were all factors that increased risk of having persisting concussion symptoms at 28 days.[7] There are multiple factors that likely play a role in the persistence of concussion symptoms, ranging from injury characteristics to individual genetic predispositions. Other factors that have also been associated with prolonged symptomatology following concussion include higher initial symptom burden, female sex, presence of ADHD, dizziness at time of injury and earlier pubertal stage at injury, migraines, anxiety and depression, sleep disturbance, and visual and vestibular deficits; however, some studies are conflicting.[24] In addition, the presence of visiovestibular deficits following concussion has been found to be predictive of prolonged recovery as well.[2]

The approach to persistent symptoms has evolved over the last decade to include more active management with targeted rehabilitation therapies that address the causes of these persistent symptoms, thereby improving quality of life. In particular, the assessment of various domains of function is essential to determine which systems are at the root of persistent symptomatology. Interventions are then targeted toward those specific domains. In particular, vestibular deficits are commonly observed in children after concussion[26] and, when persistent in nature, appear to improve with vestibular rehabilitation therapy.[16] Patients often complain of dizziness, motion sickness, and poor motion tolerance after injury. Standard courses of vestibular therapy, which involve habituation training and increasing tolerance to motion over time with balance, VOR and VMS retraining, may be effective over the course of weeks to months at improving these symptoms.[15,18] Balance rehabilitation may be particularly important as there is increasing evidence that athletes with concussion are at higher risk of sustaining musculoskeletal injuries in the subsequent months following recovery, which may result from detraining after concussion or potentially unrehabilitated balance and vestibular deficits.[1]

Visual disorders are also common in children after concussion and should be assessed in anyone with prolonged symptomatology. There is evidence that children may not always recognize that they have vision problems after concussion,[3] so clinician index of suspicion is essential for detecting oculomotor problems or monocular or binocular vision deficits. In children who have abnormal screening assessments for these vision and oculomotor problems, further evaluation by a developmental optometrist trained in vision therapy is indicated. Rehabilitation of the visual system may include retraining saccades and smooth pursuits, as well as accommodation and convergence, with specific exercises designed to promote the fusing of two images into one in the case of convergence insufficiency and to improve binocular eye tracking.[14] An additional feature of persisting concussion symptomatology may be dysautonomia which may manifest as exercise intolerance.[35] This is effectively treated with subsymptom threshold aerobic exercise training designed to gradually increase aerobic activity based on heart rate targets associated with symptom exacerbation. Aerobic exercise in patients with exercise intolerance helps retrain injured patients and return them to a preinjury level of function.[35]

In addition to vestibular, vision, and aerobic rehabilitation, additional targets for intervention include cognition, mood, and sleep. With regard to cognitive rehabilitation, the main approach has been to utilize the school setting as a rehabilitative setting.[4] In a practical way, modified school activities function as cognitive rehabilitation for children recovering from concussion. If accommodations can be made through the subacute and chronic phases for patients with prolonged symptomatology, school work, along with tutoring and study skills coaching, may serve as a highly effective means by which children rehabilitate their cognitive challenges after concussion. If executive function deficits are more profound or long-lasting, comprehensive neuropsychological testing may be undertaken to identify areas of need and an individualized plan for support may be developed, which may include speech and occupational therapy for memory, retention, and recall issues. Working with an educational psychologist or "college coach" may be helpful to students with persistent cognitive symptoms in order to improve study and testing habits. Some clinicians may prescribe medication, stimulant or otherwise, to students manifesting attentional deficits following concussion. The evidence to support this is limited, but if the student meets criteria for attention deficit after a concussion, appropriate treatment is indicated.[12]

Similarly, anxiety and depression are common both in adolescence and following concussion. In light of this fact, treatment with known effective interventions, such as cognitive behavioral therapy and, for some, medication management may be indicated in certain cases.[36] In addition, persistent sleep problems are an important issue to monitor in children with prolonged symptoms that may also exacerbate cognitive and mood issues. Sleep hygiene measures, such as consistent bedtime and routine, as well as limiting electronics, food, and exercise right before bed may be helpful. Melatonin is sometimes used for sleep issues, but there are limited data to support its use.[37] Cognitive behavioral therapy for insomnia may also be helpful, but warrants further investigation.[33] For younger children, all of these therapies are valid options. Younger children have successfully completed rehabilitation using modified approaches for young children,[14,16] so those who are identified should be treated in the same manner as older teens and young adults, but with developmental adjustments to the approach.

CONCLUSION

Concussion is a common injury that occurs across childhood from the preschool years to young adulthood. As such, it is important for any clinician who interacts with children across the age span to be familiar with the diagnosis and management of concussion in the various developmental stages when they may occur. Clinical acumen in diagnosis and management remains essential, with advances in our understanding informing our acute management of injury and gradual return to all life activities, including school, sports, and life. Recognizing the various domains that may be affected by concussion will enable the clinician to tailor management during recovery to ameliorate the effects of such deficits as seen in the visiovestibular, cognitive, and mood domains. Such interventions will invariably improve the quality of life for children as they recover from this common injury and return to full participation in their life activities. For the substantial minority of children who experience persisting concussion symptoms, there is promising evidence that active management with targeted rehabilitation therapies mitigates the impact of prolonged recovery on pediatric quality of life and returns children back to full functioning in a timely fashion. For children and young adults across the age span, there is great promise that concussion need not have a prolonged negative impact on their experience of childhood if careful attention is paid to the recognition, diagnosis, and active management of this injury.

REFERENCES

1. Brooks MA, Peterson K, Biese K, Sanfilippo J, Heiderscheit BC, Bell DR. Concussion increases odds of sustaining a lower extremity musculoskeletal injury after return to play among collegiate athletes. *Am J Sports Med.* 2016;44(3):742−747.
2. Haarbauer-Krupa J, Arbogast KB, Metzger KB, et al. Variations in mechanisms of injury for children with concussion. *J Pediatr.* 2018;197:241−248 e241.
3. Arbogast KB, Curry AE, Pfeiffer MR, et al. Point of health care entry for youth with concussion within a large pediatric care Network. *JAMA Pediatr.* 2016:e160294.
4. Grady MF, Master CL. Return to school and learning after concussion: tips for pediatricians. *Pediatr Ann.* 2017;46(3):e93−e98.
5. Henry LC, Elbin RJ, Collins MW, Marchetti G, Kontos AP. Examining recovery trajectories after sport-related concussion with a multimodal clinical assessment approach. *Neurosurgery.* 2016;78(2):232−241.
6. Nelson LD, Guskiewicz KM, Barr WB, et al. Age differences in recovery after sport-related concussion: a comparison of high school and collegiate athletes. *J Athl Train.* 2016;51(2):142−152.
7. Zemek R, Barrowman N, Freedman SB, et al. Clinical risk score for persistent postconcussion symptoms among children with acute concussion in the ED. *JAMA.* 2016;315(10):1014−1025.
8. Pardini D, Stump J, Lovell M, Collins M, Moritz K, Fu F. The post-concussion symptom scale (PCSS): a factor Analysis. *Br J Sports Med.* 2004;38(5):661−662.
9. Corwin DJ, Propert KJ, Zorc JJ, Zonfrillo MR, Wiebe DJ. Use of the vestibular and oculomotor examination for concussion in a pediatric emergency department. *Am J Emerg Med.* 2018.
10. Darby DG, Master CL, Grady MF. Computerized neurocognitive testing in the medical evaluation of sports concussion. *Pediatr Ann.* 2012;41(9):371−376.
11. Giza CC, Hovda DA. The new neurometabolic cascade of concussion. *Neurosurgery.* 2014;75(suppl 4):S24−S33.
12. Brown NJ, Mannix RC, O'Brien MJ, Gostine D, Collins MW, Meehan 3rd WP. Effect of cognitive activity level on duration of post-concussion symptoms. *Pediatrics.* 2014;133(2):e299−304.
13. Majerske CW, Mihalik JP, Ren D, et al. Concussion in sports: postconcussive activity levels, symptoms, and neurocognitive performance. *J Athl Train.* 2008;43(3):265−274.
14. Gallaway M, Scheiman M, Mitchell GL. Vision therapy for post-concussion vision disorders. *Optom Vis Sci.* 2017;94(1):68−73.

15. Aligene K, Lin E. Vestibular and balance treatment of the concussed athlete. *NeuroRehabilitation*. 2013;32(3):543–553.

16. Master CL, Master SR, Wiebe DJ, et al. Vision and vestibular system dysfunction predicts prolonged concussion recovery in children. *Clin J Sport Med*. 2018;28(2):139–145.

17. Leddy JJ, Cox JL, Baker JG, et al. Exercise treatment for postconcussion syndrome: a pilot study of changes in functional magnetic resonance imaging activation, physiology, and symptoms. *J Head Trauma Rehabil*. 2013;28(4):241–249.

18. Alsalaheen BA, Mucha A, Morris LO, et al. Vestibular rehabilitation for dizziness and balance disorders after concussion. *J Neurol Phys Ther*. 2010;34(2):87–93.

19. Quinn DK, Mayer AR, Master CL, Fann JR. Prolonged postconcussive symptoms. *Am J Psychiatry*. 2018;175(2):103–111.

20. Kuppermann N, Holmes JF, Dayan PS, et al. Identification of children at very low risk of clinically-important brain injuries after head trauma: a prospective cohort study. *Lancet*. 2009;374(9696):1160–1170.

21. Papa L, Brophy GM, Welch RD, et al. Time course and diagnostic accuracy of glial and neuronal blood biomarkers GFAP and UCH-L1 in a large cohort of trauma patients with and without mild traumatic brain injury. *JAMA Neurol*. 2016;73(5):551–560.

22. McCrea M, Guskiewicz K, Randolph C, et al. Effects of a symptom-free waiting period on clinical outcome and risk of reinjury after sport-related concussion. *Neurosurgery*. 2009;65(5):876–882. discussion 882-873.

23. Asken BM, Bauer RM, Guskiewicz KM, et al. Immediate removal from activity after sport-related concussion is associated with shorter clinical recovery and less severe symptoms in collegiate student-athletes. *Am J Sports Med*. 2018;46(6):1465–1474.

24. Iverson GL, Gardner AJ, Terry DP, et al. Predictors of clinical recovery from concussion: a systematic review. *Br J Sports Med*. 2017;51(12):941–948.

25. Sady MD, Vaughan CG, Gioia GA. Psychometric characteristics of the postconcussion symptom inventory in children and adolescents. *Arch Clin Neuropsychol*. 2014;29(4):348–363.

26. Corwin DJ, Wiebe DJ, Zonfrillo MR, et al. Vestibular deficits following youth concussion. *J Pediatr*. 2015;166(5):1221–1225.

27. Mucha A, Collins MW, Elbin RJ, et al. A brief vestibular/ocular motor screening (VOMS) assessment to evaluate concussions: preliminary findings. *Am J Sports Med*. 2014;42:2479–2486.

28. Davis GA, Purcell L, Schneider KJ, et al. The child sport concussion assessment tool 5th edition (child SCAT5): background and rationale. *Br J Sports Med*. 2017;51(11):859–861.

29. Williams J, Crowe LM, Dooley J, et al. Developmental trajectory of information-processing skills in children: computer-based assessment. *Appl Neuropsychol Child*. 2016;5(1):35–43.

30. Bangirana P, Sikorskii A, Giordani B, Nakasujja N, Boivin MJ. Validation of the CogState battery for rapid neurocognitive assessment in Ugandan school age children. *Child Adolesc Psychiatr Ment Health*. 2015;9:38.

31. McCrory P, Meeuwisse W, Dvorak J, et al. Consensus statement on concussion in sport—the 5th international conference on concussion in sport held in Berlin, October 2016. *Br J Sports Med*. 2017. bjsports-2017-097699.

32. Buckley TA, Munkasy BA, Clouse BP. Acute cognitive and physical rest may not improve concussion recovery time. *J Head Trauma Rehabil*. 2016;31(4):233–241.

33. Wickwire EM, Schnyer DM, Germain A, et al. Sleep, sleep disorders, and circadian health following mild traumatic brain injury in adults: review and research agenda. *J Neurotrauma*. 2018;35(22):2615–2631.

34. MacDonald J, Wilson J, Young J, et al. Evaluation of a simple test of reaction time for baseline concussion testing in a population of high school athletes. *Clin J Sport Med*. 2015;25(1):43–48.

35. Leddy J, Baker JG, Haider MN, Hinds A, Willer B. A physiological approach to prolonged recovery from sport-related concussion. *J Athl Train*. 2017;52(3):299–308.

36. Ellis MJ, Ritchie LJ, Koltek M, et al. Psychiatric outcomes after pediatric sports-related concussion. *J Neurosurg Pediatr*. 2015;16(6):709–718.

37. Meehan 3rd WP. Medical therapies for concussion. *Clin Sports Med*. 2011;30(1):115–124. ix.

CHAPTER 13

Assessment and Treatment of Concussion in Service Members and Veterans

ROBERT D. SHURA, PSYD, ABPP-CN • ERICA L. EPSTEIN, PSYD •
PATRICK ARMISTEAD-JEHLE, PHD, ABPP-CN •
DOUGLAS B. COOPER, PHD, ABPP-CN • BLESSEN C. EAPEN, MD

BACKGROUND

Incidence of traumatic brain injury (TBI) in active duty service members (SMs) steadily increased from approximately 11,000 in the year 2000 to a peak of nearly 33,000 in 2011, with subsequent decline.[1] Between the years of 2000 to the first quarter of 2018 there are 383, 947 SMs diagnosed with TBI, with 82.3% falling in the mild range of severity.[1] The rise in TBI is seen primarily in the Army, and even though there is an increase of TBI awareness, mild TBI (mTBI; used interchangeably here with concussion) can easily go undiagnosed, overlooked, or underreported. The diagnostic criteria for mTBI according to the Department of Defense (DoD) and Veterans Administration (VA) is defined as having an alteration in consciousness for less than 24 h and normal results on brain imaging. If there is any loss of consciousness it lasts less than 30 min, and if there is any post-traumatic amnesia it lasts less than 24 h.[2] Due to the lack of noticeable physical wounds and normal results on brain imaging, mTBI is considered by many to be the "silent" or "invisible" injury.[3] Nonetheless, others have considered TBI to be the "signature injury" of recent conflicts, highlighting the increase in injury incidence.[4]

The incidence and outcome of TBI has evolved over the course of military conflicts. Namely, recent conflicts in Iraq and Afghanistan have seen a dramatic increase in the use of explosive devices such as improvised explosive devices (IEDs), rockets, and mortars. Although the use of explosive devices is not new to warfare, one major difference between past conflicts and todays' is the survivability of blasts. Blast-related injuries were more likely to be deadly to SMs in the past, and today's SMs benefit from advanced tactical gear designed to withstand ballistic weaponry and adapted to a number of warfare situations. Many of today's SMs are able to walk away from assaults that would have caused irreparable bodily damage in the past.[5] This has led to an increase in blast-related injuries and the emerging problem of combat-based concussion.[6]

Anyone who previously served in the military is considered a veteran. Whereas assessment and management of concussion for SMs is predominantly handled by the DoD through the Military Healthcare System (MHS), veterans utilize the Veterans Health Administration (VHA)[1] or other forms of civilian care: the different contexts lead to differences in approaching concussion assessment and management. For example, even at the level of tracking concussion, self-report consistency is an issue. Currently, self-report is the main method of reporting an mTBI and sequela. However, research has found that self-report of TBI-related symptoms in the DoD is inconsistent with the VHA, such that veterans are likely to report significantly more TBI-related symptoms when in the VHA.[7] Although this may indicate validity issues concerning self-report, it may also reflect the difference between the mission of the DoD versus the VA. The mission of the DoD focuses on fitness for duty with priority for protecting the country: "To provide the military forces needed to deter war and to protect the security of our country,"[8] and the VA mission is veteran focused and centers on healthcare and disability: "To care for him who shall have borne the battle."[9]

---

[1]MHS refers to the healthcare system within the larger DoD. Similarly, the VHA and VBA are two of the three subdepartments in the larger VA system, focusing on healthcare and benefits, respectively.

Concussion. https://doi.org/10.1016/B978-0-323-65384-8.00013-4
Copyright © 2020 Elsevier Inc. All rights reserved.

These differing missions lead to differences in treatment interventions and goals, and is important to note when conceptualizing TBI across the two contexts.

Immediately after sustaining mTBI, many individuals experience physical, emotional, and cognitive symptoms; however, most individuals experience a full and fast recovery, with deficits typically resolving in days to weeks, though some may take up to 3 months.[10] Due to the short recovery period, evaluating mTBI in isolation can make it seem like a simple injury, but in the context of deployment, the picture of mTBI becomes much more complicated. Current literature has evaluated the long-term effects of mTBI during deployment and has found a host of associated consequences that are not commonly found in civilians, which includes poorer long-term outcomes.[11] Veterans who experienced an mTBI with loss of consciousness are more likely to be diagnosed with post-traumatic stress disorder (PTSD), report poor health, and have persisting postconcussive symptoms.[11,12] In fact for veterans, mTBI often co-occurs with PTSD and chronic pain, termed the "polytrauma clinical triad."[13–15] Iraq and Afghanistan veterans may accumulate numerous physical, emotional, and cognitive problems, including polytrauma clinical triad disorders, which potentially lead to a negative trajectory of general well-being, including an increased risk for suicide.[13,16] In other words, evaluation and both acute and chronic management of concussion for SMs and veterans is arguably more complex than in other contexts.

It is still unclear if mTBI has a causative relationship with PTSD and health symptoms, or if repeated exposure to blasts and head injuries leave the veteran vulnerable to co-occurring conditions; however, what is clear is that mTBI rarely occurs in isolation for the Iraq/Afghanistan veteran, and treatment for the veteran with mTBI will often include other areas of health and psychological functioning. This chapter will review aspects of blast injury, which comprise the majority of deployment-based TBI, discuss assessment and rehabilitation efforts following acute and chronic mTBI, and outline barriers to recovery following mTBI for SMs and veterans.

THE UNIQUE CASE OF BLAST INJURY

Historically, TBI has been considered predominantly a result of blunt-force trauma. However, somewhat unique to combat and especially the recent conflicts in Iraq and Afghanistan is the phenomenon of blast forces due to the increased use of IEDs, mortars, and rockets. While the majority of SM TBIs occur in garrison

and are secondary to similar causes as the general population (e.g., falls, motor vehicle accidents, and assaults),[17] the majority of *combat-related* TBI in Iraq and Afghanistan involve blast-related forces.[6] Studies have found around 81% of sustained injuries from Iraq and Afghanistan veterans are due to explosions as opposed to gunshots.[6] Although this number is higher than past conflicts, use of explosive devices is not a new war tactic, and past wars saw 65% explosion injuries in Vietnam, 73% in WWII, and 35% in WWI.[6]

The term blast injury refers to a broad array of injuries incurring either directly or indirectly from a blast. There are up to 5 separate types of injuries resulting from a blast, including primary injury of the pressure wave force, the possible secondary injury involving blunt trauma, tertiary translation force injuries, quaternary heat and burn injuries, and quinary indirect injuries such as hypoxia or chemical exposure.[18] Additionally, increasing research has begun to focus on non–combat-related blast injuries, such as are incurred in training of breachers.[19–21] A significant blast exposure event may not result in acute symptoms to meet criteria for mTBI, but may potentially lead to significant physiological disruption, the so-called subconcussive blast exposure.

Recent research has turned toward evaluating if there are unique physiologic disruptions follow blast exposure, and if there are clinically significant impairments in functional outcomes involving physical, cognitive, and emotional domains. Physiologically, there is mixed research indicating possible neuroanatomical disruption from blast. For example, Newsome and colleagues[22] found reduced functional connectivity in the right globus pallidus after covarying for age and psychiatric symptoms. A recent case series found changes in white matter hyperintensities related to severity of blast exposure, but not functional outcomes.[23] Postmortem, a case series of blast-exposed SMs found astroglial scarring at the boundary zones between tissue and fluid, as well as between white and gray matter.[24] However, a review by Mu and colleagues[25] highlighted vast variability in methodology across studies, and definitive conclusions regarding physiological disruption in blast injury remain elusive.

Even if there is unique brain disruption caused by blast forces, functional outcomes are generally nonsignificant. A systematic review of blast versus nonblast TBI in SMs and veterans found similar rates across a variety of health outcomes when comparing the two groups; however, there were inconsistent results for headache, hearing loss, PTSD, and cognitive symptoms.[26] Regarding chronic symptoms, there were no significant differences between blast and nonblast TBI in a sample of veterans greater than 1 month post injury, with the exception of greater hearing complaints in the blast group.[27] Lange and colleagues[28] found no additive effect of a blast plus blunt trauma injury beyond a blunt trauma injury on cognitive measures after covarying for psychiatric symptoms. In contrast, Walker and colleagues[29] found higher rates of nonspecific, self-reported symptoms in a blast mTBI group with post-traumatic amnesia compared to the nonblast group, though symptom validity was not assessed. Although some studies find functional effects related to blast exposure, clinical relevance is questionable in most cases. In sum, there generally do not appear to be significant functional deficits unique to blast,[28,30,31] with the possible exception of hearing impairment, and where deficits are noted, clinical relevance is unclear.

ASSESSMENT AND REHABILITATION IN THE DOD

In considering the assessment and treatment of SMs with a history of concussion, there are a handful of military-specific instruments and protocols that providers working with SMs could benefit from understanding. Within the DoD, during the acute and subacute time of injury SMs are commonly administered the Military Acute Concussion Evaluation (MACE).[32] This instrument was designed as a screening tool to for the acute assessment of SMs involved in a potentially concussive event. It was originally published in 2008, and in 2012 the clinical algorithms were updated to improve accuracy and expand on concussion management. The MACE consists of a history and three evaluation components. The history component is comprised of targeted questions to confirm the diagnosis of mTBI. If positive, the evaluation components are administered, which consist of a brief neurologic evaluation, cognitive assessment, and symptom report. The neurologic examination assesses ocular functioning (pupil response to light and tracking), speech (fluency and word finding), motor functioning (grip strength and pronator drift), and balance (tandem Romberg Test). If any of these four items are abnormal the MACE is coded Red, and if all are normal it is coded Green. The cognitive assessment portion of the MACE is based on the Standardized Assessment of Concussion (SAC) and assesses the following domains: orientation, immediate memory, concentration, and delayed memory. A maximum score of 30 can be attained and the suggested cut score of <25 has been established to indicate abnormal cognitive functioning. Finally, the MACE consists of a symptom screening which is based on self-reported difficulties that frequently follow a concussion (i.e., headache, dizziness, nausea, etc.).

The MACE was designed to be administered by medics and corpsman. An SM with a verified concussion and abnormality in any area is referred to a higher-level provider. In October 2018, a second edition of the MACE was released. The MACE-2 holds a similar structure to the original version; however, it adds a single leg stance to the balance portion of the neurological examination and includes the Vestibular Ocular Motor Screening (VOMS). Currently, the validity of the original MACE has been established in the military population,[33] but at the time of this publication there has been no validity studies on the MACE-2. For the outside provider treating an SM or veteran, there is value in understanding the nature of the patient's injury and initial presentation when diagnosing mTBI and understanding their injury. The MACE and MACE-2 can provide this information.

Another instrument that is relatively unique to the DoD is the Automated Neuropsychological Assessment Metrics (ANAM). The ANAM is a computer-based library of cognitive tests designed to assess various aspects of cognition. The US Military currently employs the fourth version of this instrument (ANAM-4), which is comprised of seven subtests: Simple Reaction Time, Procedural Reaction Time, Code Substitution Learning, Code Substitution Delayed, Mathematical Processing, Matching to Sample, and Simple Reaction Time Second Administration. Per current regulation, this measure is to be administered prior to deployment so that an individual baseline can be obtained for each SM. This baseline can then be compared to postinjury administration to assist in return-to-duty decisions. Each ANAM administration should be referred to a centralized database so that multiple longitudinally obtained scores can be compared as necessary. Providers working with SMs and/or veterans may find this previous cognitive testing useful in assessment and treatment planning.

Next, the Defense Center of Excellence (DCoE) and the Defense and Veterans Brain Injury Center (DVBIC) have established progressive return to activity clinical recommendation protocols following acute mTBI for the primary care and rehabilitation providers.[34] The guidance for primary care managers is a self-guided, provider-supervised staged recovery, whereas the guidance for the rehabilitation providers is a clinician-directed and daily monitored staged recovery. Protocols provide 6 stages of progression from rest to preinjury activities and measure three domains (physical, cognitive, and vestibular/balance) as parameters for ongoing management. The protocols also employ the Neurobehavioral Symptom Inventory (NSI) for ongoing symptom evaluation. Each protocol begins with a mandatory 24-hour rest period (stage 1). Depending on the patient's response and results from initial exertional testing, the protocol then progresses through light routine activity (stage 2), light occupational-oriented activity (stage 3), moderate activity (stage 4), intense activity (stage 5), and unrestricted activity (stage 6). Criteria for progression in the primary care protocol are essentially successful completion of the task with no NSI items >1. If the patient does not recover as expected, is symptomatic after exertional testing following stage 5, or has had two concussions in the last 12 months and has any NSI items >1 after 24 h of rest, then he/she is to be referred to a rehabilitation provider and the rehabilitation protocol is to be engaged.

The rehabilitation protocol utilizes additional instruments to measure progress, which consist of Borg's rate of perceived exertion, theoretical maximum heart rate during activity, resting heart rate, and resting blood pressure. Each stage of recovery has suggested maximum heart rates and rates of perceived exertion, as well as suggested activities across domains and prescribed work to rest ratios. A detailed outline of the cognitive, physical, and vestibular/balance activities associated with each stage are beyond the scope of this review, but can be found at the DVBIC website.[35] For providers working with active duty SMs, understanding and application of these protocols will be important to demonstrate that the SM is ready for a return to unrestricted duties. For the providers working with veterans who may have had chronic symptoms potentially related to previous concussions, understanding how these SMs progressed through these stages of recovery closer to the time of injury may help to inform current treatment planning.

ASSESSMENT AND REHABILITATION IN THE VA

The Polytrauma System of Care (PSC) was developed in 2004 from the existing infrastructure of the VHA brain injury centers in response to the increasing number of SMs returning with severe combat injuries and thereafter with the "invisible injures" of war. The VA defines polytrauma as "two or more injuries to physical regions or organ systems, one of which may be life threatening, resulting in physical, cognitive, psychological, or psychosocial impairments and functional disability" (p. 3).[36] The PSC is an integrated tiered rehabilitation network,[37,38] which provides a continuum of care from coma-to-community reintegration for patients with brain injury. The tiered network includes comprehensive inpatient rehabilitation, residential brain injury programs, and comprehensive outpatient TBI clinics with over 110 access points. The PSC also utilizes interdisciplinary care teams in order to provide a holistic approach to the management of these polymorbid conditions.

In order to identify veterans for potential PSC, the VHA has developed a national TBI clinical reminder and a 4-question screening tool to assess deployment-related TBI exposure and symptomology in post 9/11 veterans. The VHA has screened over 1 million veterans for potential TBI with over 20% referred on for a comprehensive TBI evaluation (CTBIE). The overarching goal of the CTBIE is to assess a veteran for TBI using the VA/DoD criteria for diagnosis of TBI. In addition, the CTBIE assesses for neurobehavioral symptoms using the NSI, targeted physical examination, and development of treatment plan. If treatment is indicated for sequalae of TBI and comorbid conditions, the veteran is then referred the PSC interdisciplinary team. Once TBI care has been established, progress in therapies, care coordination, and community reintegration are tracked using the Individualized Rehabilitation and Community Reintegration (IRCR) plan of care.

EVIDENCE-BASED TREATMENTS FOR CHRONIC MTBI

In response to the large number of SMs and veterans seeking treatment for chronic postconcussive symptoms, several significant advancements have occurred in the development of evidence-based rehabilitation treatments. Treatment approaches that have been examined for postconcussive symptoms following mTBI include psychoeducation, cognitive rehabilitation (CR), and psychotherapeutic approaches. Systematic reviews of these interventions have been completed in both civilian[39–41] and military/veteran populations[42] and have concluded that psychoeducational interventions have substantial support in the acute phase of recovery after a concussion, but more limited support in the chronic phase. Studies have also shown support for psychotherapeutic approaches in the chronic phase of recovery from mTBI, particularly in individuals with co-occurring psychological conditions such as depression and PTSD. Finally, several recent studies have shown that CR interventions can be effective in reducing functional cognitive difficulties in this population. The evidence underlying these conclusions is described in more depth below.

Psychoeducation

A fairly robust literature has demonstrated that psycho-educational interventions provided in the acute or sub-acute phase of recovery from a concussion can reduce the severity of symptoms and the duration of symptoms.[41,43] The intervention, which has been replicated in several trials, includes providing patients with education about common symptoms after concussion, strategies to manage these symptoms, positive expectations of recovery, and guidance about returning to preinjury roles and functions. Studies have shown that this intervention is effective when provided in one-on-one formats, through written handouts, as well as in group sessions, provided that the intervention includes the critical components described above.[40,44,45] No additional benefit has been shown with more intensive interventions during the acute period of recovery.[46,47] Although favorable initial findings were found for the effectiveness of an adapted psychoeducational intervention for SMs and veterans with chronic postconcussive symptoms,[48] a subsequent randomized controlled trial (RCT) of a computer-based psychoeducational intervention in veterans with chronic symptoms failed to replicate those findings.[49] Given that education should be a core component of treatment for any chronic condition, and in the absence of data suggesting a harmful effect, psychoeducation should likely be included in any treatment plan and considered a standard of care in concussion clinics,[2] particularly when adapted to include the multiple potential causes for emotional, cognitive, and physical symptoms in patients with chronic symptoms after mTBI.

Cognitive Rehabilitation

Cognitive complaints are ubiquitous in postdeployment treatment settings, and many SMs and veterans attribute these symptoms to a personal history of mTBI. As such, CR interventions have been studied extensively in this population. Unlike CR for severe TBI or stroke, which focuses on restorative techniques and addresses objective cognitive impairments, CR interventions for individuals with mTBI typically include compensatory strategies for subjective, functional, cognitive complaints.

CogSMART is one of the most widely studied and implemented CR interventions in SMs and veterans with chronic mTBI.[50] The intervention includes both psychoeducational didactics and strategy training on compensatory techniques to manage functional cognitive complaints. The intervention has been adapted for both individual and group interventions and is typically organized in cognitive modules.[51,52] Twamley

et al. showed reductions in both postconcussive symptoms and improved prospective memory in their initial RCT,[50] with treatment gains continuing at 1 year follow-up.[53] The CogSMART CR intervention has been replicated in other independent samples and has been utilized in combined approaches using both CR and psychotherapy conjointly.[54–56] Additionally, studies with veterans have shown that baseline mental health comorbid symptoms did not moderate the efficacy of this intervention in a sample of veterans.[57]

The largest CR trial to date, the SCORE clinical trial,[58] compared four, 6-week treatment arms in a sample of 126 SMs with combat-related mTBI and ongoing cognitive complaints. Subjects were randomized to one of four treatment arms: (1) psychoeducation and medical management; (2) independent self-administered computer-based CR; (3) therapist-directed manualized CR; and (4) therapist-directed CR integrated with cognitive-behavioral psychotherapy (CBT). Significant reductions in functional cognitive difficulties were shown in both treatment arms that included therapist-directed CR (Arms 3 and 4) when compared with treatment arms without therapist-directed rehabilitation (Arms 11 and 2). The addition of psychotherapy in Arm 4 was associated with improved psychological outcomes but was not significantly better than therapist-directed CR without CBT.[58] A post hoc analysis of factors that influenced treatment responsiveness in the SCORE trial showed that comorbid depression and individuals assigned to a team-treatment milieu were associated with positive treatment responsiveness in CR interventions.[59] An unexpected, but important additional finding was that self-administered use of computerized CR interventions failed to show a positive outcome and also negatively impact treatment outcomes. In fact, this study suggested that computerized CR may be harmful to subjects. Follow-up studies are currently underway to determine ways to optimize the SCORE trial using reduced dosage/number of treatment sessions and alternate platforms to expand access to CR services throughout the MHS and VHA.

Psychotherapeutic Approaches

A high rate of psychological comorbidity, such as PTSD and depression, after mTBI has been well documented in military and veteran populations.[2] Given the likely interactive effect between postconcussive symptom reporting and PTSD,[60] several investigators have focused on providing evidence-based PTSD treatments to individuals with a history of mTBI and PTSD. Studies of prolonged exposure not only have demonstrated effectiveness in PTSD symptom reduction but also have shown a more generalized effect on patient outcomes through reductions in overall postconcussive symptoms.[61–64] Similar findings have been shown with cognitive processing therapy.[54,65] A recent post hoc investigation of a subsample of patients with co-morbid PTSD and mTBI demonstrated that exposure therapy obtained considerably greater outcomes than CR and the effect could be produced with less treatment sessions.[66] However, a caveat to the study that should be noted is that not all individuals are ready or willing to engage in exposure therapy, which will likely affect the reproducibility of these findings in other clinic samples.

In order to enhance outcomes and reduce the potential stigma of mental health treatment, several studies have examined integrated psychotherapy in addition to compensatory CR in SMs and veterans dually diagnosed with mTBI and PTSD.[54–56] Using a 7-week intensive residential treatment program model, studies have shown statistically significant reductions in postconcussive symptoms with combined treatment to reduce PTSD symptoms. Outcomes were substantial even in individuals who are also diagnosed with depression.[55] This finding is consistent with prior studies of factors that influence treatment responsiveness from the SCORE clinical trial,[59] as well as in a prior RCT in a civilian sample,[67] providing support for the use of combined psychotherapeutic and CR interventions in military SMs and veterans with chronic postconcussive symptoms.

BARRIERS TO REHABILITATION UNIQUE TO DOD AND VA

Even though a large research base suggests full and fast recovery from mTBI,[68–73] and considerable efforts have increased to identify, evaluate, and rehabilitate SMs and veterans with a history of mTBI, a percentage continue to report chronic postconcussive symptoms and extended recovery periods. A number of situational factors are potentially at play, such as misattribution of nonspecific and unrelated symptoms to a head injury, the uniqueness of blast injury, the stressors of war (e.g., PTSD, sleep deprivation), and premorbid factors likely related to individuals who volunteer to serve in the military compared to those who do not. However, both the DoD and VA have additional potential barriers to recovery inherent in the military and VA contexts. For example, during active duty many SMs may experience a TBI but not report such or downplay the felt effects in order to return to the mission. Such could lead to premature return to duty. In the combat theater, possible repeat injury within the acute time frame may

potentially complicate or extend recovery. This effect was highlighted in two case examples used to present ethical dilemmas encountered by psychologists who evaluate and make return to duty recommendations for concussed SMs.[74]

Another potential mechanism to prolonged recovery involves the initiation of mass TBI screenings in both active duty and VA settings. In the DoD, TBI screening occurs as part of Periodic Health Assessments and Post Deployment Health Assessment and Re-Assessment evaluations. In the VA, a 4-item TBI screen occurs as part of a postdeployment screening, which can trigger a consult for the second-level TBI evaluation with the PSC. Hoge and colleagues[75] warned against the idea of mass screening for remote concussion due to the possibility of instilling an iatrogenic effect whereby an individual misattributes nonspecific symptoms to an injury event, indicating to a patient that the symptoms are unresolvable due to permanent brain damage. Others have echoed similar concerns: "population screening for mild TBI is unnecessary at best and potentially harmful at worst" (p. 211).[38,76] However, the iatrogenesis of TBI screening remains untested, in part due to the difficulty of operationalizing iatrogenesis, and many who screen positive do likely benefit from treatment of nonspecific symptoms that would have otherwise gone unnoticed, even if unrelated to mTBI.

Bridging both DoD and VA are the processes of a medical separation from service via Medical Evaluation Board (MEB) and consideration of service connection (SC) via a Compensation and Pension (C&P) evaluation. In short, when an SM is deemed unable to meet medical retention standards and is unlikely within the next year to reach a point of recovery where medical standards will be met, he/she is referred into the Integrated Disability Evaluation System (IDES). This process not only determines medical fitness but also includes VA evaluations to determine any degree of SC for medical conditions. The outcome of this evaluation will be a determination of whether or not the SM can continue with military service and if not what percentage of SC the SM will be awarded for various medical conditions. Increasing percentage of SC (0% −100%) corresponds to increasing monetary compensation based on severity of symptoms and level of functional impairment.

As the MEB process essentially becomes a disability evaluation, secondary gain and associated symptom exaggeration can be a factor in select patients. Previous research has demonstrated that SMs engaged in this process have significantly higher rates of performance and symptom validity test failure than those seen in the context of clinical care.[77–79] Research has also demonstrated similar findings in military veterans.[80] It is of further note that when an SM or veteran presents for an MEB or C&P evaluation, all previous medical records are considered in making corresponding decisions. To this end, secondary gain has been considered potentially omnipresent in these populations and treating providers should be cognizant of this factor, particularly if symptom reports appear inconsistent and/or aphysiologic in nature.

Service-connected disability evaluations can be embedded in the IDES process, but may also occur following discharge and transition to the VA system, where the mission is to care for those who served as opposed to combat and combat support. Under the Veterans Benefits Association (VBA), veterans who have physical or psychiatric conditions that were "incurred or aggravated during active military service" may be entitled to disability payments.[81] The evaluation process involves submitting a claim with supporting documents, a forensic evaluation (C&P exam), and final determination by a VBA rater, resulting in a percentage rating for qualified conditions that is predominantly based on lost occupational productivity due to the additive effects of all rated conditions (0%–100%). By the availability of a very clear external incentive in a large system where veterans may easily conflate healthcare treatment and disability entitlement, some have suggested that the VA has incentivized the sick role, probably most argued for PTSD, to where motivation for successful rehabilitation, or at least to report symptom improvement, might be an issue.[82–84] Specific to concussion, systematic reviews and meta-analyses have found litigation to be the most prominent factor in those reporting persisting symptoms following concussion.[70,85] Dismuke-Greer and colleagues[86] found a relationship between a history of concussion and percentage of SC disability in a sample of nearly 500 Iraq and Afghanistan veterans; with each TBI reported there was a corresponding 3.6% increase in SC disability, with blast injuries incurring the highest percentage. Given this systemic presence of external incentive, malingering is a concern. One study[87] used a VA C&P sample to extrapolate nationwide estimates of malingered cognitive deficits among those assessed for cognitive complaints related to a history of mTBI (i.e., not accounting for other TBI sequela such as headache). Results suggested that approximately $235 million per year in lost revenue was being distributed to those likely to be malingering cognitive deficits attributed to remote mTBI, an injury in which cognitive deficits are typically expected to resolve after days to several weeks.

A case study published by Roth and Spencer[88] synthesizes many of these barriers with a 35-year-old veteran. The case illustrates a variety of systemic issues as the SM progressed through a medical discharge following a blast mTBI, repeated referral to specialty clinics and related iatrogenesis, failed validity performance on neuropsychological testing, and ultimate achievement of 100% SC disability rating. The authors suggested that those factors led to an investment in the sick role by the veteran, one that will likely be maintained despite the history of what appeared to be a successful recovery from the concussion. Ultimately, such situations can negatively affect both the individual veteran, as well as the larger VA system.

CONCLUSIONS

The evolution of warfare and technologies has in part led to increased mTBI incidence among SMs. Specified treatment and management has emerged both within the MHS and VHA. Assessment and management of concussion with both SMs and veterans can be arguably more complex than for civilians and lead to barriers in treatment, especially in the cases of blast-induced mTBI and when numerous comorbidities stemming from the combat deployment context are present. Nonetheless, both the MHS and VHA have large system-wide screening procedures and complex integrative rehabilitation systems in both acute and chronic stages following mTBI. Evidenced-based treatment approaches examine for postconcussive symptoms and include psychoeducation, CR, psychotherapeutic approaches, and community reintegration.

Despite the increased research on mTBI in these populations, there is still much to learn. Ongoing and future studies should continue to focus on the effects of blast exposure, including blast plus blunt trauma, subconcussive blast, and noncombat blast. Some have also suggested a potential for iatrogenic effects of mass TBI screenings, and future studies should test that hypothesis due to the potential for such to impede the recovery process. Additionally, when considering treatment and recovery, attention should be given to the potential of reinforcing effects of external incentives in large systems, which may further prevent or prolong recovery for SMs and veterans. Overall, mTBI in the military context includes unique factors with regard to the concussing event, environment, and SM characteristics, which play an important role in mTBI diagnosis and treatment in both the MHS and VHA.

DISCLAIMER

The views expressed in this chapter are those of the authors and do not necessarily reflect the position or policy of the Department of Veterans Affairs, the Department of Defense, or the U.S. Government.

REFERENCES

1. Defense and Veterans Brain Injury Center (DVBIC). *Total DoD TBI worldwide numbers*. 2018.
2. The Management of Concussion/mTBI Working Group. VA/DoD clinical practice guideline for management of concussion/mTBI. In: *Affairs DoV*. 2016:1–109. Version 2.0.
3. Helmick KM, Spells CA, Malik SZ, Davies CA, Marion DW, Hinds SR. Traumatic brain injury in the US military: epidemiology and key clinical and research programs. *Brain Imag Behav*. 2015;9(3):358–366.
4. DePalma RG, Hoffman SW. Combat blast related traumatic brain injury (TBI): decade of recognition; promise of progress. *Behav Brain Res*. 2018;340:102–105.
5. Wallace D. Improvised explosive devices and traumatic brain injury: the military experience in Iraq and Afghanistan. *Australas Psychiatr*. 2009;17(3):218–224.
6. Owens BD, Kragh Jr JF, Wenke JC, Macaitis J, Wade CE, Holcomb JB. Combat wounds in operation Iraqi freedom and operation enduring freedom. *J Trauma*. 2008;64(2):295–299.
7. Russo AC, Fingerhut EC. Consistency of self-reported neurocognitive symptoms, post-traumatic stress disorder symptoms, and concussive events from end of first deployment to veteran health administration comprehensive traumatic brain injury evaluation by operations enduring freedom/Iraqi freedom/new dawn veterans. *Arch Clin Neuropsychol*. 2017;32(2):184–197.
8. U.S. Department of Defense. U.S. Department of Defense. 2018. https://www.defense.gov/.
9. U.S. Department of Veterans Affairs. Department of Veterans Affairs. 2018. https://www.va.gov/.
10. Boyle E, Cancelliere C, Hartvigsen J, Carroll LJ, Holm LW, Cassidy JD. Systematic review of prognosis after mild traumatic brain injury in the military: results of the International Collaboration on Mild Traumatic Brain Injury Prognosis. *Arch Phys Med Rehabil*. 2014;95(3 suppl):S230–S237.
11. Mac Donald CL, Johnson AM, Wierzechowski L, et al. Outcome trends after US military concussive traumatic brain injury. *J Neurotrauma*. 2017;34:2206–2219.
12. Hoge CW, McGurk D, Thomas JL, Cox AL, Engel CC, Castro CA. Mild traumatic brain injury in U.S. Soldiers returning from Iraq. *N Engl J Med*. 2008;358(5):453–463.
13. Finley EP, Bollinger M, Noel PH, et al. A national cohort study of the association between the polytrauma clinical triad and suicide-related behavior among US Veterans who served in Iraq and Afghanistan. *Am J Public Health*. 2015;105(2):380–387.
14. Lew HL, Otis JD, Tun C, Kerns RD, Clark ME, Cifu DX. Prevalence of chronic pain, posttraumatic stress disorder, and persistent postconcussive symptoms in OIF/OEF veterans: polytrauma clinical triad. *J Rehabil Res Dev*. 2009;46(6):697–702.
15. Pugh MJ, Finley EP, Copeland LA, et al. Complex comorbidity clusters in OEF/OIF veterans: the polytrauma clinical triad and beyond. *Med Care*. 2014;52(2):172–181.
16. Brenner LA, Vanderploeg RD, Terrio H. Assessment and diagnosis of mild traumatic brain injury, posttraumatic stress disorder, and other polytrauma conditions: burden of adversity hypothesis. *Rehabil Psychol*. 2009;54(3):239–246.
17. DVBIC. *TBI & the Military*; 2018. https://dvbic.dcoe.mil/tbi-military.
18. Cernak I. Understanding blast-induced neurotrauma: how far have we come? *Concussion*. 2017;2(3):CNC42.
19. Carr W, Polejaeva E, Grome A, et al. Relation of repeated low-level blast exposure with symptomology similar to concussion. *J Head Trauma Rehabil*. 2015;30(1):47–55.
20. Carr W, Stone JR, Walilko T, et al. Repeated low-level blast exposure: a descriptive human subjects study. *Mil Med*. 2016;181(5 suppl):28–39.
21. Tate CM, Wang KKW, Eonta S, et al. Serum brain biomarker level, neurocognitive performance, and self-reported symptom changes in soldiers repeatedly exposed to low-level blast: a breacher pilot study. *J Neurotrauma*. 2013;30:1–11.
22. Newsome MR, Mayer AR, Lin X, et al. Chronic effects of blast-related TBI on subcortical functional connectivity in veterans. *J Int Neuropsychol Soc*. 2016;22:631–642.
23. Martindale SL, Rowland JA, Shura RD, Taber KH. Longitudinal changes in neuroimaging and neuropsychiatric status of post-deployment veterans: a CENC pilot study. *Brain Inj*. 2018;32(10):1208–1216.
24. Shively SB, Horkayne-Szakaly I, Jones RV, Kelly JP, Armstrong RC, Perl DP. Characterisation of interface astroglial scarring in the human brain after blast exposure: a post-mortem case series. *Lancet Neurol*. 2016;15(9):944–953.
25. Mu W, Catenaccio E, Lipton ML. Neuroimaging in blast-related mild traumatic brain injury. *J Head Trauma Rehabil*. 2017;32(1):55–69.
26. Greer N, Sayer N, Koeller E, Velasquez T, Wilt TJ. Outcomes Associated With Blast Versus Nonblast-Related Traumatic Brain Injury in U.S. Military Service Members and Veterans: a systematic review. *J Head Trauma Rehabil*. 2018;33(2). E16–E29.
27. Belanger HG, Proctor-Weber Z, Kretzmer T, Kim M, French LM, Vanderploeg RD. Symptom complaints following reports of blast versus non-blast mild TBI: does mechanism of injury matter? *Clin Neuropsychol*. 2011;25(5):702–715.
28. Lange RT, Pancholi S, Brickell TA, et al. Neuropsychological outcome from blast versus non-blast: mild traumatic brain injury in U.S. Military service members. *J Int Neuropsychol Soc*. 2012;18(3):595–605.

29. Walker WC, Franke LM, Sima AP, Cifu DX. Symptom trajectories after military blast exposure and the influence of mild traumatic brain injury. *J Head Trauma Rehabil.* 2017;32(3):E16−e26.

30. Belanger HG, Kretzmer T, Yoash-Gantz RE, Pickett T, Tupler LA. Cognitive sequelae of blast-related versus other mechanisms of brain trauma. *J Int Neuropsychol Soc.* 2009;15:1−8.

31. Cooper DB, Chau PM, Armistead-Jehle P, Vanderploeg RD, Bowles AO. Relationship between mechanism of injury and neurocognitive functioning in OEF/OIF service members with mild traumatic brain injuries. *Mil Med.* 2012;177(10):1157−1160.

32. French L, McCrea M, Baggett M. The military acute concussion evaluation (MACE). *J Spec Oper Med.* 2008;8(1):68−77.

33. McCrea M, Guskiewicz K, Doncevic S, et al. Day of injury cognitive performance on the Military Acute Concussion Evaluation (MACE) by US military service members in OEF/OIF. *Mil Med.* 2014;179(9):990−997.

34. McCulloch KL, Goldman S, Lowe L, et al. Development of clinical recommendations for progressive return to activity after military mild traumatic brain injury: guidance for rehabilitation providers. *J Head Trauma Rehabil.* 2015;30(1):56−67.

35. DVBIC. *Progressive Return to Activity Following Acute Concussion/Mild TBI Clinical Suite;* 2018. https://dvbic.dcoe.mil/material/progressive-return-activity-following-acute-concussion-mild-tbi-clinical-suite.

36. U.S. Department of Veterans Affairs. Polytrauma rehabilitation procedures. In: *Administration VH.* 2005:1−26.

37. Sigford BJ. "To care for him who shall have borne the battle and for his widow and his orphan" (Abraham Lincoln): the Department of Veterans Affairs polytrauma system of care. *Arch Phys Med Rehabil.* 2008;89(1):160−162.

38. Belanger HG, Uomoto JM, Vanderploeg RD. The Veterans Health Administration's (VHA's) Polytrauma System of Care for mild traumatic brain injury: cost, benefits, and controversies. *J Head Trauma Rehabil.* 2009;24(1):4−13.

39. Al Sayegh A, Sandford D, Carson AJ. Psychological approaches to treatment of postconcussion syndrome: a systematic review. *J Neurol Neurosurg Psychiatry.* 2010;81(10):1128−1134.

40. Comper P, Bisschop SM, Carnide N, Tricco A. A systematic review of treatments for mild traumatic brain injury. *Brain Inj.* 2005;19(11):863−880.

41. Snell DL, Surgenor LJ, Hay-Smith EJC, Siegert RJ. A systematic review of psychological treatments for mild traumatic brain injury: an update on the evidence. *J Clin Exp Neuropsychol.* 2009;31(1):20−38.

42. Cooper DB, Bunner AE, Kennedy JE, et al. Treatment of persistent post-concussive symptoms after mild traumatic brain injury: a systematic review of cognitive rehabilitation and behavioral health interventions in military service members and veterans. *Brain Imag Behav.* 2015;9(3):403−420.

43. Mittenberg W, Tremont G, Zielinski RE, Fichera S, Rayls KR. Cognitive-behavioral prevention of postconcussion syndrome. *Arch Clin Neuropsychol.* 1996;11(2):139−145.

44. Wade DT, King NS, Wenden FJ, Crawford S, Caldwell FE. Routine follow up after head injury: a second randomised controlled trial. *J Neurol Neurosurg Psychiatry.* 1998;65(2):177−183.

45. Ponsford J, Willmott C, Rothwell A, et al. Impact of early intervention on outcome following mild head injury in adults. *J Neurol Neurosurg Psychiatry.* 2002;73(3):330−332.

46. Paniak C, Toller-Lobe G, Durand A, Nagy J. A randomized trial of two treatments for mild traumatic brain injury. *Brain Inj.* 1998;12(12):1011−1023.

47. Paniak C, Toller-Lobe G, Reynolds S, Melnyk A, Nagy J. A randomized trial of two treatments for mild traumatic brain injury: 1 year follow-up. *Brain Inj.* 2000;14(3):219−226.

48. King EG, Kretzmer TS, Vanderploeg RD, Asmussen SB, Clement VL, Belanger HG. Pilot of a novel intervention for postconcussive symptoms in active duty, veterans, and civilians. *Rehabil Psychol.* 2013;58(3):272−279.

49. Belanger HG, Barwick F, Silva MA, Kretzmer T, Kip KE, Vanderploeg RD. Web-based psychoeducational intervention for postconcussion symptoms: a randomized trial. *Mil Med.* 2015;180(2):192−200.

50. Twamley EW, Jak AJ, Delis DC, Bondi MW, Lohr JB. Cognitive Symptom Management and Rehabilitation Therapy (CogSMART) for veterans with traumatic brain injury: pilot randomized controlled trial. *J Rehabil Res Dev.* 2014;51(1):59−70.

51. Huckans M, Pavawalla S, Demadura T, et al. A pilot study examining effects of group-based Cognitive Strategy Training treatment on self-reported cognitive problems, psychiatric symptoms, functioning, and compensatory strategy use in OIF/OEF combat veterans with persistent mild cognitive disorder and history of traumatic brain injury. *J Rehabil Res Dev.* 2010;47(1):43−60.

52. Storzbach D, Twamley EW, Roost MS, et al. Compensatory cognitive training for operation enduring freedom/operation Iraqi freedom/operation new dawn veterans with mild traumatic brain injury. *J Head Trauma Rehabil.* 2017;32(1):16−24.

53. Twamley EW, Thomas KR, Gregory AM, et al. CogSMART compensatory cognitive training for traumatic brain injury: effects over 1 year. *J Head Trauma Rehabil.* 2015;30(6):391−401.

54. Chard KM, Schumm JA, McIlvain SM, Bailey GW, Parkinson RB. Exploring the efficacy of a residential treatment program incorporating cognitive processing therapy-cognitive for veterans with PTSD and traumatic brain injury. *J Trauma Stress.* 2011;24(3):347−351.

55. Walter KH, Barnes SM, Chard KM. The influence of comorbid MDD on outcome after residential treatment for veterans with PTSD and a history of TBI. *J Trauma Stress.* 2012;25(4):426−432.

56. Walter KH, Kiefer SL, Chard KM. Relationship between posttraumatic stress disorder and postconcussive symptom improvement after completion of a posttraumatic stress disorder/traumatic brain injury residential treatment program. *Rehabil Psychol.* 2012;57(1):13−17.

57. Pagulayan KF, O'Neil M, Williams RM, et al. Mental health does not moderate compensatory cognitive training efficacy for veterans with a history of mild traumatic brain injury. *Arch Phys Med Rehabil.* 2017;98(9):1893−1896. e1892.

58. Cooper DB, Bowles AO, Kennedy JE, et al. Cognitive rehabilitation for military service members with mild traumatic brain injury: a randomized clinical trial. *J Head Trauma Rehabil.* 2017;32(3):E1−e15.

59. Vanderploeg RD, Cooper DB, Curtiss G, Kennedy JE, Tate DF, Bowles AO. Predicting treatment response to cognitive rehabilitation in military service members with mild traumatic brain injury. *Rehabil Psychol.* 2018;63(2):194−204.

60. Cooper DB, Kennedy JE, Cullen MA, Critchfield E, Amador RR, Bowles AO. Association between combat stress and post-concussive symptom reporting in OEF/OIF service members with mild traumatic brain injuries. *Brain Inj.* 2011;25(1):1−7.

61. Wolf GK, Kretzmer T, Crawford E, et al. Prolonged exposure therapy with veterans and active duty personnel diagnosed with PTSD and traumatic brain injury. *J Trauma Stress.* 2015;28(4):339−347.

62. Wolf GK, Mauntel GJ, Kretzmer T, et al. Comorbid posttraumatic stress disorder and traumatic brain injury: generalization of prolonged-exposure PTSD treatment outcomes to postconcussive symptoms, cognition, and self-efficacy in veterans and active duty service members. *J Head Trauma Rehabil.* 2018;33(2):E53−e63.

63. Wolf GK, Strom TQ, Kehle SM, Eftekhari A. A preliminary examination of prolonged exposure therapy with Iraq and Afghanistan veterans with a diagnosis of posttraumatic stress disorder and mild to moderate traumatic brain injury. *J Head Trauma Rehabil.* 2012;27(1):26−32.

64. Sripada RK, Rauch SA, Tuerk PW, et al. Mild traumatic brain injury and treatment response in prolonged exposure for PTSD. *J Trauma Stress.* 2013;26(3):369−375.

65. Davis JJ, Walter KH, Chard KM, Parkinson RB, Houston WS. Treatment adherence in cognitive processing therapy for combat-related PTSD with history of mild TBI. *Rehabil Psychol.* 2013;58(1):36−42.

66. Vanderploeg RD, Belanger HG, Curtiss G, Bowles AO, Cooper DB. Re-conceptualizing rehabilitation of individuals with chronic symptoms following mild traumatic brain injury. *Rehabil Psychol.* 2019;64(1):1−12.

67. Tiersky LA, Anselmi V, Johnston MV, et al. A trial of neuropsychologic rehabilitation in mild-spectrum traumatic brain injury. *Arch Phys Med Rehabil.* 2005;86(8):1565−1574.

68. Boyle E, Cancelliere C, Hartvigsen J, Carroll LJ, Holm LW, Cassidy JD. Systematic review of prognosis after mild traumatic brain injury in the military: results of the international collaboration on mild traumatic brain injury prognosis. *Archiv Phys Med Rehab.* 2014;95(3 suppl 2):5230−5237.

69. Carroll LJ, Cassidy JD, Cancelliere C, et al. Systematic review of the prognosis after mild traumatic brain injury in adults: cognitive, psychiatric, and mortality outcomes: results of the International Collaboration on Mild Traumatic Brain Injury Prognosis. *Archiv Phys Med Rehab.* 2014;95(3 suppl):S152−S173.

70. Carroll LJ, Cassidy JD, Peloso PM, et al. Prognosis for mild traumatic brain injury: results of the WHO collaborating centre task force on mild traumatic brain injury. *J Rehabil Med.* 2004;(43 suppl):84−105.

71. Cassidy JD, Cancelliere C, Carroll LJ, et al. Systematic review of self-reported prognosis in adults after mild traumatic brain injury: results of the International Collaboration on Mild Traumatic Brain Injury Prognosis. *Arch Phys Med Rehab.* 2014;95(3 suppl):S132−S151.

72. Cassidy JD, Carroll LJ, Peloso PM, et al. Incidence, risk factors and prevention of mild traumatic brain injury: results of the WHO collaborating centre task force on mild traumatic brain injury. *J Rehabil Med.* 2004;(43 suppl):28−60.

73. Donovan J, Cancelliere C, Cassidy JD. Summary of the findings of the international collaboration on mild traumatic brain injury prognosis. *Chiropr Man Ther.* 2014;22(38):1−9.

74. Armistead-Jehle P. Ethical considerations in the management of military related concussion. *Mil Psychol.* 2018;30(6):487−494.

75. Hoge CW, Goldberg HM, Castro CA. Care of war veterans with mild traumatic brain injury–flawed perspectives. *N Engl J Med.* 2009;360(16):1588−1591.

76. Vanderploeg RD, Belanger HG. Screening for a remote history of mild traumatic brain injury: when a good idea is bad. *J Head Trauma Rehabil.* 2013;28(3):211−218.

77. Armistead-Jehle P, Buican B. Evaluation context and symptom validity test performances in a U.S. Military sample. *Arch Clin Neuropsychol.* 2012;27(8):828−839.

78. Armistead-Jehle P, Cole WR, Stegman RL. Performance and symptom validity testing as a function of medical board evaluation in US Military service members with a history of mild traumatic brain injury. *Arch Clin Neuropsychol.* 2018;33(1):120−124.

79. Grills CE, Armistead-Jehle P. Performance validity test and neuropsychological assessment battery screening module performances in an active-duty sample with a history of concussion. *Appl Neuropsychol Adult.* 2016;23(4):295−301.

80. Nelson NW, Hoelzle JB, McGuire KA, Ferrier-Auerbach AG, Charlesworth MJ, Sponheim SR. Evaluation context impacts neuropsychological performance of OEF/OIF veterans with reported combat-related concussion. *Arch Clin Neuropsychol.* 2010;25(8):713−723.

81. U.S. Department of Veterans Affairs. *Types of Compensation*; 2018. https://www.benefits.va.gov/COMPENSATION/types-compensation.asp.

82. McNally RJ, Frueh BC. Why we should worry about malingering in the VA system: comment on Jackson et al (2011). *J Trauma Stress*. 2012;25(4):454–456.

83. McNally RJ, Frueh BC. Why are Iraq and Afghanistan War veterans seeking PTSD disability compensation at unprecedented rates? *J Anxiety Disord*. 2013;27(5):520–526.

84. Mossman D. Veterans Affairs disability compensation: a case study in countertherapeutic jurisprudence. *Bull Am Acad Psychiatry Law*. 1996;24(1):27–44.

85. Belanger HG, Curtiss G, Demery JA, Lebowitz BK, Vanderploeg RD. Factors moderating neuropsychological outcomes following mild traumatic brain injury: a meta-analysis. *J Int Neuropsychol Soc*. 2005;11(3):215–227.

86. Dismuke-Greer CE, Nolen TL, Nowak K, et al. Understanding the impact of mild traumatic brain injury on veteran service-connected disability: results from Chronic Effects of Neurotrauma Consortium. *Brain Inj*. 2018;32(10):1178–1187.

87. Denning JH, Shura RD. Cost of malingering mild traumatic brain injury-related cognitive deficits during compensation and pension evaluations in the veterans benefits administration. *Appl Neuropsychol Adult*. 2017:1–16.

88. Roth RS, Spencer RJ. Iatrogenic risk in the management of mild traumatic brain injury among combat veterans: a case illustration and commentary. *Int J Phys Med Rehab*. 2013;1(1):1–7.

CHAPTER 14

Gender and Sex Considerations in Traumatic Brain Injury

KATHERINE LIN, MD • LINDSAY MOHNEY, DO • REBECCA TAPIA, MD

INTRODUCTION

In current practice, there are little or no differences in assessment and treatment of brain injury with regard to gender. Until recently, the norm in research has been overabundant use of male rodents and male subjects. This combined with the increased incidence of traumatic brain injury (TBI) in males across the age continuum[1–3] has contributed to limited research examining the effects of gender and sex on etiology and outcomes on TBI. Nonetheless, a growing body of literature suggests incidence, clinical presentation, and functional outcomes for male and female patients with TBI may differ. By improving the understanding of sex-based differences, the treatment team may be better equipped to care for patients with TBI and its sequelae.

Before discussing the implications of sex and gender on TBI, it is necessary to define each of these terms. Often, sex and gender are used interchangeably in current literature; however, it should be noted that these terms are not synonymous. Sex is defined as the biological characteristics, including anatomy, physiology, hormones, and genetics, that distinguish male bodies from female. Gender is a social construct encompassing masculine or feminine factors like behavioral norms, identities, and relationships.[3] Due to the ambiguous classification in literature and the complexity of the relationship between sex and gender, these terms will be used interchangeably throughout this chapter.

ETIOLOGY AND EPIDEMIOLOGY

Historically, male gender is a risk factor for sustaining TBI, regardless of age, with higher emergency department visits, hospitalization rates, and deaths when compared to females. However, females represent a significant number of patients with head injury, sustaining approximately 1/3 of TBIs based on epidemiologic studies.[1] Additionally, the rate of individuals seeking medical attention for head trauma continues to increase with an estimated 2.8 million people sustaining TBI in the United States in 2013 alone, of which approximately 1.3 million were females.[2] For both males and females, rates are highest among those aged 0–4 and over 75 years.[1]

Falls remain the number one cause of head injury across all age groups, regardless of sex and injury severity. Falls also account for the most common mechanism of head injury among females.[1,2,4] TBI in males is typically attributed to societal roles, engagement in high-risk activities, and male-dominated professions (i.e., professional contact sports, construction, or military occupations), whereas females are more susceptible to TBI caused by intimate partner violence.[3,5] Occupational settings are also important as females make up more than 40% of injuries within the workplace with highest rates among government workers, in particular those in education and healthcare. While not exclusive to females, one-fourth to one-third of females report lifetime physical and/or sexual intimate partner violence with TBI rates of up to 80% in survivors.[5]

While differences within gendered occupations are noted in the literature, the impact of head injury among females in the military deserves special discussion as well. The role of females in the military has been steadily changing throughout the years. With the onset of Operation Enduring Freedom and Operation Iraqi Freedom (OEF/OIF), more than 300,000 female service members were deployed between the years 2001 and 2013, an unprecedented number from prior conflicts, placing females in increasingly hostile environments. In 2013, the repeal of the Department of Defense policy which previously excluded females from serving in combat roles further placed females at an increased risk for combat-related health issues. With the increased use of explosive weaponry during OEF/OIF, the number

Concussion. https://doi.org/10.1016/B978-0-323-65384-8.00014-6
2020 Published by Elsevier Inc.

of service members exposed to blast-related injuries has also risen.[6]

Sports-related injuries are well represented in TBI literature and remain a major cause of mild TBI (mTBI) in adolescent and young adult females. Recent research shows females competing in sex-comparable sports have a higher incidence of concussion, up to double the number sustained by their male counterparts[7–12]. Moreover, type of sport may also result in increased risk for concussion. Please refer to Table 14.1 for a list of "at-risk" sports with known injury rate in females and males.

PATHOPHYSIOLOGY

The relationship of gender and pathophysiology of brain injury remains controversial. Several theories have been postulated. Both direct/primary damage and secondary biochemical cascade may play a role in gender differences after TBI; however, this is mostly based off conjecture and beyond the scope of this chapter. Gender differences in concussion susceptibility primarily focus on anatomic, biomechanical, and hormonal differences. Social considerations may also play an important factor in rate of concussion, which will be discussed later.

Research within sports at greatest risk of head injury has determined that disparities in neck musculature and head/neck stability leave females more susceptible to injury; females typically have more slender necks and a smaller head-to-ball ratio than males. This contributes to increased reactive forces and up to 50% more head acceleration in females when head trauma is sustained[7,8,10]. Furthermore, it has also been proposed that females have lower biomechanical thresholds, thus a similar force applied to both males and females will produce more injuries in a female.[6]

Hormonal factors, including menstrual phase cycle, are an emerging area of research and may impact recovery outcomes. In short, estrogen may be detrimental, while progesterone may confer a favorable effect on the brain after trauma[7,8]. The serum concentration of progesterone at time of injury may influence overall outcomes due to a neuroprotective effect that inhibits secondary injury cascades in the central nervous system. In addition to the absolute concentration of progesterone at the time of injury, the change in concentration of progesterone following the injury may influence outcome as well. TBI occurring in the setting of high progesterone may result in a sudden decrease in serum progesterone concentration and worse outcomes compared to TBI occurring in the setting of low progesterone.[9] Though promising, studies on this topic are relatively small with low-quality evidence and further clinical trials are needed to determine the effects of hormones on neurologic outcome.[13,14]

PROGNOSIS

Due to the heterogenous nature of TBI including the diverse population of injured patients, outcomes following head injury are difficult to gauge. Animal studies have demonstrated improved survival and cognitive function among females after TBI compared to males. However, several observational studies in humans have reported mixed results related to outcome after moderate to severe TBI between males and females.[4,10,15,16] Specific to sports concussion, females

---

TABLE 14.1
"At-Risk" Sports With Incidence of Concussion.

	INCIDENCE (PER 10,000)					
	HOOTMAN ET AL[11]		MARAR ET AL[12]		COVASSIN ET AL[9]	
Type of Sport	Females	Males	Females	Males	Females	Males
Softball	1.4		1.6		2.34	
Baseball		0.7		0.5		1.2
Basketball	2.2	1.6	2.1	1.6	4.67	3.34
Lacrosse					4.99	5.44
Soccer	4.1	2.8	3.4	1.9	6.45	4.19
Ice hockey	9.1	4.1			6.75	5.94

are more likely to experience prolonged symptoms after sustaining injury.[10] Many factors including mode of primary injury, injury severity, development of secondary complications, and preinjury considerations impact recovery post brain injury which may account for the lack of consistent findings.

Quality of Life

Further complicating evaluation of prognosis after TBI is difficulty with measurement of quality of life; what is profoundly disabling to one person may be vastly different for another. Some studies show no difference between males and females related to quality of life after TBI, while others report better quality of life for females compared to males. Married individuals report increased quality of life following TBI with females having greater marital stability after injury.[17]

Employment

Although data support higher symptom loads long term after mTBI in females, community integration and perceived disability are less adversely affected. The frequency of marked/extreme global disability is approximately 36% in females compared to 65% in males.[6] However, multiple factors can impact this, many of which will be discussed in the medical complications section.

Studies that have investigated the relationship between sex and employment have found mixed results. In one study comparing outcomes after mTBI, males and females did not significantly differ with respect to number of days to return to normal daily activities after concussion. In this same study, males had reduced odds of being in a "higher missed days at work" category, though the results did not reach statistical significance.[18] Another large-scale study utilizing the Traumatic Brain Injury Model Systems (TBIMS) national dataset showed females are more likely to decrease hours of employment or stop working than males; this decreased employment is most evident for married females. However, females showed better employment outcomes as age increased, with females in the oldest age group (55−64) less likely to be unemployed than males.[19] Causation is speculative but may be related to social factors, such as preinjury occupational type and financial need with males more likely to be the primary wage earner and females more likely to have a premorbid caretaker/homemaker role. Along these lines, family roles (parent, spouse, caretaker) can further complicate loss of occupational identity when they are no longer able to fulfill these responsibilities.[17]

Symptom Reporting

There are several hypotheses regarding importance of social factors on outcome after TBI; however, there is little evidence that directly explores this topic. Increased symptom reporting by females has been demonstrated in other disease states, such as coronary artery disease and hypertension.[18] This reporting bias is seen in the athlete population as well. Further adding to increased reporting, societal pressure may increase reluctance to report symptoms in males who may fear ineligibility in a sporting event, are encouraged to "tough it out" despite ongoing symptoms, or who want to appear "manly."[7,8,10]

In addition to gender differences, age may further account for social factors and community reintegration after head trauma. Adult females often occupy multiple personal and professional roles and as a result sometimes neglect their own health. Perhaps minors are more likely than adults to receive follow-up medical care after mTBI because parents or guardians are responsible for pursuing their care.

MEDICAL COMPLICATIONS

There are several well-studied medical complications following TBI: post-traumatic seizures, postconcussive syndrome, neuroendocrine dysfunction, autonomic instability, deep vein thrombosis, heterotopic ossification, osteopenia/osteoporosis, and bowel/bladder dysfunction. This section will look specifically at the medical complications that are unique to females or where gender differences have been noted in the literature.

Postconcussive Syndrome

Following acute mTBI, most symptoms resolve within the first 1−3 months. When symptoms persist months to years after injury they are known as postconcussion syndrome, a constellation of complaints that include headache, dizziness, poor sleep, poor concentration, and irritability.[17,20]

Gender-based differences in postconcussive syndrome are recognized in the literature but still poorly understood. Studies suggest that females with mTBI experience greater cognitive decline, higher postconcussive symptom scores, and take longer to return to baseline compared to men.[19,21,22] Headache, dizziness, fatigue, irritability, and concentration problems were areas where females with mTBI struggled more than males in sports-related injury.[22]

In recent years, with the increasing role of females in the military, more research has focused on this unique subset of the population. Studies suggest female service members are more likely to report persistent somatic symptoms following mTBI relative to their male counterparts, which is consistent with the current literature in the civilian population. These findings have been closely linked to coexistent post-traumatic stress disorder (PTSD)[6,23] which will further be discussed in the mental health section. Gender-based differences in postconcussive syndrome may partially be attributed to increased symptom reporting in females compared to males, as discussed earlier.

Mental Health
Coexisting life stressors and psychiatric illness such as depression and PTSD can negatively impact recovery from TBI from both a brain health perspective and a post-TBI community reintegration perspective.

PTSD and sexual trauma
In the general population, females are twice as likely to have a depressive episode and two to three times as likely to experience PTSD than men.[24,25] Partially accounting for this increased prevalence is the fact that females are more likely to experience sexual assault than males and are more likely to encounter chronic ongoing trauma in their intimate relationships. Within the military setting females experience substantially higher rates of military sexual assault and harassment than males.[26,27]

Earlier studies have focused more on the male experience of trauma and PTSD, but as more studies emerge an interesting finding is being noted. While males experience higher rates of trauma exposure, the prevalence of PTSD is higher in females; these findings suggest females may have an increased vulnerability to processing trauma or experience trauma that is higher risk for developing PTSD. One of the highest risks for developing PTSD is sexual trauma.[27] In one study, females were found to have similar rates of PTSD and depressive symptoms as males, suggesting that military sexual trauma may be more highly associated with the development of PTSD than combat exposure.[26] The coexistence of PTSD and TBI has been correlated with increased somatosensory symptoms in females relative to males.[23]

Depression
It is known that individuals with TBI are at increased risk for development of depression compared to the general population.[28] Depression has also been linked to adverse outcomes, including increased social isolation, hostility, and ongoing cognitive deficits. In the general population, females are more than twice as likely as males to experience depressive episodes; however, within the TBI population the consensus is unclear. Studies have either shown males to be at increased risk,[4] females to be at increased risk,[29] or no gender-based differences in risk of depression.[30]

Several studies in the TBI population have shown that while there may be no difference among males and females in the development of depression, gender impacted the manifestation of depressive symptoms. Females tended to experience more psychosomatic symptoms resulting in poor sleep while males tended to experience greater cognitive symptoms presenting as poor concentration.[30,31]

Cognition and Neuropsychological Test Performance
Neuropsychological assessment is a useful tool to assess the functional integrity of the brain following TBI. It examines several different cognitive domains: memory, attention, processing speed, reasoning, judgment, problem-solving, spatial and language functions, and executive function.

While studies in the literature are mixed, females tend to outperform males in tests of executive functioning,[32–34] working memory,[35] and written language.[36] Males tend to score higher on tests of verbal and visual memory.[10,36] Impaired executive functions, which encapsulates self-awareness, planning, and the ability to regulate one's own behavior, confer a negative prognostic sign for successful community reintegration along with caregiver burden.[37] These findings provide one explanation for why despite higher symptom loads long term after mTBI in females, community integration and perceived disability are less adversely affected as previously noted.

Endocrine/Reproductive Dysfunction
Development of neuroendocrine dysfunction secondary to hypopituitarism following TBI is well cited. In females with TBI, a transient disturbance in the hypothalamic pituitary ovarian (HPO) axis can lead to a period of amenorrhea or menstrual cycle irregularity.[38,39] High cortisol levels from increased physical and emotional strain following TBI can also further suppress the HPO axis leading to anovulation in some women.[40] More severe injury has been found to be predictive of a longer duration of amenorrhea, with studies finding an average duration of around 60 days to 6 months.[38,39]

Abnormal menstrual patterns can be associated with low estrogen levels which can have a significant health impact in females. Low estrogen has been associated with decreased bone mineral density, increased risk of cardiovascular disease, infertility, and depression. In young adolescent females, estrogen is especially important in the development of secondary sexual characteristics and development of adequate bone mineral density which peaks during late adolescence.[41]

There is some evidence that a shorter duration of amenorrhea is predictive of better global outcome ratings, community participation, and increased quality of life post injury.[38] Given the significant health implications of neuroendocrine dysfunction, females should be closely monitored for abnormal menstrual patterns following TBI. In premenopausal females, evidence of an abnormal menstrual cycle should prompt further investigation with serum levels of follicle stimulating hormone, luteinizing hormone, and estradiol.

Despite the evidence to support a transient period of menstrual irregularity following head injury, reproductive research in females with TBI is still limited. Studies to date have found no changes in fertility and ability to conceive; however, females with TBI tended to have increased postpartum difficulties compared to their controls. The most common postpartum findings encompassed increased fatigue, depression, mobility problems, and inability to concentrate.[39]

Osteopenia/Osteoporosis

TBI in both males and females has been associated with decreased bone mineral density secondary to prolonged immobilization as well as hormonal changes secondary to disruption of the hypothalamic pituitary axis. Deficiencies in growth hormone and thyroid-stimulating hormone can alter bone metabolism leading to increased skeletal fragility and increased risk for fracture.[42]

Females may be at further increased risk for osteopenia/osteoporosis relative to males. This is clinically significant as it increases the risk for fracture following a fall. Female gender and older age have been identified as major risk factors for fracture following a fall.[43]

As previously discussed in the endocrine section, females with TBI may experience transient irregularities in their menstrual cycle due to disruptions in the HPO axis. These disturbances can result in decreased estrogen production which has also been linked to decreased bone mineral density. This is especially significant in young females who may not yet have reached their peak bone mineral density. Studies have shown that females younger than 20 years with menstrual irregularity are three times more likely to have bone mineral density below normal for their age compared to those who develop menstrual irregularity at older than 20 years.[44]

In the first few years following menopause, females go through a period of rapid bone loss secondary to loss of estrogen which continues into the postmenopausal years. A higher peak bone density reduces the risk of osteoporosis later in life and this protective factor may be lost in young females with neuroendocrine dysfunction following TBI.

Sexuality

Traumatic brain injury can negatively impact sexual functioning in both males and females. In addition to the direct impact of the injury itself and concurrent physiologic and hormonal changes, there is often also a psychological component of altered self-esteem, self-image, and emotional complexity that plays a role in sexual dysfunction. There is a tendency to view females as more asexual than males and an even greater tendency to overlook the importance of sexuality in females with disabilities.

It has been noted that females with TBI often present with decreased desire, decreased vaginal lubrication, and greater difficulty with achieving orgasm.[45] Fatigue has also been reported as a significant barrier to engagement in sexual activity following TBI in females.[46]

A large TBIMS multicenter study by Sander et al.[47] sought to determine predictors of sexual functioning and satisfaction 1 year following TBI. The study found older age, female gender, and severity of injury to be associated with greater sexual dysfunction at 1 year following injury. In addition, females were found to have a 2.5 increase in odds of sexual impairments compared to males.[47]

Sexual dysfunction has been shown to correlate with greater global disability as measured by the Glasgow Outcome Scale and with greater physical and psychosocial dysfunction on the Sickness Impact Profile.[48] It has also been linked to increased rates of depression in persons with TBI.[47,48] Inability to engage in a healthy sex life negatively impacts intimate partner relationships, creating distance and loss of emotional connection.

Routine Medical Screening

Females with TBI are still susceptible to the same medical needs as females without TBI and require long-term management. However, females with TBI often face unique challenges and barriers when it comes to their healthcare needs. Limited access to care places females at greater risk for developing preventable health conditions and comorbid diseases such as diabetes, hypertension, and heart disease.

Females with TBI use less conception and maternity services than females without TBI[49] and are less likely to have their pap smear within the recommended time frame.[3] These findings are similar to those noted in females with physical and cognitive disabilities who were found to be less likely to undergo routine cervical cancer screening.[50] Structural and logistical barriers have been cited as potential obstacles to care among those with disabilities. These include transportation access, building access, poorly designed examination rooms/equipment, difficulty with wheelchair transfers, and proper positioning due to spasticity.[50,51]

Communication barriers and provider bias may also come into play when treating females with TBI. They may incorrectly assume that females with TBI are not sexually active and forgo sexual transmitted disease testing and birth control counseling. Greater education to both patients and providers about the importance of preventative health services and screening should be an area of greater focus in females with TBI. Providers should advocate for these individuals who may lack the cognitive and/or physical capacity to understand the health information they are receiving.

PHARMACOLOGY

Medications are often used in TBI patients to manage the medical complications and symptomatic sequelae. The literature is lacking when it comes to gender-based pharmacological management specifically in TBI; however, there is a significant amount of information regarding pharmacology considerations in pregnant females. The same guidelines that govern medication use during pregnancy in the general population should be extended to pregnant females with TBI, with a risk versus benefit analysis applied.

CONCLUSION

Though there remains a paucity of reporting, limited research suggests incidence, etiology, and prognosis of concussion are subject to gender differences. Data on moderate to severe TBI is lacking, but females with mTBI typically present with more severe injury, greater deficits, different symptom constellation, and delayed resolution of symptoms. Ongoing studies are needed to explore why such differences occur, though likely multifactorial. More research is also needed regarding the epidemiologic and clinical aspects of TBI, which may impact guidelines for practice as well as prognosis post injury.

REFERENCES

1. Faul M, Xu L, Wald MM, Coronado VG. *Traumatic Brain Injury in the United States: Emergency Department Visits, Hospitalizations and Deaths 2002-2006*. Atlanta: Centers for Disease control and Prevention, National Center for Injury Prevention and Disease Control; 2010.
2. Taylor CA, Bell JM, Breiding MJ, Xu L. Traumatic brain injury — related emergency department visits, hospitalizations, and deaths — United States, 2007 and 2013. *MMWR Surveill Summ*. 2017;66(SS-9):1—16. https://doi.org/10. 15585/mmwr.ss6609a1.
3. Colantonio A. Sex, gender, and traumatic brain injury: a commentary. *Arch Phys Med Rehabil*. 2016;97(2 suppl 1): S1—S4.
4. Albrecht J, McCunn M, Stein D, Simoni-Wastila L, Smith G. Sex Differences in Mortality following isolated traumatic brain injury. *J Trauma Acute Care Surg*. 2016; 81(3):486—492.
5. Iverson K, Pogoda T. Traumatic brain injury among females veterans: an invisible wound of intimate partner violence. *Med Care*. 2015;53:S112—S119.
6. Brickell TA, Lippa SM, French LM, Kennedy JE, Bailie JM, Lange RT. Female service members and symptom reporting after combat and non-combat-related mild traumatic brain injury. *J Neurotrauma*. 2017;34(2):300—312.
7. Mollayeva T, El-Khechen-Richandi G, Colantonio A. Sex & gender considerations in concussion research. *Concussion*. 2018;03(01):CNC51.
8. Carter C, Ireland M, Johnson A, Levine W. Sex-Based Differences in common sports injuries. *J Am Acad Orthop Surg*. 2018;26(13):447—454.
9. Covassin T, Moran R, Elbin RJ. Sex differences in reported concussion injury rates and time loss from participation: an update of the National Collegiate Athletic Association injury surveillance program from 2004-2005 through 2008-2009. *J Athl Train*. 2016;51(3):189—194.
10. Dick R. Is there a gender difference in concussion incidence and outcomes? *Br J Sports Med*. 2009;43:i46—i50.
11. Hootman JM, Dick R, Agel J. Epidemiology of collegiate injuries for 15 sports: summary and recommendations for injury prevention initiatives. *J Athl Train*. 2007;42(2): 311—319.
12. Marar M, McIlvain NM, Fields SK, Comstock RD. Epidemiology of concussions among United States high school athletes in 20 sports. *Am J Sports Med*. 2012;40(4): 747—755.
13. Wunderle K, Hoeger K, Wasserman E, Bazarian J. Menstrual Phase as a Predictor of outcome after mild traumatic brain injury in females. *J Head Trauma Rehabil*. 2014;29(5): E1—E8.
14. Ma J, Huang S, Qin S, You C, Zeng Y. Progesterone for acute traumatic brain injury. *Cochrane Database Syst Rev*. 2016;(12):CD008409. https://doi.org/10.1002/146518 58.CD008409.pub4.

15. Renner C, Hummelsheim H, Kopczak A, et al. The influence of Gender on the injury severity, course, and outcome of traumatic brain injury. *Brain Inj.* 2012; 26(11):1360–1371.

16. Ratcliff J, Greenspan A, Goldstein F, et al. Gender and traumatic brain injury: do the sexes fare differently? *Brain Inj.* 2007;21(10):1023–1030.

17. Tapia RN, Eapen B. Rehabilitation of persistent symptoms after concussion. *Phys Med Rehabil Clin.* 2017;28(2): 287–299.

18. Barsky A, Peekna H, Borus J. Somatic symptom reporting in females and males. *J Gen Intern Med.* 2001;16:266–275.

19. Bazarian JJ, Blyth B, Mookerjee S, He H, McDermott MP. Sex differences in outcome after mild traumatic brain injury. *J Neurotrauma.* 2010;27(3):527–539. PubMed: 19938945.

20. Corrigan JD, Lineberry LA, Komaroff E, Langlois JA, Salassie AW, Wood KD. Employment after traumatic brain injury: differences between males and females. *Arch Phys Med Rehabil.* 2007;88:1400–1409.

21. Preiss-Farzanegan SJ, Chapman B, Wong TM, Wu J, Bazarian JJ. The relationship between gender and postconcussion symptoms after sport-related mild traumatic brain injury. *Pharm Manag PM R.* 2009;1(3):245–253.

22. Broshek DK, Kaushik T, Freeman JR, Erlanger D, Webbe F, Barth JT. Sex differences in outcome following sports-related concussion. *J Neurosurg.* 2005;102(5):856–863.

23. Lippa SM, Brickell TA, Bailie JM, French LM, Kennedy JE, Lange RT. Postconcussion symptom reporting after mild traumatic brain injury in female service members: impact of gender, post traumatic stress disorder, severity of injury and associated bodily injury. *J Head Trauma Rehabil.* 2018; 33(2):101–112.

24. Brody DJ, Pratt LA, Hughes J. *Prevalence of Depression Among Adults Aged 20 and Over: United States, 2013–2016. NCHS Data Brief, No 303.* Hyattsville, MD: National Center for Health Statistics; 2018.

25. Kimerling R, Weitlauf JC, Iverson KM, Karpenko JA, Jain S. Gender issues in PTSD. In: Friedman MJ, Keane TM, Resick PA, eds. *Handbook of PTSD: Science and Practice.* New York: Guilford Press; 2013.

26. Afari N, Pittman J, Floto E, Owen L. Differential impact of combat on Postdeployment symptoms in female and male veterans of Iraq and Afghanistan. *Mil Med.* 2015;180(3): 296.

27. Resnick EM, Mallampalli M, Carter CL. Current challenges in female veterans' health. *J Womens Health.* 2012;21: 895–900.

28. Scholten AC, Haagsma JA, Cnossen MC, Olff M, van Beeck EF, Polinder S. Prevalence of and risk factors for anxiety and depressive disorders after traumatic brain injury: a systematic review. *J Neurotrauma.* 2016;33:1969–1994.

29. Iverson KM, Hendricks AM, Kimerling R, et al. Psychiatric diagnoses and neurobehavioral symptom severity among OEF/OIF VA patients with deployment-related traumatic brain injury: a gender comparison. *Wom Health Issues.* 2011;21(4 suppl):S210–S217.

30. Lavoie S, Sechrist S, Quach N, et al. Depression in males and females one year following traumatic brain injury (TBI): a TBI model systems study. *Front Psychol.* 2017;8: 634. https://doi.org/10.3389/fpsyg.2017.00634.

31. Alexandrino-Silva C, Wang YP, Carmen Viana M, Bulhoes RS, Martins SS, Andrade LH. Gender differences in symptomatic profiles of depression: results from the Sao Paulo megacity mental health Survey. *J Affect Disord.* 2013;147:355–364.

32. Barr WB. Neuropsychological testing of high school athletes. Preliminary norms and test-retest indices. *Arch Clin Neuropsychol.* 2003;18(1):91–101.

33. Niemeier JP, Marwitz JH, Lesher K, Walker WC, Bushnik T. Gender differences in executive functions following traumatic brain injury. *Neuropsychol Rehabil.* 2007;17(3): 293–313.

34. Putukian M, Echemendia RJ, Mackin S. The acute neuropsychological effects of heading in soccer: a pilot study. *Clin J Sport Med.* 2000;10(2):104–109.

35. Liossi C, Wood R. Gender as a moderator of cognitive and affective outcome after traumatic brain injury. *J Neuropsychiatry Clin Neurosci.* 2009;21:43–45.

36. Bounds TA, Schopp L, Johnstone B, Unger C, Goldman H. Gender differences in a sample of vocational rehabilitation clients with TBI. *NeuroRehabilitation.* 2003;18:189–196.

37. Bogdanova Y, Verfaellie M. Cognitive sequelae of blast-induced traumatic brain injury: recovery and rehabilitation. *Neuropsychol Rev.* 2012;22:4–20.

38. Ripley DL, Harrison-Felix C, Sendroy-Terrill M, Cusick CP, Dannels-McClure A, Morey C. The impact of female reproductive function on outcomes after traumatic brain injury. *Arch Phys Med Rehabil.* 2008;89:1090–1096.

39. Colantonio A, Mar W, Escobar M, et al. Females's health outcomes after traumatic brain injury. *J Womens Health.* 2010;19:1109–1116.

40. Ranganathan P, Kumar R, Davis K, et al. Longitudinal sex and stress hormone profiles among reproductive age and post-menopausal females after severe TBI: a case series analysis. *Brain Inj.* 2016;30:452–461.

41. Henry YM, Fatayerji D, Eastell R. Attainment of peak bone mass at the lumbar spine, femoral neck and radius in males and females: relative contributions of bone size and volumetric bone mineral density. *Osteoporos Int.* 2004;15(4):263–273.

42. Bajwa NM, Kesavan C, Mohan S. Long-term consequences of traumatic brain injury in bone metabolism. *Front Neurol.* 2018;9:115. https://doi.org/10.3389/fneur.2018. 00115.

43. Kantayaporn C. Fall with and without fracture in elderly: what's different? *J Med Assoc Thail.* 2012;95(suppl 10): S109–S112.

44. Popat VB, Calis KA, Vanderhoof VH, et al. Bone mineral density in estrogen-deficient young females. *J Clin Endocrinol Metab.* 2009;94(7):2277–2283.

45. Hibbard MR, Gordon WA, Flanagan S, Haddad L. Sexual Dysfunction after traumatic brain injury. *Neurol Rehabil.* 2000;15:107–120.

46. Goldin Y, Canto J, Tsaousides T, et al. Sexual functioning and the effect of fatigue in traumatic brain injury. *J Head Trauma Rehabil.* 2014;5:418–426.

47. Sander AM, Maestas KL, Nick TG, et al. Predictors of sexual functioning and satisfaction 1 year following traumatic brain injury: a TBI model systems multicenter study. *J Head Trauma Rehabil.* 2013;28:186–194.

48. Kreuter M, Dahllof AG, Gudjonsson G, Sullivan M, Siosteen A. Sexual adjustment and its predictors after traumatic brain injury. *Brain Inj.* 1998;12:349–368.

49. Toor G, Harris J, Scobar M, et al. Long term service outcomes among females with traumatic brain injury. *Arch Phys Med Rehabil.* 2016;97:54–63.

50. Rivera Drew J, Short S. Disability and pap smear receipt among U.S. females 2000 and 2005. *Perspect Sex Reprod Health.* 2010;42:4.

51. Dejong G, Palsbo SE, Beatty PW, Jones GC, Knoll T, Neri MT. The organization and financing of health services for persons with disabilities. *Milbank Q.* 2002;80(2): 261–301.

CHAPTER 15

A Look Ahead: Cutting Edge Research in the Diagnosis, Assessment, Rehabilitation Management, and Prevention of Concussion and Its Sequelae

SAMUEL CLANTON, MD, PHD • XIN LI, DO • CAROLINE SIZER, MD • GARY GOLDBERG, BASC, MD

INTRODUCTION: CUTTING-EDGE RESEARCH ADVANCING CONCUSSION MEDICINE

This chapter will focus on a highly selective review of some of the state-of-the-art emerging research on the leading edge of Concussion Medicine that is currently being published with regard to various aspects of concussion diagnosis, assessment, rehabilitation management, and prevention. This is not intended to be a comprehensive review of the emerging literature but is comprised of carefully selected areas of research that are thought to be particularly promising and of immanent clinical value. The authors have performed a thorough literature review of recently published relevant research and have evaluated the emerging literature for significant trends as well as the application of new approaches and technologies in Concussion Medicine. Additional active areas of research extending beyond those reviewed in the text are listed in the four supplemental tables. A general review paper on "research frontiers in traumatic brain injury" provides a broad overview of the many different areas of ongoing brain injury research.[1]

NEW DEVELOPMENTS IN CONCUSSION DIAGNOSIS

Concussion is a clinical diagnosis made by a licensed health professional. This section will focus on acute diagnosis of adult concussion. For the purpose of this section, concussion and mild traumatic brain injury (mTBI) will be used interchangeably. In 1993, the American Congress of Rehabilitation Medicine (ACRM) defined mTBI as "a traumatically induced physiological disruption of brain function, as manifested by at least one of the following: (1) any period of loss of consciousness (LOC); (2) any loss of memory for events immediately before or after the accident; (3) any alteration in mental state at the time of the accident (e.g., feeling dazed, disoriented, or confused); and (4) focal neurological deficit(s) that may or may not be transient; but where the severity of the injury does not exceed the following: loss of consciousness of approximately 30 minutes or less; after 30 minutes an initial Glasgow Coma Scale (GCS) of 13−15; and posttraumatic amnesia (PTA) not greater than 24 hours"[2] The 2017 Berlin Concussion in Sport Group Consensus Statement provided additional mandatory and discretionary signs to aid in the diagnosis of concussion. Specific mandatory signs identified by this group require removal of an athlete from play for mandatory assessment. These signs include "LOC; lying motionless >5 seconds; confusion/disorientation; amnesia, vacant look; motor incoordination; tonic posturing; impact seizure; ataxia."[3] Athletes exhibiting discretionary signs should stop playing and be evaluated. These signs include "clutching the head; being slow to get up; suspected facial fracture; possible ataxia; behavior change; other clinical suspicion."[3] An athlete who presents with these signs in addition to a mechanism of injury

Concussion. https://doi.org/10.1016/B978-0-323-65384-8.00015-8
2020 Published by Elsevier Inc.

to either the head, neck, and/or body would have a higher chance of having a concussion diagnosis. The American Academy of Neurology, in addition to the Berlin consensus statement, also notes slurred speech, emotional lability, vomiting, vision changes, headache, and photosensitivity as possible symptoms of concussion after an identified mechanism of injury.[4] Definitive diagnostic fluid biomarkers and imaging tools are still under investigation in research studies.

Fluid Biomarkers

Wang et al. listed some attributes needed for fluid biomarkers that range from sensitivity, specificity, and readily accessible bodily fluids (blood and/or CSF) that reflect the severity of injury (mild to severe TBI); the biomarker levels should also reflect treatment.[5] The majority of fluid biomarker studies have been carried out in sports-related concussions. Studies have found the following biomarkers to be elevated in blood after concussion compared with controls: S100 calcium binding protein B6,[6-9] total tau,[7] plasma soluble cellular prion protein,[10] glial fibrillary acidic protein,[11] neuron-specific enolase (NSE),[11] α-amino-3-hydroxy-5-methyl-4-isoxazolepropionic acid receptor (AMPAR),[12] marinobufagenin,[13] calpain-derived α II-spectrin N-terminal fragment (SNTF),[14] and metabolomics profiling.[15] Shan et al. also found elevated levels of galectin 3 (LGALS3), matrix metalloproteinase 9 (MMPG), and occluding (OCLN) and decreased copeptin 8 hours post injury. Limitations to these studies are limited to sports concussions, small sample size, majority being young males, and short follow-up periods. Another barrier for implementation of the use of biomarkers is the complexity of the assays. The utility of these biomarkers for diagnosis of concussion is currently low. Ideally, serial fluid biomarkers would allow for not only aid in diagnosis of concussion/mTBI but also for improvement in management and prognostication.[16]

Imaging Studies

Conventional MRI and CT scans are most often unable to show abnormalities after concussion. Advanced MRI techniques such as diffusion tensor imaging (DTI), functional MRI (fMRI), along with other techniques have been able to reveal subtle changes in the brain after concussion. DTI can measure axonal changes although studies have been both positive and negative.[17-21] Magnetic resonance spectroscopy measures brain metabolite concentrations. One metabolite that is reduced after concussion is N-acetylaspartate.[22,23] fMRI studies, similar to DTI studies, have reported contradictory

results. This is likely due to the variability in methodologies used across studies.[24-27] Limitations to these studies are small N and inconsistencies with methodologies to help establish protocol. As research continues, both fluid biomarkers and imaging studies may become an important component of concussion diagnosis, prognosis, and measuring treatment effectiveness.

A list of some active areas of research in concussion diagnosis is provided in Table 15.1.

NEW DEVELOPMENTS IN CONCUSSION ASSESSMENT

The research literature on emerging techniques for the assessment of effects of concussion is extensive and no attempt will be made to cover it here in a comprehensive manner. There are many different means of functional assessment of the effects of concussion. These include rapid sideline assessment of sports-related

TABLE 15.1
Some Active Areas of Research in Concussion Diagnosis.

1. Development of imaging biomarkers and protocols for concussion diagnosis
2. Development and evaluation of serum biomarkers for concussion diagnosis
3. Development and evaluation of neurophysiological biomarkers for concussion diagnosis
3. Development and refinement of various clinical instruments for rapid and accurate sideline assessment and diagnosis of sports-related concussion
4. Development of clinical indications for justifying performance of neuroimaging in the emergency department
5. Concussion differential diagnosis in pediatric versus adult populations
6. Improvement in diagnostic protocols and determinations of severity of injury with prognostic significance
7. Improved recognition of neuropsychiatric factors and stress response aspects in concussion diagnosis
8. Recognition of sex-related variation in vulnerability to effects of concussion
9. Recognition of genetic factors that predispose to effects of concussion
10. Evaluation of recurrent concussion and accumulated effects of brain trauma
11. Noninvasive methods for diagnosis of Chronic Traumatic Encephalopathy in the presence of a history of recurrent concussion

concussion,[28] neuropsychological assessment, computerized neurocognitive assessment, structural imaging, functional imaging, vestibular and vestibulo-ocular testing, gait analysis, oculomotor function, exertional tolerance, and a wide variety of other approaches to the evaluation of the effects of concussion and the application of such means of assessment to questions of concussion management and prognosis as well as the objective tracking of concussion recovery. In fact, it is not yet clear exactly what domains of clinical function would be most fruitful to assess after a concussion.[29]

In this section, we will briefly highlight three specific areas of research in concussion assessment:

1. The effects of concussion on neuro-autonomic regulation in the general context of 'Stress Medicine,' and the autonomic response to stress—or 'allostatic load'—utilizing heart rate variability (HRV) as an objective measure of cardiac autonomic regulation in postconcussion assessment;
2. Changes in the functional brain connectome and the pathodynamics of functional brain network disruption associated with concussion;
3. Assessment of the pathophysiology of persistent post-traumatic headache (PPTH) with respect to emerging information regarding autonomic dysfunction; particularly, the participation of the trigeminovascular system (TVS) in the neural regulation of cerebral blood flow, as well as the role of calcitonin gene-related peptide (CGRP) in migraine headache, cerebral blood flow autoregulation, and the concussion-related pathophysiology of blood flow regulation associated with PPTH and second impact syndrome (SIS).

Heart Rate Variability in Concussion Assessment

The general role of the central nervous system in the response to perceived threat or "allostatic load" has been proposed to occur in accordance with the "free energy principle."[30] Stress is argued to be associated with uncertainty of potential existential significance. The role of the central nervous system (CNS) is the "mastering" of this challenge through the strategic reduction of uncertainty.[31] The orchestration of how a person copes with stressful experience then occurs such that "within the brain, a distributed, dynamic, and plastic neural circuitry coordinates, monitors and calibrates behavioral and physiological stress response systems to meet the demands imposed by particular stressors."[32] To accomplish this, the brain must exert control over energy flows throughout the body, a feat

primarily accomplished through the autonomic nervous system (ANS). The unique challenge in concussion and, for that matter, in acquired brain injury in general, is the fact that the stress of the trauma itself is associated with injury to the organ system primarily responsible for the management and amelioration of stress and the reduction in uncertainty. It has been suggested that dysfunction in the ability of the CNS to manage energy flows in the body through ANS control is a potential biomarker for the effects of concussion[33] and can correlate with functional outcomes after moderate and severe TBI, as well.[34] A potent biomarker for ANS dysfunction is HRV, a measure of cardiac autonomic regulation which can be viewed as reflecting the interaction between sympathetic and parasympathetic influences on the heart.[35] A recent study of 23 concussed collegiate athletes showed that HRV high-frequency power (HRV-HF) recorded within the first few days following injury was significantly reduced at rest compared to nonconcussed controls. While HRV-HF did not change significantly between rest and cognitive challenge with performance of a 2-Back working memory task in the nonconcussed control subjects, it rose significantly with cognitive activation from the lowered level of resting HRV-HF in the concussed athletes.[36] Asymptomatic concussed athletes may continue to exhibit significant alteration in cardiac autonomic regulation as shown by decreased HRV-HF, particularly with physical exertion for extended periods of time following concussion.[37] Athletes with multiple concussions showed persisting cardiac autonomic dysregulation manifested through HRV measures for even longer periods of time often extending beyond the point at which they were cleared to return to play.[38] With the advent of highly reliable wearable physiological recorders capable of long-term stable recording of the electrocardiogram, together with advances in signal processing and nonlinear analytical methods for examining HRV, research into cardiac autonomic dysregulation following concussion is likely to advance concussion science and provide guidance for medical management strategies.[39–41] HRV studies performed serially after a concussion in a recent prospective study of 29 young concussed athletes demonstrated that HRV dropped acutely initially for the first 30—40 days following a significant injury, and then increased above baseline during subsequent recovery up to approximately 75 days post injury before returning back down to baseline.[42] Those with higher postacute HRV elevations had greater persistent postconcussion symptom complaints. This suggests that recovery from concussion and the development of postconcussion complications is associated with an attendant *biphasic* stress response that may be reflected in the occurrence of somewhat chaotic "dysregulated shifts" between the sympathetic and parasympathetic components of the ANS throughout the period of recovery.[42]

Functional Brain Network Pathodynamics following Concussion

Concussion can be understood as inducing a pathological disturbance in the dynamics of the functional connectome of the human brain underlying normal conscious cognition, both "at rest" and during active cognitive engagement. With the advent of "network neuroscience" and dynamic functional brain imaging including the application of complex network analysis and graph theory methods to resting state functional MRI (rs-fMRI) data, these dynamics can be directly interrogated and studied. In normal "resting" adult brain, rs-fMRI demonstrates dynamic shifting between several major functional brain networks, including the "default mode network," the "salience network," and the "executive network" (also called the "bifrontal network"), among several others—reflective of baseline cognitive flexibility.[43] Furthermore, using time-resolved functional connectivity fMRI (trFC-fMRI) analysis of data obtained during active cognitive task performance, network dynamics have been shown to rapidly fluctuate adaptively between "integrated cognitive states" (ICSs) characterized by low modularity with broad areal integration accompanied by pupillary dilatation, and partitioned cognitive states (PCSs) characterized by segregated nodes and high network modularity.[44] When functional connectivity demonstrates an "integrated network topology," structural and functional connectivity have been found to be more tightly linked suggesting that one role of normal structural connectivity is to facilitate the dynamic emergence of such integrative cognitive states.[45] Another feature of functional brain network architecture is that certain critical cortical nodes serving as "hubs" are particularly endowed with copious interconnections and tend to interconnect strongly with each other as a result, forming what have been called "rich clubs."[46] One identified presumably protective response to brain injury that may enhance resilience and resistance to the deleterious effects of recurrent TBI, at least in the short term, is the development of functional hyperconnectivity between rich club hubs,[47] noted, for example, between posterior cingulate and cortical association areas and between occipital and frontal rich club nodes.[48] However, increased coupling within the default mode network has been shown to correlate with increased postconcussion symptomatology, possibly due to a reduction in cognitive flexibility.[49]

How does this all relate to the study of concussion? TBI can be understood as a problem that can be examined in the context of systems neuroscience.[50] It would stand to reason that exploration of disturbances in functional connectivity and disruption of network dynamics at rest and during cognitive activation could serve as a rich source of potential biomarkers for concussion. While computationally intensive, functional brain imaging methods are essentially noninvasive and can be repeated serially in the same concussed subject over the course of their clinical recovery and used as biomarkers to longitudinally track the postconcussion recovery process and predict clinical outcomes.[51] Recent studies utilizing rs-fMRI data have demonstrated that various alterations in the functional connectome may indeed serve as useful biomarkers correlated with symptom severity in individuals with sports-related concussion and mild TBI.[52–56] The impact of concussion on cognitive flexibility and the capacity to dynamically shift between integrated low-modularity and parcellated high-modularity network topologies in the context of active performance of cognitive tasks using trFC-fMRI methods[57] is also an area of active investigation.

Pathophysiological Assessment of Persistent Posttraumatic Headache

The most common sequela of concussion is PPTH often accompanied by photophobia.[58] Recent research suggests that the pathophysiology of PPTH overlaps with that of migraine and that individuals with PPTH have higher vasomotor domain autonomic dysfunction.[59] Furthermore, there is growing evidence to suggest that PPTH after mTBI is associated with trigeminal hypernociception.[60,61] Given that the trigeminal system is not only involved in intracranial nociception, but also in the regulation of cerebral blood flow, it has been hypothesized that the TVS may become pathologically activated in mTBI leading to an increased risk of "reactive hyperaemia" in intracranial structures.[62] It is of significant interest that CGRP is expressed in high concentration throughout the TVS[63] and that CGRP-dependent pain and headache-related behaviors along with significantly elevated CGRP levels in the TVS have been demonstrated to occur in a rat model of concussion.[64,65] This leads to a number of questions that are being actively explored: the overlap between the pathophysiology of PPTH and migraine, the potential for treatment of PPTH with anti-CGRP monoclonal antibodies developed for the prevention of migraine

TABLE 15.2
Some Active Areas of Research in Concussion Assessment.

1. New methods for sideline acute assessment of sports-related concussion
2. New approaches to neuropsychological assessment of neurocognitive and affective response effects of concussion
3. Computerized neurocognitive performance assessment application and limitations
4. Structural brain imaging effects of concussion (e.g., on white matter tracts using DTI-MRI)
5. Functional brain imaging (e.g., fMRI) of effects of concussion on the dynamics of functional brain networks using complex network analysis theory
6. Balance and vestibular function testing after concussion
7. Vestibulo-ocular reflex testing after concussion
8. Oculomotor control testing (e.g., visual tracking) after concussion
9. Exertional effects on neurocognitive performance after concussion and effects of concussion on exercise tolerance
10. Neuro-autonomic effects of concussion (e.g., heart rate variability, cardiorespiratory coupling, etc)
11. Path Analysis linkages between different postconcussion symptoms and associated conditions and syndromes (e.g., PTSD, sleep disturbance, headache, chronic pain, mood disorders)
12. Effects of concussion on the strategic response to stress (i.e., 'allostatic load') in the context of the Free Energy Principle (i.e., the role of the CNS in uncertainty reduction)
13. Neuropsychiatric, neuroendocrine, and neuroimmune effects of concussion
14. Pathophysiological effects of concussion on cerebral blood flow autoregulation and post-traumatic headache mechanisms including overlap with migraine pathogenesis and pathophysiology of Second Impact Syndrome
15. Cumulative effects of repeated concussion and the risk of developing chronic traumatic encephalopathy (CTE)
16. Characterization of potentially beneficial adaptive responses to concussion

headaches, as well as a potential role for TVS pathophysiology and, with it, the release of CGRP in the etiology of SIS.[66,67]

A list of some active areas of research in concussion assessment is provided in Table 15.2.

NEW DEVELOPMENTS IN CONCUSSION REHABILITATION MANAGEMENT

Initial concussion rehabilitation in the acute phase follows three major principles: identification of concussion (see section on diagnosis), relative physical and cognitive rest after an initial period of 24–48 hours of strict physical and cognitive rest (see below), and injury prevention during the critical period of recovery (see section on prevention), during which a second injury could produce more permanent or severe and prolonged injury, and potentially have catastrophic consequences, as in the cases of SIS.

Relative Rest

Considering the multitude of postconcussive symptoms and the well-described physiologic and emotional impacts of social isolation,[68] sensory deprivation,[69] and deconditioning[70] on human beings, the harm of prolonged complete cognitive and physical rest cannot be overemphasized. Recent research has focused on the potential risks and benefits of strict physical and cognitive rest for treatment of concussion and has revealed that extended strict rest prolongs concussion symptoms.[71,72] Further research has shown that early introduction of supervised graded aerobic exercise is both safe in sport-related concussion and mTBI, and quite effective, significantly shortening postconcussive symptom duration.[73–76] In response to these findings, recommendations have changed to emphasize *relative*, rather than strict *absolute*, physical and cognitive rest for concussion recovery. This approach places greater emphasis on initiating a progressive and graded return to normal activities after the initial 24–48 hours period of rest. These recommendations are recognized as standard practice internationally in multiple recently published clinical practice guidelines for management of mTBI and sports concussion,[77,78] including the high-profile consensus statement from the 5th International Conference on Concussion in Sport, held in Berlin in 2016.[79] When there are exacerbations with progression to the next step in the return to learn/work/play protocol, a 24 hour period of rest is prescribed, and the patient returns to the previous level of activity that they could tolerate without severely exacerbating their symptoms, and is then progressed as tolerated. Naturally, treatment focuses first on return to everyday mobility and activities of daily living, second on graded return to learning or working, and third on graded return to play in the case of sports-related concussion.

Systematic Approach to Persistent Postconcussive Symptoms

As discussed in detail in prior sections, concussion can present with a wide array of symptoms, signs, and impairments, an understandable reflection of its complex pathophysiology. In the face of so many undifferentiated and interconnected symptoms, a systematic (evidence-based and often interdisciplinary) approach to concussion rehabilitation and recovery takes on the greatest practical importance in the clinic. Concussion symptom inventories can provide a means to organize the plethora of symptoms into approachable symptom domains to focus therapeutic interventions (examples include the Neurobehavioral Symptom Inventory, the Rivermead Post Concussion Symptoms Questionnaire, or the SCAT-5 concussion symptom form). Many concussion care providers conceptualize the major intersecting concussion symptom domains as falling into four major categories: somatic, affective, sleep, and cognitive. Though most patients will present with symptoms in more than one domain, identification of the primary symptom domain helps to focus initial treatment. Consideration of the social and environmental background in which a patient recovers should inform clinicians when they develop treatment recommendations, set goals with the patient and their stakeholders, and set expectations and timelines for outcomes, as psychosocial context and conditions strongly impact recovery.

The Interdisciplinary Team

Interdisciplinary approaches to treatment show superior outcomes in the management of concussion, particularly in cases of prolonged symptoms.[80–83] The following sections will address rehabilitation and treatment of the four major concussion symptom domains with discussion of the major contributions of each of the typical members of the interdisciplinary treatment team to the recovery of the concussed patient, but many more disciplines may also contribute to concussion recovery, depending upon recovery complexity. Based upon their clinical expertise, treating physicians make these referrals when appropriate in order to optimize and speed recovery and community reintegration. Regardless of the primary symptom domain, patient and stakeholder education serve as the building blocks for state-of-the-art concussion care and treatment.

Postconcussive Symptoms: The Somatic Domain

This broad category of symptoms also tends to be the most approachable for healthcare providers. Somatic symptoms and impairments in concussion include vestibular dysfunction (peripheral and central), vestibulo-ocular dysfunction, cervical myofascial pain, postconcussive headaches, and autonomic dysfunction (measurable by HRV changes postconcussion, discussed in more detail in the Assessment section above). These symptoms and impairments can overlap in clinical presentation, and identification of the major source of somatic complaints takes precedence in the clinic. Examination includes both a neurologic examination, which involves specific examination of balance. The most commonly used balance test for concussion is called the Balance Error Scoring System (BESS). Validated normative values for men and women by age have been evaluated and published for reference.[84] The concussion provider tailors evaluation and treatment approach to the primary somatic symptom. To give examples, a patient presenting with vestibular dysfunction receives a referral for vestibular therapy; a patient presenting with exertional symptoms completes Buffalo Concussion Treadmill Testing and embarks on a supervised progressive aerobic exercise program for autonomic post concussive symptoms[85–87]; a patient presenting with postconcussive headaches participates with education on proper sleep hygiene, dangers of medication overuse headaches complicating treatment, and appropriate medication prescription to address the headaches by headache type and comorbidities. Specific treatment approaches to the subsets of the somatic domain of postconcussive symptoms receive dedicated focus in specific research articles, book chapters, and clinical practice guidelines.[77,78]

Postconcussive Symptoms: the Sleep Domain

Sleep dysfunction frustrates recovery in many recovering from concussion, and receives a great deal of research attention, particularly in the military population, as a domain that strongly impacts all other concussion domains.[88–90] In fact, persistent symptoms frequently associate with undiagnosed and untreated sleep disorders in those with mTBI.[88] Further, sleep dysfunction observed in acute concussion has been demonstrated to persist in individuals beyond 1 month to even years postconcussion, which should raise its consideration as a serious contributor to postconcussive symptom severity, education on proper sleep hygiene, and referral for sleep evaluation in the setting of persistent symptoms.[91]

Postconcussive Symptoms: The Affective Domain

Mood complaints frequently present after concussion, and can magnify other symptom domain complaints, as well as worsen with suboptimal treatment of the other symptom domains. Careful medication, social and medical history review will inform providers of contributing factors that can worsen mood after concussion (e.g., βblockers for headaches, premorbid PTSD or depression, substance use disorder such as alcohol, chronic opioid dependence, etc.). In mild or moderate mood dysfunction, education, sleep hygiene, regular social and physical activity, and cognitive behavioral therapy can provide sufficient symptom control. However, severe symptoms require a combination of pharmacologic and nonpharmacologic treatment, and likely involvement of a psychologist and/or psychiatrist. When considering pharmacotherapy, the prescriber should exercise caution to avoid side effects, minimize polypharmacy, use the lowest effective doses, change one medication at a time, and follow up regularly. Several scales exist to measure severity of depression (PHQ-2, PHQ-9, Beck Depression Inventory, Major Depression Index)[92] and anxiety (GAD-7, Hamilton anxiety scale, PC-PTSD-5, PCL-5).[93–95] First-line agents frequently include "multitasker" medications that can address both sleep disturbance and mood, or sleep, pain, and mood. The best described agents for treatment of concussion include amitriptyline, used frequently for its beneficial effects at low doses for sleep, pain, and mood. Selective serotonin reuptake inhibitor therapy remains first-line therapy for isolated mood symptoms. Finally, nonpharmacologic integrative approaches continue to present new and interesting approaches to address mood symptoms, particularly irritability, and include various mindfulness techniques[96] and light therapies.[97]

Postconcussive Symptoms: the Cognitive Domain

Clinicians employ many different strategies to assess cognition after concussion. Typical areas of greatest clinical interest include attention, orientation, and short-term memory. Computerized neuropsychological testing (such as ImPACT) have gained popularity in their use due to their ease of administration, and ability to be utilized with serial measurements to track progress and assess for changes from baseline or recovery measurements in the event of future concussions. However, cost and time can limit its use clinically, and proper interpretation of results still frequently suffers when not performed by a neuropsychologist.[98] Standardized cognitive testing tools such as SCAT-5, Montreal Cognitive Assessment Test, and Folstein Mini Mental Status Examination can also demonstrate impairments in various domains of cognitive functioning. However,

the gold standard for formal evaluation of neuropsychological functioning, particularly in situations when a learning disability or other premorbid cognitive impairment predate an individual's concussion, or in situations with strong social pressures that impede progress such as litigation or other compensation or other forms of secondary gain associated with injury, remains formal pencil and paper neuropsychological testing.[98] The benefits of formal neuropsychological testing abound, as neuropsychologists can provide highly individualized education and accommodation recommendations based on testing and evaluation, which often proves an invaluable asset for successful return-to-learn, -play, and -work efforts and processes.[99] However, access to this testing remains a challenge from financial, time, and provider access perspectives. Consideration of pharmacologic interventions should occur only after confounding comorbid issues are addressed first (sleep, pain, sedating medications, mood disorders), and should follow a highly individualized and systematic approach, ideally measuring performance both before and after medication trials.

Community Reintegration
Return to learn
Return to learn receives priority in the management of concussion in children. Typically, this graduated process follows a similar approach to return to play, with progressive levels of participation until full return to learning commences. Specific accommodations to allow a child to progress through these phases requires close monitoring and individualized recommendations, which can come from the treating provider, speech therapist, physical therapist, occupational therapist, or neuropsychologist. In the ideal interdisciplinary approach, input from all specialties involved is combined into formal recommendations from the entire treatment team, with a consensus recommendation by the primary concussion provider (typically a physiatrist, neurologist, or sports medicine specialist). If a child moves to the next level, but has exacerbation of their symptoms with the new level of intensity, they may often take 24 hours of rest to recover, and then restart school at the previous level of intensity and progress from there as tolerated.[100]

Return to work
Return to work follows a similar graduated and progressive process as return to learn with specific accommodations individualized to the worker's job requirements and symptoms. In these cases, a job description proves particularly helpful in individualizing return to work

recommendations. Proper implementation of the specific requirements and graduated return to full duty improves the likelihood of successful return to work. A recent meta-analysis evaluating return to work after mTBI showed that more than half of individuals with concussion return to work by 1 month post injury, and 80% by 6 months post injury.[101]

Return to play

Return to play guidelines for sports-related concussion have received particular focus in the mainstream media due to the increasing public awareness of the importance of recognition of sports-related concussion and the potential catastrophic effects of SIS. Consequently, formal international guidelines for return to play recommendations have been developed and continue to undergo regular updates, with the most recent consensus statement coming from the 5th international conference on concussion in sport, held in Berlin in 2016.[79] Recommendations from this landmark conference include immediate removal from play when a concussion is suspected and no return to play the same day as a concussion occurs. In children, students complete a return to learn program prior to initiating the graduated return to play protocol.

A list of some active areas of research in concussion rehabilitation management is provided in Table 15.3.

TABLE 15.3
Some Active Areas of Research in Concussion Rehabilitation Management.

1. Specificity and clinical utility of concussion symptom questionnaires for guiding rehabilitative treatment by concussion symptom domain or subtype.
2. Impact of the specialized interdisciplinary concussion rehabilitation team on outcome in persistent postconcussive symptoms.
3. Role of active rehabilitation in concussion recovery.
4. Role of aerobic exercise in the treatment of persistent postconcussive symptoms.
5. Exploration of graded combined aerobic and resistance exercise for persistent postconcussive symptoms.
6. Proper identification and access to treatment of vision and oculomotor dysfunction in concussion rehabilitation.
7. Efficacy of standardized education for concussion rehabilitation.
8. Effects of interventions to increase awareness of concussion recovery in the lay population.
9. Disparities in access to timely concussion education and rehabilitative care after discharge from emergency room settings.
10. Application of emerging neurotechnologies for the management of postconcussion symptoms
11. Application of neuro-autonomic biofeedback in postconcussion symptom management

NEW DEVELOPMENTS IN CONCUSSION PREVENTION

In this section we report on recent research, organizational, and commercial efforts in the primary prevention of concussion. Currently, the major public area of focus in the prevention of mTBI/concussion in particular is in risk reduction in sports that involve player-to-player contact.

Concussion has become a very popular topic recently with an increase in media attention paid to the incidence and potential long-term sequelae of sports concussion in particular among athletes in many contact sports. This is in line with increasing public awareness and concern among athletes and their families, who are in many individual cases are now deciding if the risk of concussion is worth the potential benefits of engaging in individual sports. There are two major types of concussion prevention efforts; first in changing sports rules and training to prevent the incidence of head injuries, and second in engineering efforts to reduce concussion through changes in protective equipment including helmets. These efforts have been covered to some extent within the scientific literature;[102,103] however, many efforts in prevention

of sports concussion are being undertaken by independent or private entities (e.g., sports leagues or equipment companies) and do not operate on the basis of public evidence. Given the disparate nature of different researchers, companies, and organizations involved in different activities related to prevention of head injury, we can only present a snapshot of a subset of recent and ongoing efforts.

Changes in Sports Rules, Participant Conduct, and Training

Most states have passed sports concussion laws aimed at general reduction of concussion-related harm, starting with the Washington State "Zackery Lystedt Law" of 2009.[104] This and similar laws passed in most states are primarily concerned with return-to-play guidelines rather than prevention. Most current governmental efforts regarding prevention are mainly intended to increase awareness among athletes and parents. CDC publications regarding concussion prevention primarily revolve around education rather than specific preventative strategies.[105] Efforts aimed at actually preventing concussions are generally sport-specific and originate with governing bodies or authorities within each sport, with a loose relationship to public or private research.

In the United States, American football has received perhaps the most attention in terms of the results of head injury and its prevention, but there have been a number of attempts to change rules, regulations, and training mechanisms in other full- and partial-contact sports intended to prevent head injury. Likely the most well-known football rule changes are in the NFL (professional) American football league, in which new rule development has to some degree focused on the reduction of head injuries over the past 10 years. This began in 2009[106] with increasing limitations on head and neck contact on players and progressed most recently to a 2018 rule making it illegal to initiate contact with the helmet.[107] Increasing penalties in the form of fines and expulsion have been instituted to enforce these rule changes. Unfortunately, tightening of these rules has not resulted in a reduction in incidence of concussion within the league, which has in fact increased from 2012−17.[108] These data are notable for the fact that they include self-reported concussions, which increased significantly during this period in terms of concussions reported during practice sessions as well as with self-referral for concussion evaluation within games. This result is reported by media sources[109,110] as the data are being accumulated and analyzed by the private company IVQIA and not available publicly. Therefore the apparent increase in concussions may be a reflection of the increase in public awareness and acceptance of reporting concussion symptoms within the league. It is worth noting that similar NFL concussion database information from a previous period has provoked criticism as publicly acknowledged concussions (in one case prompting player retirement) were not reflected in the data that were revealed to the public.[111] Given this history and the private nature of the data and their analysis, it is difficult to determine if rule changes within the NFL have had a positive or negative impact on the incidence of concussion.

There have been efforts at changing training methods for American football players at all levels intended to decrease the number of concussions. These efforts include the "Heads Up Football" and similar programs intended to reduce injuries, including concussion within youth, middle-, and high-school age football players through coach and player training and certification. Although studies regarding the effectiveness of these programs are limited, existing studies show mildly positive results, interestingly in some research showing a reduction of head injuries in practice but not in games.[112] Different youth football leagues

have also implemented contact restriction guidelines limiting player-to-player contact football during practices, which also clearly limits the number of head injuries sustained during practice, but points toward reducing head injuries sustained in games as well.[113,114] As data regarding these interventions are currently severely limited, more public research in this area is needed.

Efforts aimed at concussion prevention are also common within other sports, primarily involving reduction of the amount of player-to-player contact. One example of this is in youth and development league hockey, which in some cases is seeking to reduce concussion risk through systematically stricter interpretation of existing rules or changing rules to reduce risky collisions.[115] Organizing bodies of sports including soccer/international football have also implemented rules to prevent potential head injuries including the banning of intentional headers in players under the age of 11 years in United States Soccer as a part of their 2016 Concussion Initiative Guidelines.[116] World Rugby has recently trialed modifications to tackling rules in an effort to reduce head injuries.[117] The impact of regulatory changes regarding concussion in these sports is not yet known. These and other contact sports generally have launched initiatives to increase concussion awareness within the sport and have implemented policies regarding removal from play and return to play guidelines, but explicit concussion prevention measures within these activities have been less well publicized.[118]

Of note some there are a few investigations into concussion prevention measures that are not intended to affect the nature of how these sports are played. For example, one set of efforts is aimed at the reduction of concussion in sports is based on the fact that neck strength has been found to be inversely related to concussion incidence[119] and intends to systematically train neck strength into student athletes[120] to reduce sports-related concussion. A neck strengthening intervention has been shown to improve tested neck strength and reduce neck muscle fatigue,[121] but clearly more research is needed in measuring the effectiveness of neck strengthening in reducing concussions.

Other sports in which concussion has been a concern are full-contact martial arts including and especially boxing, in which the explicit goal of the sport is to score a knockout against an opponent. The meaning of this the term in itself indicates that a TBI has occurred and is in most actual cases associated with any definition of a mTBI. Preventative efforts in these sports appear to be aimed more aimed at the prevention of cumulative injury, which is beyond the scope of this chapter. In general, there remains little hard evidence for any particular risk reduction strategy for sports concussion without changing the nature and appeal of many sports in which player-to-player contact has traditionally been part of the game.[118]

The Use and Governance of Protective Equipment

The primary protective device associated with prevention of concussion is naturally the helmet. Helmets have been clearly shown to reduce the incidence of head injury in bicycling[122,123] and motorsports including all-terrain vehicles[124] and motorcycles,[125] and the implementation of motorcycle helmet laws to increase helmet wearing is associated with reduction of rider head injury.[126] In contrast, helmets are less clearly associated with risk reduction in other sporting/recreational activities in which they have been more widely adopted recently such as alpine sports[127,128] despite prospective and earlier reports that incidence of concussion is reduced with helmet use.[129,130] Similarly, among different sports there has been some mild controversy regarding the actual utility of helmets in preventing concussion.[131,132] Along these lines, there has been some efforts to actually remove helmets and protective gear in American football practices in order to influence tackling technique in order to reduce head injury.[133] Currently, public and regulatory sentiment appears to be in favor of increasing helmet use in any sports or recreational activities involving the potential for head injury.

Helmet Standards

There has been a good deal of attention among commercial companies and the media regarding prevention and harm reduction of sports concussion through engineering efforts to improve protective gear. Laws governing minimum standards for helmets intended for on-road motorcycle use are covered by the US Department of Transportation in US DOT standard FMVSS218.[134] Similarly, bicycle helmets have been regulated under the Consumer Product Safety Commission CSPC standard.[135] Sports and recreational helmets are regulated by standards published by different certification organizations including ASTM (American Society for Testing and Materials), ANSI (American National Standards Institute), NOCSAE (National Operating Committee on Standards for Athletic Equipment) and the Snell Memorial Foundation. Compliance by standards set by these organizations is on a per-league or voluntary basis.

Innovations in Helmet and Equipment Design

More recently, increased attention has been given to specific helmet design in order to prevent concussion. The effect of helmets the ability to protect the wearer from different types of head injury is currently under investigation,[136] and there is an increasing understanding that different types of impacts, e.g., those causing linear versus rotational acceleration has a role in the assessment of concussion severity.[137] With this understanding, there have been efforts to rate commercially available helmets in terms of protection from linear and rotational impacts[138,139] and more sophisticated modeling of specific impacts on the brain.[140] More recently, a reportedly similar but closed analysis was performed on NFL football helmets and the results of these tests were published by the NFL in the form of a poster.[141] While there has been some public research focused on helmet design for concussion prevention,[139,142–144] the state of the art is represented by different manufacturers and engineering firms are independently constructing helmets to improve testing and real-world performance based on proprietary designs.[145]

Other efforts to improve helmets with new technology have been based on potential concussion-preventive constituents such as non-Newtonian fluids and other smart materials.[146,147] A very interesting series of efforts has been the application of biological models to protective equipment based on animals such as the woodpeckers who are subjected to repeated head injury in nature.[148] Proposed helmet designs have been based on the shock dispersion and absorption properties of their beaks and skull structure.[149] Another mechanism in which woodpeckers ameliorate head injury has involved mild cervical compression collars aimed at compressing the jugular vein and producing mild cerebral engorgement and reduction of the effect of the brain moving inside the skull.[150] However, the use of woodpeckers as a model for concussion/TBI prevention design has been called under question as stigmata of brain injury such as axonal injury and tau protein deposits have been found in the brains of deceased woodpeckers.[151]

In summary, preventive efforts aimed at reducing mTBI in particular have generally been focused on either strategies to reduce the amount of contact in contact sports or on engineering innovations in helmets and other devices intended to reduce head injury. Despite changes in rules and conduct in sports, as well as the development of new devices intended to reduce concussion, a concomitant reduction in the

TABLE 15.4
Some Active Areas of Research in Concussion Prevention.

1. Incidence tracking and understanding of factors involved in concussion risk.
2. Changes in public knowledge regarding concussion and concussion diagnosis/assessment.
3. Rule or conduct changes within different sports and the effect on concussion incidence/severity.
4. Changes in training methods intended to reduce concussion incidence.
5. Understanding the cumulative effects of concussion and harm reduction in sports in which concussion is inherent (e.g., boxing).
6. Changes in laws and rules governing the use of protective equipment/helmets.
7. Changes in standards regulating the development of helmets and protective equipment.
8. Research into specific factors involved in collisions leading to differential risk of concussion.
9. Optimization of helmet design intended to reduce head injury.
10. Research into smart and novel materials that could enhance concussion prevention.
11. Alternative devices intended to prevent concussion (e.g., cervical compression collars).
12. Bio-inspired modeling of concussion prevention measures.

of significant general interest in terms of having the potential to substantially impact the clinical care and understanding of concussion. It is very likely, however, that there may be significant breakthroughs over the next few years in areas outside of those surveyed here.

Because concussion is such a common condition affecting a complex organ system of such broad and unquestionable significance both at a personal and cultural level, it has received a great deal of media coverage over the past several years for a variety of reasons, both helpful and not quite as helpful. As a result, significant resources have been directed toward an improved understanding of concussion and its sequelae as well as improved means of preventing significant injuries in the contexts in which they occur most frequently—particularly in the context of high-profile injuries taking place in popular contact sports and blast injuries sustained by military personnel in theater. This raises the hope and the expectation that, through the supporting of such ongoing research efforts, the field of Concussion Medicine will continue to advance and needed insights and innovations into how we may best not only minimize the prevalence and deleterious impact of this common condition, but also fully recognize the adaptive response to such injuries from a comprehensive systems science perspective,[152] will be forthcoming.

actual incidence of sports-related head injuries has not been seen. While this research is heavily confounded by the evolution in the diagnosis and public sentiment toward the long-term effects of concussion that affects incidence tracking, it is likely that the efforts underway to prevent concussion have in some measure been effective in reducing the impact of significant head injury. Considering the current state of the number of private efforts in concussion prevention research currently underway, an increasing intersection between public and closed efforts can only increase their utility.

A list of some active areas of research in concussion prevention is provided in Table 15.4.

CONCLUSION. MOVING CONCUSSION MEDICINE FORWARD

Concussion Medicine advances through research that extends across a vast swath of related fields, the comprehensive coverage of which would be impossible to complete in this limited space. We have attempted here to provide the reader with a limited glimpse of some highlights of this research that we feel is most promising and

REFERENCES

1. Gardner AJ, Shih SL, Adamov EV, Zafonte RD. Research frontiers in traumatic brain injury. Defining the injury. *Phys Med Rehabil Clin.* 2017;28:413−431.
2. American Congress of Rehabilitation Medicine. Brain injury interdisciplinary special interest group, mild traumatic brain injury task force definition of mild traumatic brain injury. *J Head Trauma Rehabil.* 1993;8:86−87.
3. Patricios JS, Ardern CL, Hislop MD, et al. Implementation of the 2017 Berlin Concussion in Sport Group Consensus Statement in contact and collision sports: a joint position statement from 11 national and international sports organisations. *Br J Sports Med.* 2018; 52(10):635−641.
4. AAN Sports Concussion. https://www.aan.com/tools-and-resources/practicing-neurologists-administrators/patient-resources/sports-concussion-resources/.
5. Wang KK, Yang Z, Zhu T, et al. An update on diagnostic and prognostic biomarkers for traumatic brain injury. *Expert Rev Mol Diagn.* 2018;18(2):165−180. https://doi.org/10.1080/14737159.2018.1428089. Epub 2018 Jan 23. PubMed PMID: 29338452.
6. Kiechle K, Bazarian JJ, Merchant-Borna K, et al. Subject-specific increases in serum S-100B distinguish sports-related concussion from sports-related exertion. *PLoS One.* 2014;9:e84977.

7. Shahim P, Tegner Y, Wilson DH, et al. Blood biomarkers for brain injury in concussed professional ice hockey players. *JAMA Neurol.* 2014;71:684−692.

8. Bouvier D, Duret T, Abbot M, et al. Utility of S100B serum level for the determination of concussion in male rugby players. *Sports Med.* 2017;47(4):781−789. https://doi.org/10.1007/s40279-016-0579-9.

9. Shahim P, Mattsson N, Macy EM, et al. Serum visinin-like protein-1 in concussed professional ice hockey players. *Brain Inj.* 2015;29(7−8):872−876.

10. Pham N, Akonasu H, Shishkin R, et al. Plasma soluble prion protein, a potential biomarker for sport-related concussions: a pilot study. *PLoS One.* 2015;10:e0117286.

11. Schulte S, Rasmussen NN, McBeth JW, et al. Utilization of the clinical laboratory for the implementation of concussion biomarkers in collegiate football and the necessity of personalized and predictive athlete specific reference intervals. *EPMA J.* 2015;7:1.

12. Dambinova SA, Shikuev AV, Weissman JD, et al. AMPAR peptide values in blood of nonathletes and club sport Athletes with concussions. *Mil Med.* 2013;178:285−290.

13. Oliver J, Abbas K, Lightfoot JT, et al. Comparison of neurocognitive testing and the measurement of marinobufagenin in mild traumatic brain injury: a preliminary report. *J Exp Neurosci.* 2015;9:67−72.

14. Siman R, Shahim P, Tegner Y, et al. Serum SNTF increases in concussed professional ice hockey players and relates to the severity of postconcussion symptoms. *J Neurotrauma.* 2015;32:1294−1300.

15. Daley M, Dekaban G, Bartha R, et al. Metabolomics profiling of concussion in adolescent male hockey players: a novel diagnostic method. *Metabolomics.* 2016;12.

16. Shan R, Szmydynger-Chodobska J, Warren OU, Mohammad F, Zink BJ, Chodobski A. A new panel of blood biomarkers for the diagnosis of mild traumatic brain injury/concussion in adults. *J Neurotrauma.* 2016; 33:49−57. https://doi.org/10.1089/neu.2014.3811.

17. Lancaster MA, Olson DV, McCrea MA, et al. Acute white matter changes following sport-related concussion: a serial diffusion tensor and diffusion kurtosis tensor imaging study. *Hum Brain Mapp.* 2016;37:3821−3834.

18. Borich M, Makan N, Boyd L, et al. Combining whole-brain voxel-wise analysis with in vivo tractography of diffusion behavior after sports-related concussion in adolescents: a preliminary report. *J Neurotrauma.* 2013; 30:1243−1249.

19. Virji-Babul N, Borich MR, Makan N, et al. Diffusion tensor imaging of sports-related concussion in adolescents. *Pediatr Neurol.* 2013;48:24−29.

20. Cubon VA, Putukian M, Boyer C, et al. A diffusion tensor imaging study on the white matter skeleton in individuals with sports-related concussion. *J Neurotrauma.* 2011;28:189−201.

21. Murugavel M, Cubon V, Putukian M, et al. A longitudinal diffusion tensor imaging study assessing white matter fiber tracts after sports-related concussion. *J Neurotrauma.* 2014;31:1860−1871.

22. Henry LC, Tremblay S, Boulanger Y, et al. Neurometabolic changes in the acute phase after sports concussions correlate with symptom severity. *J Neurotrauma.* 2010;27: 65−76.

23. Johnson B, Gay M, Zhang K, et al. The use of magnetic resonance spectroscopy in the subacute evaluation of athletes recovering from single and multiple mild traumatic brain injury. *J Neurotrauma.* 2012;29: 2297−2304.

24. Zhang K, Johnson B, Pennell D, et al. Are functional deficits in concussed individuals consistent with white matter structural alterations: combined FMRI & DTI study. *Exp Brain Res.* 2010;204:57−70.

25. Chen JK, Johnston KM, Collie A, et al. A validation of the post concussion symptom scale in the assessment of complex concussion using cognitive testing and functional MRI. *J Neurol Neurosurg Psychiatry.* 2007;78: 1231−1238.

26. Keightley ML, Saluja RS, Chen JK, et al. A functional magnetic resonance imaging study of working memory in youth after sports-related concussion: is it still working? *J Neurotrauma.* 2014;31:437−451.

27. Slobounov SM, Zhang K, Pennell D, et al. Functional abnormalities in normally appearing athletes following mild traumatic brain injury: a functional MRI study. *Exp Brain Res.* 2010;202:341−354.

28. Echemendia RJ, Meeuwisse W, McCrory P, et al. The sport concussion assessment tool 5th edition (SCAT5): background and rationale. *Br J Sports Med.* 2017;51: 848−850. https://doi.org/10.1136/bjsports-2017-097506.

29. Fedderman-Demont N, Echemendia RJ, Schneider KJ, et al. What domains of clinical function should be assessed after sport-related concussion? A systematic review. *Br J Sports Med.* 2017;51:903−918. https://doi.org/10.1136/bjsports-2016-097403.

30. Friston K. The free-energy principle: a unified brain theory? *Nat Rev Neurosci.* 2010;11:127. https://doi.org/10.1038/nm2787.

31. Peters A, McEwen B, Friston K. Uncertainty and stress: why it causes diseases and how it is mastered by the brain. *Prog Neurobiol.* 2017;156:164−188. https://doi.org/10.1016/j.pneurobio.2017.05.004.

32. McEwen BS, Gianaros PJ. Stress- and allostasis-induced brain plasticity. *Annu Rev Med.* 2011;62:431−445. https://doi.org/10.1146/annurev-med-052209-100430.

33. Esterov D, Greenwald BD. Autonomic dysfunction after mild traumatic brain injury. *Brain Sci.* 2017;7:100. https://doi.org/10.3390/brainsci7080100.

34. Pertab JL, Merkley TL, Cramond AJ, et al. Concussion and the autonomic nervous system: an introduction to the field and the results of a systematic review. *NeuroRehabilitation.* 2018;42:397−427. https://doi.org/10.3233/NRE-172298.

35. Shaffer F, Ginsberg JP. An overview of heart rate variability metrics and norms. *Front Public Health.* September 28, 2017. https://doi.org/10.3389/fpubh.2017.00258.

36. Huang M, Frantz J, Moralez G, et al. Reduced resting and increased elevation of heart rate variability with cognitive task performance in concussed athletes. *J Head Trauma Rehabil.* 2019;34:45–51. https://doi.org/10.1097/HTR.0000000000000409.

37. Abaji JP, Curnier D, Moore RD, Ellemberg D. Persisting effects of concussion on heart rate variability during physical exertion. *J Neurotrauma.* 2016;33:811–817. https://doi.org/10.1089/neu.2015.3989.

38. Senthinathan A, Mainwaring LM, Hutchison M. Heart rate variability of athletes across concussion recovery milestones: a preliminary study. *Clin J Sport Med.* 2017;27:288–295. https://doi.org/10.1097/JSM.0000000000000337.

39. Blake TA, McKay CD, Meeuwisse WH, Emery CA. The impact of concussion on cardiac autonomic function: a systematic review. *Brain Inj.* 2016;30:132–145. https://doi.org/10.3109/02699052.2015.1093659.

40. Paniccia M, Taha T, Keightley M, et al. Autonomic function following concussion in youth athletes: an exploration of heart rate variability using 24-hour recording methodology. *J Vis Exp.* 2018;139:e58203. https://doi.org/10.3791/58203.

41. Bishop SA, Dech RT, Guzik P, Neary JP. Heart rate variability and implication for sport concussion. *Physiol Funct Imaging.* 2018;38:733–742. https://doi.org/10.1111/cpf.12487.

42. Paniccia M, Verweel L, Thomas SG, et al. Heart rate variability following youth concussion: how do autonomic regulation and concussion symptoms differ over time postinjury? *BMJ Open Sport Exerc Med.* 2018;4:e000355. https://doi.org/10.1136/bmjsem-2018-000355.

43. Papo D, Zanin N, Pineda-Pardo JA, et al. Functional brain networks: great expectations, hard times and the big leap forward. *Phil Trans R Soc B.* 2014;369:20130525. https://doi.org/10.1098/rstb.2013.0525.

44. Shine JM, Bissett PG, Bell PT, et al. The dynamics of functional brain networks: integrated network states during functional task performance. *Neuron.* 2016;32:544–554. https://doi.org/10.1016/j.neuron.2016.09.018.

45. Fukushima M, Betzel RF, He Y, et al. Structure-function relationships during segregated and integrated network states of human brain functional connectivity. *Brain Struct Funct.* 2018;223:1091–1106. https://doi.org/10.1007/s00429-017-1539-3.

46. Griffa A, van den Heuvel MP. Rich-club neurocircuitry: function, evolution, and vulnerability. *Dialogues Clin Neurosci.* 2018;20:121–131. PMCID: PMC6136122.

47. Hillary FG, Rajtmajer SM, Roman CA, et al. The rich get richer. Brain injury elicits hyperconnectivity in core subnetworks. *PLoS One.* 2014;9:e104021. https://doi.org/10.1371/journal.pone.0104021.

48. Iraji A, Chen H, Wiseman N, et al. Compensation through functional hyperconnectivity. A longitudinal connectome assessment of mild traumatic brain injury. *Neural Plast.* 2016;2016:4072402. https://doi.org/10.1155/2016/4072402.

49. Dunkley BT, Urban K, Da Costa L, et al. Default mode network oscillatory coupling is increased following concussion. *Front Neurol.* 2018;9:280. https://doi.org/10.3389/fneur.2018.00280.

50. Chen H-CI, Burke JF, Cohen AS. Editorial: traumatic brain injury as a systems neuroscience problem. *Front Syst Neurosci.* 2016;10:100. https://doi.org/10./3389/fnsys.2016.00100.

51. Madhavan R, Joel SE, Mullick R, Cogsil T, Niogi SN, Tsiouris AJ, Mukherjee P, Masdeu JC, Marinelli L, Shetty T. Longitudinal Resting State Functional Connectivity Predicts Clinical Outcome in Mild Traumatic Brain Injury. *J Neurotrauma.* 2019;36(5):650–660. Published online. https://doi.org/10.1089/neu.2018.5739. Epub 2018 Oct 3.

52. Zhu DC, Covassin T, Nogle S, et al. A potential biomarker in sports-related concussion: brain functional connectivity alteration of the default-mode network measured with longitudinal resting-state fMRI over thirty days. *J Neurotrauma.* 2015;32:327–341. https://doi.org/10.1089/neu.2014.3413.

53. Churchill NW, Hutchison MG, Graham SJ, Schweizer TA. Connectomic markers of symptom severity in sport-related concussion: whole-brain analysis of resting-state fMRI. *Neuroimage Clin.* 2018;18:518–528. https://doi.org/10.1016/j.nicl.2018.02.011.eCollection 2018.

54. van der Horn HJ, Scheenen ME, de Koning ME, et al. The default mode network as a biomarker of persistent complaints after mild traumatic brain injury: a longitudinal functional magnetic resonance imaging study. *J Neurotrauma.* 2017;34:3262–3269. https://doi.org/10.1089/neu.2017.5185.

55. van der Horn HJ, Liemburg EJ, Scheenen ME, et al. Graph analysis of functional brain networks in patients with mild traumatic brain injury. *PLoS One.* 2017;12:e0171031. https://doi.org/10.1371/journal.pone.0171031.

56. Stephens JA, Salorio CF, Barber AD, et al. Preliminary findings of altered functional connectivity of the default mode network linked to functional outcomes one year after pediatric traumatic brain injury. *Dev Neurorehabil.* 2018;21:423–430. https://doi.org/10.1080/17518423.2017.1338777.

57. Fukushima M, Betzel RF, He Y, et al. Fluctuations between high- and low-modularity topology in time-resolved functional connectivity. *Neuroimage.* 2018;180:406–416. https://doi.org/10.1016/j.neuroimage.2017.08.044.

58. Mares C, Dagher JH, Harissi-Dagher M. Narrative review of the pathophysiology of headaches and photosensitivity in mild traumatic brain injury and concussion. *Can J Neurol Sci.* 2018:1–9. https://doi.org/10.1017/cjn.2018.361.

59. Howard L, Dumkrieger G, Chong CD, et al. Symptoms of autonomic dysfunction among those with persistent posttraumatic headache attributed to mild traumatic brain injury: a comparison to migraine and healthy controls. *Headache.* 2018;58:1397–1407. https://doi.org/10.1111/head.13396.

60. Benromano T, Defrin R, Ahn AH, et al. Mild closed head injury promotes a selective trigeminal hypernociception: implications for the acute emergence of post-traumatic headache. *Eur J Pain*. 2015;19:621–628. https://doi.org/10.1002/ejp.583.

61. Daiutolo BV, Tyburski A, Clark SW, Elliott MB. Trigeminal pain molecules, allodynia, and photosensitivity are pharmacologically and genetically modulated in a model of traumatic brain injury. *J Neurotrauma*. 2016;33:748–760. https://doi.org/10.1089/neu.2015.4087.

62. Sakas DE, Whitwell HL. Neurological episodes after minor head injury and trigeminovascular activation. *Med Hypotheses*. 1997;48:431–435.

63. Messlinger K. The big CGRP flood - sources, sinks and signalling sites in the trigeminovascular system. *J Headache Pain*. 2018;19:22. https://doi.org/10.1186/s10194-018-0848-0.

64. Tyburski AL, Chen L, Assari S, et al. Frequent mild head injury promotes trigeminal sensitivity concomitant with microglial proliferation, astrocytosis, and increased neuropeptide levels in the trigeminal pain system. *J Headache Pain*. 2017;18:16. https://doi.org/10.1186/s10194-017-0726-1.

65. Bree D, Levy D. Development of CGRP-dependent pain and headache related behaviours in a rat model of concussion: implications for mechanisms of post-traumatic headache. *Cephalgia*. 2018;38:246–258. https://doi.org/10.1177/0333102416681571.

66. Sakas DE, Whittaker KW, Whitwell HL, Singounas EG. Syndromes of posttraumatic neurological deterioration in children with no focal lesions revealed by cerebral imaging: evidence for a trigeminovascular pathophysiology. *Neurosurgery*. 1997;41:661–667.

67. Squier W, Mack J, Green A, Aziz T. The pathophysiology of brain swelling associated with subdural hemorrhage: the role of the trigeminovascular system. *Childs Nerv Syst*. 2012;28:2005–2015. https://doi.org/10.1007/s00381-012-1870-1.

68. Leigh-Hunt N, Bagguley D, Bash K, et al. An overview of systematic reviews on the public health consequences of social isolation and loneliness. *Publ Health*. 2017;152:157–171.

69. Mohan A, Vanneste S. Adaptive and maladaptive neural compensatory consequences of sensory deprivation-from a phantom percept perspective. *Prog Neurobiol*. 2017;153:1–17.

70. Hughson RL, Shoemaker JK. Autonomic responses to exercise: deconditioning/inactivity. *Auton Neurosci*. 2015;188:32–35.

71. Buckley TA, Munkasy BA, Clouse BP. Acute cognitive and physical rest may not improve concussion recovery time. *J Head Trauma Rehabil*. 2016;31(4):233–241.

72. Grool AM, Aglipay M, Momoli F, et al. Association between early participation in physical activity following acute concussion and persistent postconcussive symptoms in children and adolescents. *J Am Med Assoc*. 2016;316(23):2504–2514. https://doi.org/10.1001/jama.2016.17396.

73. Leddy JJ, Hinds AL, Miecznikowski J, et al. Safety and prognostic utility of provocative exercise testing in acutely concussed adolescents: a randomized trial. *Clin J Sport Med*. 2018;28(1):13–20.

74. Leddy JJ, Haider MN, Ellis M, Willer BS. Exercise is medicine for concussion. *Curr Sports Med Rep*. 2018;17(8):262–270.

75. Leddy JJ, Haider MN, Hinds AL, et al. A preliminary study of the effect of early aerobic exercise treatment for sport-related concussion in males. *Clin J Sport Med*. 2018. https://doi.org/10.1097/JSM.0000000000000663.

76. Hassett L, Moseley AM, Harmer AR. Fitness training for cardiorespiratory conditioning after traumatic brain injury. *Cochrane Database Syst Rev*. 2017;12:CD006123.

77. Lumba-Brown A, Yeates KO, Sarmiento K, et al. Centers for disease control and prevention guideline on the diagnosis and management of mild traumatic brain injury among children. *JAMA Pediatr*. 2018;172(11):e182853.

78. *Guidelines for Concussion/mTBI and Persistent Symptoms, Healthcare Professional Version*. 3rd ed. Ontario Neurotrauma Foundation; 2018.

79. McCrory P, Meeuwisse W, Dvorak J, et al. Consensus statement on concussion in sport—the 5th international conference on concussion in sport held in Berlin, October 2016. *Br J Sports Med*. 2017;51:838–847.

80. Kenzie ES, Parks EL, Bigler ED, et al. Concussion as a multi-scale complex system: an interdisciplinary synthesis of current knowledge. *Front Neurol*. 2017;8:513.

81. Ott SD, Bailey CM, Broshek DK. An interdisciplinary approach to sports concussion evaluation and management: the role of a neuropsychologist. *Arch Clin Neuropsychol*. 2018;33(3):319–329.

82. Pabian PS, Oliveira L, Tucker J, et al. Interprofessional management of concussion in sport. *Phys Ther Sport*. 2017;23:123–132.

83. Rytter HM, Westenbaek K, Henriksen H, Christiansen P, Humle F. Specialized interdisciplinary rehabilitation reduces persistent post-concussive symptoms: a randomized clinical trial. *Brain Inj*. 2018;30:1–16.

84. Iverson GL, Koehle MS. Normative data for the balance error scoring system in adults. *Rehabil Res Pract*. 2013;2013:846418.

85. Leddy JJ, Baker JG, Haider MN, Hinds A, Willer B. A physiological approach to prolonged recovery from sport-related concussion. *J Athl Train*. 2017;52(3):299–308.

86. Leddy JJ, Sandhu H, Sodhi V, Willer B. Rehabilitation of concussio and post-concussion syndrome. *Sport Health*. 2012;4(2):147–154.

87. Leddy JJ, Hinds A, Sirica D, Willer B. The role of controlled exercise in concussion management. *Pharm Manag PM R*. 2016;8(3 Suppl):S91–S100.

88. Mollayeva T, Pratt B, Mollayeva S, et al. The relationship between insomnia and disability in workers with mild traumatic brain injury/concussion: insomnia and disability in chronic mild traumatic brain injury. *Sleep Med*. 2016;20:157–166.

89. Mollayeva T, Mollayeva S, Shapiro CM, Cassidy JD, Colantonio A. Insomnia in workers with delayed recovery from mild traumatic brain injury. *Sleep Med.* 2016; 19:153−161.

90. Dwyer B, Katz DI. Postconcussion syndrome. *Handb Clin Neurol.* 2018;158:163−178.

91. Raikes AC, Schaefer SY. Sleep quantity and quality during acute concussion: a pilot study. *Sleep.* 2016;39(12): 2141−2147.

92. Kroenke K, Spitzer RL, Williams JB. The PHQ-9: validity of a brief depression severity measure. *J Gen Intern Med.* 2001;16(9):606−613.

93. Spitzer RL, Kroenke K, Williams JB, et al. A brief measure for assessing generalised anxiety disorder: the GAD-7. *Arch Intern Med.* 2006;166:1092−1097.

94. Prins A, Bovin MJ, Kimerling R, et al. *The Primary Care PTSD Screen for DSM-5 (PC-PTSD-5) [Measurement Instrument]*; 2015. Available from: http://www.ptsd.va.gov.

95. Weathers FW, Litz BT, Keane TM, Palmieri PA, Marx BP, Schnurr PP. *The PTSD Checklist for DSM-5 (PCL-5) − Standard [Measurement Instrument]*; 2013. Available from: http://www.ptsd.va.gov/.

96. Cole MA, Muir JJ, Cole MA, Muir JJ, Gans JJ, et al. Simultaneous treatment of neurocognitive and psychiatric symptoms in veterans with post-traumatic stress disorder and history of mild traumatic brain injury: a pilot study of mindfulness-based stress reduction. *Mil Med.* 2015; 180(9):956−963.

97. Raikes AC, Killgore WD. Potential for the development of light therapies in mild traumatic brain injury. *Concussion.* 2018;3(3):CNC57.

98. Echemendia RJ, Iverson GL, McCrea M. Advances in neuropsychological assessment of sport-related concussion. *Br J Sports Med.* 2013;47(5):294−298.

99. Echemendia RJ, Gioia GA. The role of neuropsychologists in concussion evaluation and management. *Handb Clin Neurol.* 2018;158:179−191.

100. Karlin AM. Concussion in the pediatric and adolescent population: "different population, different concerns". *Pharm Manag PM R.* 2011;3(10 Suppl 2):S369−S379.

101. Bloom B, Thomas S, Ahrensberg JM, et al. A systematic review and meta-analysis of return to work after mild Traumatic brain injury. *Brain Inj.* 2018:1−14.

102. Schneider DK, Grandhi RK, Bansal P, et al. Current state of concussion prevention strategies: a systematic review and meta-analysis of prospective, controlled studies. *Br J Sports Med.* 2017. https://doi.org/10.1136/bjsports-2015-095645.

103. Emery CA, Black AM, Kolstad A, et al. What strategies can be used to effectively reduce the risk of concussion in sport? A systematic review. *Br J Sports Med.* 2017;51(12): 978−984. https://doi.org/10.1136/bjsports-2016-097452.

104. State of Washington House Bill 1824, 61st Legislature, 2009 Regular Session. http://lawfilesext.leg.wa.gov/biennium/2009-10/Pdf/Bills/House Bills/1824.pdf.

105. CDC Injury Center. Get a Heads Up on Concussion in Sports Policies. www.cdc.gov/.

106. Health & Safety Rules Changes | NFL Football Operations. https://operations.nfl.com/football-ops/nfl-ops-honoring-the-game/health-safety-rules-changes/.

107. 2018 Rules Changes and Points of Emphasis | NFL Football Operations. https://operations.nfl.com/the-rules/2018-rules-changes-and-points-of-emphasis/.

108. 2017 Injury Data − NFL Play Smart, Play Safe. https://www.playsmartplaysafe.com/newsroom/reports/2017-injury-data/.

109. NFL concussions rise to highest level since league began sharing data. http://www.espn.com/nfl/story/_/id/22226487/nfl-concussions-rise-highest-level-league-began-sharing-data.

110. NFL concussions: Reported cases up to six-year high in 2017. https://www.usatoday.com/story/sports/nfl/2018/01/26/nfl-concussions-2017-season-study-history/1070344001/.

111. Decoding the N.F.L. Database to Find 100 Missing Concussions - The New York Times. https://www.nytimes.com/2016/03/25/sports/football/at-least-100-concussions-left-out-of-nfl-studies.html.

112. Kerr ZY, Yeargin SW, Valovich McLeod TC, Mensch J, Hayden R, Dompier TP. Comprehensive coach education reduces head impact exposure in American youth football. *Orthop J Sport Med.* 2015;3(10):1−6. https://doi.org/10.1177/2325967115610545.

113. Kerr ZY, Yeargin S, Valovich McLeod TC, et al. Comprehensive coach education and practice contact restriction guidelines result in lower injury rates in youth American football. *Orthop J Sport Med.* 2015;3(7):1−8. https://doi.org/10.1177/2325967115594578.

114. Broglio SP, Williams RM, Connor KLO, Goldstick J. Football players' head-impact exposure after limiting of full-contact practices. *J Athl Train.* 2016;51(7):511−518. https://doi.org/10.4085/1062-6050-51.7.04.

115. Black AM, Macpherson AK, Hagel BE, et al. *Policy Change Eliminating Body Checking in Non-elite Ice Hockey Leads to a Threefold Reduction in Injury and Concussion Risk in 11- and 12-Year-Old Players.* 2016:55−61. https://doi.org/10.1136/bjsports-2015-095103.

116. Head & Brain Conditions − Recognize to Recover. http://www.recognizetorecover.org/head-and-brain/#head-brain-conditions.

117. World Rugby Trial a Lower Tackle Height at U20 Competitions. https://www.world.rugby/u20/news/336546?lang=en.

118. Benson BW, McIntosh AS, Maddocks D, Herring SA, Raftery M, Dvořák J. What are the most effective risk-reduction strategies in sport concussion? *Br J Sports Med.* 2013;47(5):321−326. https://doi.org/10.1136/bjsports-2013-092216.

119. Collins CL, Fletcher EN, Fields SK, et al. Neck strength: a protective factor reducing risk for concussion in high school sports. *J Prim Prev.* 2014;35(5):309−319. https://doi.org/10.1007/s10935-014-0355-2.

120. Toninato J, Casey H, Uppal M, et al. Traumatic brain injury reduction in athletes by neck strengthening

(TRAIN). *Contemp Clin Trials Commun.* 2018;11(March): 102−106. https://doi.org/10.1016/j.conctc.2018.06.007.

121. Barrett M, McLoughlin T, Gallagher K, et al. Effectiveness of a tailored neck training program on neck strength, movement, and fatigue in under-19 male rugby players: a randomized controlled pilot study. *Open Access J Sports Med.* 2015;137. https://doi.org/10.2147/OAJSM. S74622.

122. Olivier J, Creighton P. Bicycle injuries and helmet use: a systematic review and meta-analysis. *Int J Epidemiol.* 2017;46(1):278−292. https://doi.org/10.1093/ije/ dyw153.

123. Høye A. Bicycle helmets − to wear or not to wear? A meta-analyses of the effects of bicycle helmets on injuries. *Accid Anal Prev.* 2018;117(March):85−97. https://doi.org/10.1016/j.aap.2018.03.026.

124. Benham EC, Ross SW, Mavilia M, Fischer PE, Christmas AB, Sing RF. *Injuries from All-Terrain Vehicles: An Opportunity for Injury Prevention.* 2016. https:// doi.org/10.1016/j.amjsurg.2016.11.017.

125. Rice TM, Troszak L, Ouellet J, Erhardt T, Smith GS, Tsai B-W. Motorcycle helmet use and the risk of head, neck, and fatal injury: revisiting the Hurt Study. *Accid Anal Prev.* 2016;91:200−207.

126. Peng Y, Vaidya N, Finnie R, et al. Universal motorcycle helmet laws to reduce injuries: a community guide systematic review. *Am J Prev Med.* 2017;52(6):820−832. https://doi.org/10.1016/j.amepre.2016.11.030.

127. Sulheim S, Ekeland A, Holme I, Bahr R. Helmet use and risk of head injuries in alpine skiers and snowboarders: changes after an interval of one decade. *Br J Sports Med.* 2017;51(1):44−50. https://doi.org/10.1136/bjsports-2015-095798.

128. Dickson T, Trathen S, Terweil A, Waddington G, Adams R. No reduction in head injury rates with increased helmet use: the case of Western Canadian snow sports. *J Sci Med Sport.* 2015;19:e71−e72. https:// doi.org/10.1016/j.jsams.2015.12.174.

129. Mueller BA, Cummings P, Rivara FP, Brooks MA, Terasaki RD. Injuries of the head, face, and neck in relation to ski helmet use. *Epidemiology.* 2008;19(2):270−276. https://doi.org/10.1097/EDE.0b013e318163567c.

130. Russell K, Christie J, Hagel BE. The effect of helmets on the risk of head and neck injuries among skiers and snowboarders: a meta-analysis. *Can Med Assoc J.* 2010; 182(4):333−340. https://doi.org/10.1503/cmaj.091080.

131. Benson BW, Hamilton GM, Meeuwisse WH, McCrory P, Dvorak J. Is protective equipment useful in preventing concussion? A systematic review of the literature. *Br J Sports Med.* 2009;43(suppl 1). https://doi.org/10.1136/ bjsm.2009.058271.

132. Daneshvar DH, MA C, Baugh M, et al. Helmets and mouth guards: the role of personal equipment in preventing sport-related concussions. *Clin Sports Med.* 2011;30(1): 145−163. https://doi.org/10.1016/j.csm.2010.09.006 (Helmets).

133. Swartz EE, Broglio SP, Cook SB, et al. Early results of a helmetless-tackling intervention to decrease head impacts in football players. *J Athl Train.* 2015;50(12):1219−1222. https://doi.org/10.4085/1062-6050-51.1.06.

134. Code of Federal Regulations. US DOT, NHTSA Federal Motor Vehicle Safety Standards. https://one.nhtsa.gov/ people/injury/pedbimot/NoMigrate/fmvss218.htm.

135. Committee of the Federal Register Part 1203, Subpart A. https://www.law.cornell.edu/cfr/text/16/part-1203/ subpart-A.

136. Singleton MD. Differential protective effects of motorcycle helmets against head injury. *Traffic Inj Prev.* 2017; 18(4):387−392. https://doi.org/10.1080/15389588. 2016.1211271.

137. Rowson S, Duma SM. Brain injury prediction: assessing the combined probability of concussion using linear and rotational head acceleration. *Ann Biomed Eng.* 2013;41(5):873−882. https://doi.org/10.1007/s10439-012-0731-0.

138. Football Helmet Ratings. https://www.helmet.beam.vt. edu/varsity-football-helmet-ratings.html.

139. Sproule DW, Rowson S. Comparison of impact performance between youth and varsity football helmets. *Proc Inst Mech Eng P J Sports Eng Technol.* 2017;231(4): 374−380. https://doi.org/10.1177/1754337117731989.

140. Post A, Oeur A, Hoshizaki B, Gilchrist MD. *An Examination of American Football Helmets Using Brain Deformation Metrics Associated with Concussion.* 2013. https://doi.org/ 10.1016/j.matdes.2012.09.017.

141. Helmet Laboratory Testing Performance Results - NFL Play Smart, Play Safe. https://www.playsmartplaysafe. com/resource/helmet-laboratory-testing-performance-results/.

142. Ahmadisoleymani SS, Yang J. American football helmet for preventing concussion , a literature review. *Procedia Manuf.* 2015;3(Ahfe):3796−3803. https://doi.org/ 10.1016/j.promfg.2015.07.882.

143. Rowson S, Duma SM, Greenwald RM, et al. Can helmet design reduce the risk of concussion in football? *J Neurosurg.* 2014;120(4):919−922. https://doi.org/ 10.3171/2014.1.JNS13916.

144. Zuckerman SL, Reynolds BB, Yengo-kahn AM, et al. *A Football Helmet Prototype that Reduces Linear and Rotational Acceleration with the Addition of an Outer Shell.* 2018:1−8. https://doi.org/10.3171/2018.1.JNS172733.

145. ZERO1 − VICIS. https://vicis.com/products/zero1.

146. Deshmukh SS, Mckinley GH. Related content Adaptive energy-absorbing materials using field-responsive fluid-impregnated cellular solids. *Struct.* 2007;16:106−113. https://doi.org/10.1088/0964-1726/16/1/013.

147. *Energy Absorbing Material*; 2002. https://patents.google. com/patent/US7381460.

148. May PRA, Newman P, Fuster JM, Hirschman A. Woodpeckers and head injury. *Lancet.* 1976;307(7957): 454−455. https://doi.org/10.1016/S0140-6736(76) 91477-X.

149. Wang L, CheungJason JTM, Pu F, Li D, Zhang M, Fan Y. Why do woodpeckers resist head impact injury: a biomechanical investigation. *PLoS One.* 2011;6(10):1–8. https://doi.org/10.1371/journal.pone.0026490.

150. Yuan W, Dudley J, Barber-Foss K, et al. Mild jugular compression collar ameliorated changes in brain activation of working memory after one soccer season in female high school athletes. *J Neurotrauma.* 2018;1259. https://doi.org/10.1089/neu.2017.5262. neu.2017.5262.

151. Smoliga JM. Reconsidering the woodpecker model of traumatic brain injury. *Lancet Neurol.* 2018;17(6): 500–501. https://doi.org/10.1016/S1474-4422(18) 30157-1.

152. E.S. Kenzie, E.L. Parks, E.D. Bigler, et al., The dynamics of concussion: mapping pathophysiology, persistence, and recovery with causal-loop diagramming, *Front Neurol* 9:203, 2018. https://doi.org/10.3389/fneur.2018.00203

Index

Note: Page numbers followed by "t" indicate tables and "f" indicate figures.

Printed and bound by CPI Group (UK) Ltd, Croydon, CR0 4YY

03/10/2024

01040373-0007